Assisting Survivors
of Traumatic Brain Injury

The Role of
Speech–Language Pathologists

Edited by
Karen Hux

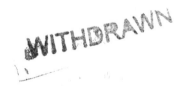
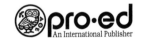
pro·ed
An International Publisher
8700 Shoal Creek Boulevard
Austin, Texas 78757-6897
800/897-3202   Fax 800/397-7633
www.proedinc.com

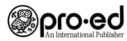

© 2003 by PRO-ED, Inc.
8700 Shoal Creek Boulevard
Austin, Texas 78757-6897
800/897-3202   Fax 800/397-7633
www.proedinc.com

Library of Congress Cataloging-in-Publication Data

Hux, Karen.
    Assisting survivors of traumatic brain injury : the role of speech–language pathologists/ Karen Hux.
        p. ; cm.
    Includes bibliographical references and index.
    ISBN 0-89079-895-8
    1. Brain damage—Patients—Rehabilitation.   2. Speech therapy.   I. Title.
    (DNLM: 1. Brain Injuries—rehabilitation.   2. Communication Disorders—rehabilitation.
    3. Brain Injuries—complications.   4. Communication Aids for Disabled.   5. Communication Disorders—etiology.   6. Speech-Language Pathology—methods.   WL 354
    H986a 2002)
    RC387.5 .H89   2002
    616.8'043—dc21   2001048730

This book is designed in Avant Garde and Goudy.

Printed in the United States of America

1 2 3 4 5 6 7 8 9 10   06 05 04 03 02

*To my daughter, Alana, who knew about TBI support groups,
disinhibition, and myoclonic jerks as a preschooler.
I love you like crazy cakes!*

Contents

─────────── **Part III** ───────────

Understanding Reintegration

Preface

About 1 year after finishing my graduate degree in speech–language pathology, I heard that one of my classmates had sustained a severe traumatic brain injury (TBI) from a car accident. At last report, she was living in a long-term care facility, was totally dependent on others for her care, and communicated only through eye blinks indicating "yes" and "no." Unfortunately, she is only one of many people I know whose life has been forever changed by TBI. Indeed, one of the hardest lessons for me to learn as a young adult was that life is not fair. TBI can happen to anyone at any time. "Playing by the rules" does not guarantee immunity, nor does knowing everything there is to know about TBI.

The effects of TBI pervade the lives of survivors, families, and communities. Physical, cognitive, communicative, and psychosocial disabilities can persist for years following injury, often never to resolve. The fact that many survivors walk, talk, and are not readily distinguishable from noninjured people is a cruel twist that only those who have experienced TBI on a personal level understand. TBI is often a hidden disability—hidden inside a survivor's perception, personality, thoughts, and feelings.

Preparing professionals to deal with the many consequences of TBI is a daunting task. Service delivery includes emergency services, hospitalization, rehabilitation, long-term care, community reentry, education, and vocational training. The variety of professionals who provide needed services is equally broad: medical personnel; social workers and case managers; physical, occupational, speech–language, and recreational therapists; clinical and educational psychologists; neuropsychologists; school administrators, staff, and educators; and vocational rehabilitation experts and job coaches.

Assisting Survivors of Traumatic Brain Injury: The Role of Speech–Language Pathologists is a tool to help prepare graduate students and practicing speech–language pathologists to serve people with TBI. The book is divided into three sections: Understanding Traumatic Brain Injury, Understanding the Role of Speech–Language Pathologists, and Understanding Reintegration.

The first section provides an overview of TBI: definitions, epidemiology, injury severity, and mechanisms of injury. Because TBI does not happen to a random sampling of the general population, professionals need to understand the subgroups of people most likely to sustain such injuries and how and when injuries are most likely to occur. Then, because most survivors of TBI begin the recovery process in a medical setting, professionals need knowledge of the medical terminology and the sequence of medical events associated with acute neurological injury. TBI causes a different pattern of brain damage than other neurological injuries, and an understanding of the nature of cortical and sub-cortical damage will help speech–language pathologists assess and treat the immediate and long-term consequences of TBI.

The second section of the book deals with the major disorders associated with TBI for which speech–language pathologists assume diagnostic and intervention responsibility: coma and posttraumatic amnesia, cognitive–communication impairments, motor speech disorders, and swallowing disorders. An additional chapter addresses the use of augmentative and alternative communication and assistive technology to compensate for various speech, language, and cognitive impairments.

The final section of the book provides information about integrating survivors of TBI into family, educational, vocational, and community settings. The impact of TBI extends beyond survivors; whole families, schools, and communities are affected. Because of this, expertise from many professionals is needed to assist in the reintegration process. Many survivors experience communication, cognitive, and physical impairments that exacerbate psychosocial challenges, breakdowns in family and peer relations, and problems related to the survivor's return to school or work environments. Speech–language pathologists who work in collaboration with professionals from fields such as psychology, neuropsychology, education, and vocational rehabilitation provide better services to survivors of TBI than ones who attempt to treat survivors in isolation.

Preparation of *Assisting Survivors of Traumatic Brain Injury* required the contributions of many people. In addition to the professionals who authored chapters, many survivors of TBI and their families contributed by sharing experiences and stories. David Beukelman deserves special thanks for his role in recruiting me for this project, providing general assistance throughout, and encouraging me during low points. I also thank Nancy Manasse for tolerating the many times I interrupted her work to discuss ideas and for taking time to proofread many of the chapters. The staff at PRO-ED—Jim Patton, Peggy Kipping, and Robin Spencer—offered encouragement, answered technical questions, and tolerated delays with admirable patience. Thank you to all of them.

Contributors

Karla Anhalt, PhD
Department of Educational Psychology
Texas A&M University
College Station, TX 77843-4225

David R. Beukelman, PhD
Barkley Memorial Center for Special
    Education and Communication
    Disorders
University of Nebraska–Lincoln
Lincoln, NE 68583-0732

Christine E. Borgelt, PhD
Quality Living, Inc.
Omaha, NE 68104

Pamela Brown, EdS
Nebraska Educational Assistive
    Technology (NEAT) Center
1910 Meridian Ave.
Cozad, NE 69130

Rebecca Burke, PhD
Communication Sciences and
    Disorders
Rockhurst University
1100 Rockhurst Rd.
Kansas City, MO 64110

Michelle Gutmann, MS
Barkley Memorial Center for Special
    Education and Communication
    Disorders
University of Nebraska–Lincoln
Lincoln, NE 68583-0731

Karen Hux, PhD
Barkley Memorial Center for Special
    Education and Communication
    Disorders
University of Nebraska–Lincoln
Lincoln, NE 68583-0738

Nancy Manasse, PhD
Department of Communication
    Disorders
California State University–
    Los Angeles
Los Angeles, CA 90032

William J. Warzak, PhD
Munroe Meyer Center for Genetics
    and Rehabilitation
University of Nebraska Medical
    Center
Omaha, NE 68198-5450

Carolyn Wright, PhD
Quality Living, Inc.
Omaha, NE 68104

Kathryn M. Yorkston, PhD
Department of Rehabilitation
    Medicine
University of Washington
Seattle, WA 98195-6490

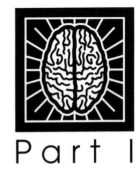

Part I

Understanding Traumatic Brain Injury

If Only I Had Known . . .

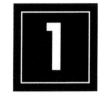

Karen Hux

Y ou never should have opened this book. That was a big mistake. Now that you have, you have brain damage, and there is nothing you can do to change that.

The time that it takes to open a book to its first page is the same amount of time that it takes for traumatic brain injury (TBI) to occur. You can die just as fast. It takes less than 1 second to die in a traffic accident in which you are travelling 55 miles per hour. Do you want to know how it happens? No? Hmm. I am going to tell you anyway. That is another thing about TBI: Survivors continually have to listen to things they do not want to hear.

> **❝** *How do I know that I'm alive. Maybe I really died in the accident, and this is what death is.* **❞**
> *—17-year-old survivor*

This is what happens in a head-on collision: In the first tenth of a second, the front bumper and grille collapse. In the second tenth, the hood crumples into the windshield and the rear of the car lifts off the ground with the wheels still spinning. The front fender starts to wrap itself around whatever object the car hit, and, although the front end of the car has stopped moving, the driver is still moving 55 miles per hour. Instinct causes the driver to stiffen the legs against the crash; that causes the knee joints to snap when the feet come in contact with the floorboard of the car. During the third tenth of a second, the driver is propelled toward the steering column. By the fourth tenth of a second, the front end of the car has 2 feet of damage, but the rear of the car is still moving at 35 miles per hour. The driver has not slowed down at all; he or she is still moving at 55 miles per hour. In the fifth tenth of a second, the steering column impales the driver's chest and blood rushes into the lungs. By the sixth tenth of a second, the driver's feet are ripped out of laced shoes, the brake pedal breaks off, the car frame buckles in the middle, and the driver's head bangs into the windshield. The rear wheels finally fall back to the ground. More structural damage occurs in the seventh tenth of a second as hinges break loose, doors open, and seats break free and strike the driver from behind. None of this matters, however, because the driver is already dead.

The implementation and enforcement of seat belt laws have greatly reduced the number of deaths and the severity if TBIs that occur during motor vehicle accidents. Figure 1.1 displays data reported by Petty (1975) about the influence of seat belt laws on the incidence of TBI in the State of Victoria, Australia. The number of severe injuries was substantially larger during 1969–1970—before legislation made seat belt use compulsory for all occupants of moving vehicles—than during 1972–1973, after enactment of the legislation. Wearing seat belts and having air bags in cars are good ideas. They save a tremendous number of lives every year.

Now, let's get back to you. You have to deal with brain damage. If you still do not believe that you can acquire brain damage from opening a book, do not worry about it. Most survivors of TBI deny their deficits initially. Eventually, you will understand that you cannot do the things you used to do. First things first, though. Right now we have to get you out of coma.

Forget about the Hollywood version of coma. People do not suddenly wake up and say, "Oh, what happened? Where am I? How long have I been here?" Coming out of coma is seldom rapid; it can be a slow, tedious, and painful

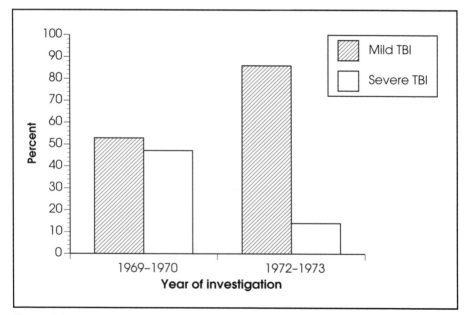

Figure 1.1. Percentage of mild and severe TBIs from motor vehicle accidents before and after enactment of legislation requiring the use of seat belts. *Note.* Based on data from Petty (1975).

process. The pain comes from three sources. First, survivors are likely to have injuries to parts of the body other than the brain, and they are likely to hurt. Second, lying in bed for days upon days causes muscles to tighten up. Physical therapists do their best to limit contractures by stretching muscles as far as possible several times a day. The survivor has no option about this; it is like an enforced exercise program. Third, the doctors, nurses, and therapists may periodically inflict pain on purpose. If it is the only way they can get the person to respond, they will do it. Being poked and prodded is part of the deal when you are in coma.

Nobody really knows what people in coma hear or comprehend. It probably differs from person to person and from day to day. The safest procedure is to assume that a person in coma understands everything; that way, people will not say things that might be upsetting. Unfortunately, not all visitors get that message. Some of your friends are so shocked by how bad you look that they cannot stop themselves from gasping at the sight of you.

Actually, you should be thrilled that your friends are visiting at all. That probably will change in the next few weeks. Try not to hold it against people for not visiting more often. Hospitals are scary places. There are all of those tubes and beeping monitors. Besides, your friends simply do not know what to do with themselves or with you when they visit. You are not responding to much of anything yet, so having a conversation is out of the question; a person can only do a limited number of monologues before running out of topics. Just sitting in the room with you is boring, and it feels awkward and unproductive; facing the members of your grief-stricken family is even worse. Your friends will soon decide that it might be better if they just stayed away for awhile—until you get better. They have

"Survivors of traumatic brain injury" or "people with traumatic brain injury" are the preferred terms to refer to individuals who have acquired brain damage and lived to tell about it. The terminology maintains a "person first" perspective, recognizing the importance of individuals before identifying their disabilities. It also avoids the problem associated with forever referring to a person as a patient. Although people who sustain TBIs may be hospital or rehabilitation patients for a period of time post-injury, they are not patients for the remainder of their lives—and should not be treated as such. Forever referring to survivors of TBI as patients may undermine their struggle for independence and recovery.

not figured out yet that TBI continues beyond hospital discharge. In fact, it lasts a lifetime.

Now, a couple weeks (or months) have passed, and you are finally becoming more responsive. You are actually acting a bit "feisty." People who work with survivors of TBI call it *agitation*. You are going to hurt yourself if you keep pulling on tubes and thrashing around in bed so much. The hospital staff cannot let that happen, so, if need be, they will put you in restraints. Although it may not feel this way, the agitation is coming from inside you—not outside. Internal agitation is like having a really high fever; your body is ultrasensitive and overly reactive to everything. Of course, being in a hospital is not helping your agitation any. Hospitals are noisy, busy places, but you are not even close to being ready to go home yet. You cannot even walk across your room to the bathroom by yourself! How are you going to manage at home? You are going to spend at least a couple months in rehabilitation, so you may as well get used to the idea.

Life in a rehabilitation center assumes dramatically different characteristics at different times of day and night. From 8:00 A.M. to 5:00 P.M., a lot of people are around. The therapists, doctors, administrators, and support staff arrive to work. You have become someone's job; actually, you have become a lot of people's jobs. In the evening, everyone except the patients and nursing staff leave and return to the real world. Suddenly the place seems deserted and a bit surreal. Is this supposed to be life?

Therapy is surprisingly hard work. Almost everything that you used to take for granted is now a part of therapy—eating, getting dressed, brushing your teeth, going to the bathroom, walking, taking a shower. Therapy, therapy, therapy. That is all you do. So we might as well do some right now. What are the steps involved in taking a shower? What do you have to do first? No, it is not time to turn the water on yet, but that is one of the steps. Let's write that down on an index card so that we can put all the steps in order later. Then, you can use the index cards to cue yourself the next time you want to take a shower. Now, think about this again. What is the first thing you need to do? No ideas? Let me give you a clue. You need to take some things into the bathroom with you. What are those things? No, the soap is already there. What else can you think of? A towel? No, the towels are already in the bathroom also. What are you going to put on after you get out of the shower? Clothes! Right! So you need to take some clothes with you into the bathroom. Good. Write that down on another index card. Hmm, it took you 20 minutes to recall and write down two steps. That is not very fast. We will have to work some more on your attention, concentration, and speed of processing. For now, let's figure out what therapy you will go to next.

No, you cannot go home yet. Please stop asking. The professionals working with you will talk to your family and let them know when you are ready. You do not have good enough judgment to make that decision for yourself. Give it a few more weeks.

> **" A major problem for survivors of TBI is that they pass rehabilitation but fail life. "**

Graduation day is finally here! You get to go home! Do not think you are going back to your old life, though. You may walk and talk, but you are still a survivor of TBI—and you always will be. When you walk out the front door of the rehabilitation center, you will leave the protected, highly structured world that has allowed you to function since you acquired brain damage. Now you are going to experience firsthand the extent of your deficits. No more therapists to catch you when you lose your balance. No more meals prepared by others and delivered to you. No more nurses reminding you to take your medication. No more professionals to talk you out of acting impulsively. No more people making decisions for you about what to do next or how to do it. In short, no more denying your deficits!

For your family, the scariest day of their lives will be the one on which they take you home from the rehabilitation hospital. How can they possibly take care of you? You are so impulsive. You seem to have no memory at all for what you are told or for the people you meet. After watching you sit around the house day after day, accomplishing nothing, your family will be convinced that you cannot do anything for yourself and can never be left alone. And what about all of those inappropriate comments you keep making? It is no wonder your friends do not want to stop by. Don't you have any tact left? How could anyone have possibly thought you were ready to go home?

Okay. So what are you going to do with the rest of your life? You have no job. You have lost all of your old friends and cannot seem to make new ones. You are not ready to go back to college. Your concentration and memory problems alone are enough to keep you from succeeding. When you add distractibility, slowed processing time, organization problems, impulsivity, poor planning and judgment, limited integration and synthesis of information, concrete reasoning, disinhibition, and fatigue, you do not stand a chance. Maybe after another year of therapy you will be ready to try one or two classes. Maybe, but no promises. This idea of yours that you are going to resume a full load of classes right away is crazy. It is not going to work. It is just another example of how you are still denying your deficits. Hey, I have an idea! Let's try learning about TBI as a part of your therapy. If you can learn the remainder of the information in this book, I will be convinced that you are ready to go back to school. Go on, give it a try. What do you have to lose? You already opened the book.

> **"** I think people should have to learn about TBI. I did crazy things before my accident. If only I had known, I wouldn't have done those things. **"**
>
> —18-year-old survivor

Reference

Petty, P. G. (1975). The influence of seat belt wearing on the incidence of severe head injury. *Medical Journal of Australia, 2,* 768–769.

Epidemiology of Traumatic Brain Injury
Who, What, When, Where, Why, and How

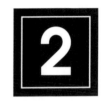

Karen Hux

Incidence and Prevalence of Traumatic Brain Injury

Traumatic brain injury (TBI) is devastating and occurs much more frequently than most people realize. Determining the incidence of TBI is a difficult task for several reasons. First, discrepancies exist in the definition of TBI. Second, some tallies include all degrees of severity, whereas others include only injuries that are severe enough to warrant hospitalization. Third, some injuries are more likely to be reported than others because of social stigmas relating to the cause of injury. Each of these factors warrants consideration before attempting to interpret incidence and prevalence reports.

Defining TBI

Traumatic brain injury is a term that can assume a very broad or a very narrow definition. In its broadest form, TBI includes both open and closed head injuries and can originate from internal or external bodily events. This definition covers a vast array of insults—such as blows to the head, gunshot wounds, brain tumors, birth traumas, cerebrovascular accidents, exposures to toxins, hypoxia, anoxia, and infections—as potential causes of TBI.

Narrow definitions of TBI limit use of the term to externally induced traumas resulting from the application of acceleration–deceleration forces to the skull. Restricting the definition in such a fashion substantially narrows the range of precipitating events that can lead to TBI. For example, limiting TBI to externally induced traumas excludes events such as brain tumors, cerebrovascular accidents, and infections, and makes inclusion of events such as near-drowning and exposure to radiation during cancer treatment questionable at best. Differences between broad and narrow definitions cause wide discrepancies in whom professionals designate as survivors of TBI and, hence, the number of TBIs tallied in epidemiological investigations.

What is the difference between incidence and prevalence?

Incidence refers to the number of times an event occurs during a specific period of time and within a specified population. For example, the annual incidence with which children and adults in the United States sustain TBIs severe enough to warrant hospitalization is around 500,000. This is the number of new cases of TBI reported to health officials each year.

Prevalence refers to the total number of existing cases of a disease at a specific moment in time and within a specified population. Thus, in any given year, the prevalence of TBI survivors in the United States includes the 500,000 who sustained injuries that year plus the hundreds of thousands who sustained injuries in previous years and are still alive. Prevalence estimates for individuals living with the consequences of TBI range from 2.5 million to 6.5 million (NIH Consensus Development Panel, 1999).

What is the difference between hypoxia and anoxia?

Hypoxia occurs when the blood supply to the brain is impeded or eliminated, and, as a result, the amount of oxygen reaching the brain is lower than normal. This would occur, for example, if a person suffered cardiac arrest and the heart failed to pump blood to the brain.

Anoxia occurs when a person's supply of oxygen is reduced or eliminated. Examples of anoxic episodes include drowning, suffocation, and inhalation of toxic fumes.

How does the federal government define TBI?

Children with TBI are eligible for special education services under the Individuals with Disabilities Education Act (IDEA; 1990, 1991). In writing this legislation the federal government adopted a narrow definition of TBI. This definition states that TBI is

> an acquired injury to the brain caused by an external physical force, resulting in total or partial functional disability or psychosocial impairment, or both, that adversely affects a child's educational performance. The term applies to open or closed head injuries resulting in impairments in one or more areas, such as cognition; language; memory; attention; reasoning; abstract thinking; judgment; problem-solving; sensory, perceptual and motor abilities; psychosocial behavior; physical functions; information processing; and speech. The term does not apply to brain injuries that are congenital or degenerative, or brain injuries induced by birth trauma. (Assistance to States for the Education of Children with Disabilities, 1992, p. 44802)

Injury Severity

Statistics about the incidence and prevalence of TBI reflect the manner in which researchers obtain reports of cases. Many researchers tally the number of people who have sought medical attention through clinics or hospital emergency rooms during specified time periods (e.g., Annegers, Grabow, Kurland, & Laws, 1980; Jennett & MacMillan, 1981; Kraus et al., 1984). Researchers may further limit tallies to include only individuals who have lost consciousness for designated lengths of time or have specific types of neurological deficits. These methods eliminate most, if not all, cases of mild injuries—a problematic scenario given that between 55% and 88% of TBIs are mild (Annegers et al., 1980; Caveness, 1979; Cohadon, Richer, & Castel, 1991; Kraus et al., 1984; Kraus, McArthur, & Silberman, 1994; Kraus & Nourjah, 1988; Miller & Jones, 1985; Rimel, Giordani, Barth, & Jane, 1982; Whitman, Coonley-Hoganson, & Desai, 1984). The likely result is the underestimation of the incidence and prevalence of TBI.

One of the reasons for not including mild TBIs in incidence and prevalence reports is that many people do not associate minor blows to the head with brain damage. The apparent insignificance of relatively minor TBIs prompts people to believe that long-term consequences will also be insignificant. However, researchers who have studied the consequences of mild TBIs have found that between 10% and 50%

Are TBIs from events such as near-drowning and exposure to radiation internally or externally induced?

The determination of whether an event is internally or externally induced is rather debatable in some instances. In a near-drowning, water external to the body prevents the person from breathing. This suggests that the resulting anoxia and brain damage are externally induced. However, many TBI definitions that use the internal/external criterion also stipulate that acceleration–deceleration forces must be present to classify an injury as externally induced. In a near-drowning, water does not exert acceleration-deceleration forces on the skull to inflict damage. So the decision about whether a near-drowning is a TBI depends on whether the definition of TBI being used stipulates that physical forces must act on the skull or head.

A similar scenario occurs when people sustain brain damage from radiation treatment. This occurs sometimes during treatment for cancers located in the head. The cancer itself may cause brain damage—as in the case of malignant brain tumors that invade or put pressure on neural structures. The damage associated directly with the tumor is always considered internally induced. The question arises when radiation treatment causes further brain damage; the radiation originates from outside of the body, suggesting the event is externally induced. However, a physical force is not present, so the classification of TBI depends on whether the definition being used stipulates the influence of an acceleration-deceleration force.

What is Shaken Baby Syndrome?

Shaken Baby Syndrome refers to a form of child abuse in which damage to the brain, spinal cord, or both results from the violent shaking of a young child. Impact to the head may occur but is not necessary to cause central nervous system damage. The rapid, violent shaking causes brain swelling, diffuse axonal injury, intracranial bleeding, and retinal hemorrhages. Medical professionals can often document intracranial damage through magnetic resonance imaging (MRI) or computerized tomography (CT) scans.

Shaken Baby Syndrome occurs most often to children under the age of 1 year and seldom occurs after age 2. Sixty percent of the victims are male, and 60% of the perpetrators are male as well. Stress related to hearing a child cry almost always precedes the abuse. About 20% to 25% of victims of Shaken Baby Syndrome die.

Symptoms of Shaken Baby Syndrome include projectile vomiting; pinpointed or dilated pupils that are unresponsive to light; pooled blood in the eyes; semiconsciousness or lethargy; difficulty breathing; seizures or spasms; and eventual swelling of the head (Alexander & Smith, 1998; Committee on Child Abuse and Neglect, 1993; Starling, Holden, & Jenny, 1995).

of survivors have long-standing memory or neurological problems (McAllister, 1992; Rimel, Giordani, Barth, Boll, & Jane, 1981; see Chapter 3).

Injury Reports

The cause of injuries and the likelihood of their being reported is another factor that makes determining the incidence and prevalence of TBI difficult. Survivors routinely seek assistance for TBIs resulting from unintentional accidents such as motor vehicle accidents or falls. However, people are less likely to report unintentional accidents relating to sporting events or to report and seek assistance for injuries resulting from intentional insults caused by assaults, domestic violence, or child abuse. For example, adolescents and young adults who sustain TBIs during sporting events may yield to social pressures from coaches and peers and not report their injuries. Furthermore, babies can sustain TBIs from violent shaking by an adult (i.e., Shaken Baby Syndrome), but because of the social and legal ramifications, parents tend not to report such incidents except in the most extreme cases.

Incidence Statistics

Disagreements in defining TBI, in deciding which cases to include and exclude in epidemiology studies, and in determining how to counteract social and legal ramifications that discourage the reporting of certain injuries cause wide variation in TBI incidence estimates. Despite these complications, a review of multiple reports suggests that between 100 and 200 people per 100,000 are hospitalized in the United States each year because of TBI (Annegers et al., 1980; Fife, Faich, Hollinshead, & Boynton, 1986; Jagger, Levine, Jane, & Rimel, 1984; Kalsbeek, McLaurin, Harris, & Miller, 1980; Klauber, Barrett-Connor, Marshall, & Bowers, 1981; Kraus et al., 1984; NIH Consensus Development Panel, 1999; Thurman & Guerrero, 1999). This means that—as a conservative estimate—between 200,000 and 500,000 new cases of TBI requiring hospitalization occur in the United States each year. Probably many more (generally mild) injuries than this actually occur. In fact, using self-reported data that included references to mild injuries, Sosin, Sniezek, and Thurman (1996) estimated that 1.5 million people sustained TBIs in the year 1991, but only 65% of these people were hospitalized for their injuries. Furthermore, an examination of trends over a 15-year period revealed a 51% decrease in hospitalization for TBI between 1980 to 1995, with the greatest drop in admissions involving mild injuries and youth between 5 and 14 years of age (Thurman & Guerrero, 1999). This trend is alarming given that it most likely reflects increasingly restrictive hospital admission practices rather than changes in the incidence of TBI.

In summary, determining the frequency of traumatic brain injury is a complicated task because of incomplete and inexact data collection procedures, ambiguities in definitions, and discrepancies in beliefs about the severity of injury necessary to cause brain damage. Despite these difficulties, determination of the incidence and prevalence of TBI is important because of the impact this information has on the provision of rehabilitation services. In addition, epidemiology information about TBI—such as identifying subgroups in the general population who sustain injuries most frequently, determining the most common causes and types of injuries, and recognizing seasonal and geographic patterns about injury occurrence—is crucial for understanding the population of survivors. The remainder of this chapter will provide information about who sustains TBIs; why some people are more susceptible to TBIs than others; how TBIs occur; when and where TBIs occur; and what identifies a TBI as mild, moderate, or severe.

Epidemiology
of TBI

TBI does not happen to a random sampling of the general population. Certain individuals are more prone to sustaining TBI than others. This does not mean that TBI cannot happen to anyone at anytime. It certainly can—and does. However, some individuals are at higher risk for sustaining a TBI than others, and some age groups are at higher risk than others.

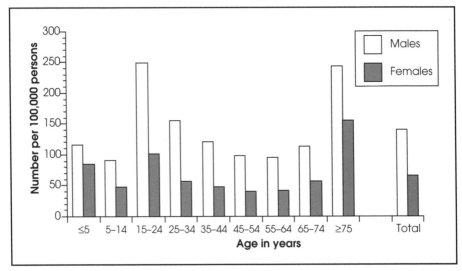

Figure 2.1. Rates of TBI across age groups and genders. *Note.* Based on data from the Centers for Disease Control and Prevention (1997).

Gender

One of the most well-documented disparities in who tends to sustain TBIs concerns gender. Throughout their lives—but especially during the teenage and young adult years—males are 2 to 3 times more likely than females to sustain TBIs (Cohadon et al., 1991; Jagger et al., 1984; Jennett & MacMillan, 1981; Kraus, 1980; Kraus et al., 1984; NIH Consensus Development Panel, 1999; Whitman et al., 1984). The primary reason for this phenomenon is the tendency for males to engage in risky behaviors—such as riding motorcycles, participating in sports such as football and wrestling, and driving recklessly—more often than females. Figure 2.1 shows the results of a 1997 report from the Centers for Disease Control and Prevention concerning the rate of TBIs for males and females throughout the life span.

Questions exist about the accuracy of the numbers showing that males are 2 to 3 times more likely than females to sustain TBIs. Investigations that included large numbers of individuals with mild TBI as well as moderate and severe TBI showed less of a discrepancy between genders. For example, Diamond (1996) performed an analysis of the medical records of all individuals who were treated and released, admitted to inpatient treatment programs, or declared "dead on arrival" at hospital emergency rooms because of TBIs and found that the male to female ratio was 1.4 to 1. Similarly, Hux, Marquardt, Skinner, and

Bond (1999) found a male to female ratio of 1.2 to 1 in a study that relied on parental reports of brain injuries, concussions, and blows to the head sustained by their middle school and high school age children.

Age

Figure 2.1 illustrates an additional imbalance in who sustains TBIs. Teenagers and young adults between 15 and 24 years of age sustain TBIs more frequently than any other age group (Centers for Disease Control and Prevention, 1997; NIH Consensus Development Panel, 1999). A second high-risk group is elderly adults, and a third high-risk group is children under the age of 5 years (Cohadon et al., 1991; NIH Consensus Development Panel, 1999). The reason for these age groups being high risk relates to social changes in the types of activities in which people engage, the incoordination of young children, and age-related degenerative changes affecting motor control.

Causes of TBI

Different causes of TBI are prominent in different age groups. As shown in Figure 2.2, the most common cause of injuries severe enough to warrant medical attention among adolescents and young adults is motor vehicle accidents (Centers for Disease Control and Prevention, 1997; NIH Consensus Development Panel, 1999). TBI occurs in approximately half of all automobile accidents (Cohadon et al., 1991) and is the cause of death in the majority of accident fatalities. In contrast to young adults, elderly adults and young children sustain the majority of their injuries from falls.

Less severe TBIs may have different patterns of etiology. In a study using parental reports of

Why are insurance rates so much higher for young male drivers than for young female drivers?

Anyone who paid for car insurance during their teenage years knows that rates are very high for new drivers. This reflects insurance companies' knowledge that inexperienced drivers have more accidents than experienced drivers. The insurance companies make a further distinction between young female drivers and young male drivers. The difference in insurance rates between teenage girls and teenage boys also has to do with the likelihood of individuals having accidents. The population at greatest risk for having car accidents is teenage boys—the same population at greatest risk for sustaining TBIs. Why do teenage boys have so many accidents? They are more likely than any other group of drivers to engage in risky behaviors such as speeding, drag-racing, and drinking and driving.

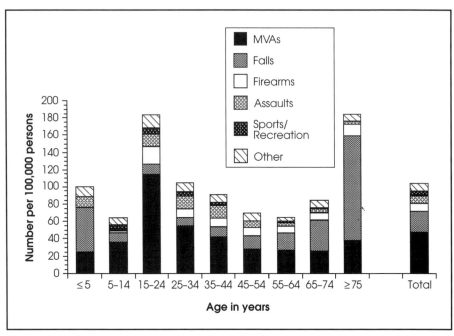

Figure 2.2. Causes of TBI severe enough to warrant medical attention across age groups. MVAs = motor vehicle accidents. *Note.* Based on data from the Centers for Disease Control and Prevention (1997).

injuries sustained by their children, 42% of youth were reported to have experienced at least one blow to the head by the time they were in middle school or high school (Hux, Bond, Skinner, Belau, & Sanger, 1998). Nearly half of the injuries were the result of sporting accidents. Motor vehicle accidents, including being thrown from a moving vehicle or sustaining a whiplash, accounted for another 26% of the injuries, and falls and fights accounted for the remaining injuries. The researchers attributed the greater frequency of sporting accidents compared to motor vehicle accidents to the severity of the sustained injuries. Specifically, more than 80% of the youth had mild injuries that did not result in changes in academic performance, behavioral or emotional control, activity level, or interactions with others. Although motor vehicle accidents are undoubtedly the cause of most moderate and severe TBIs, sporting accidents appear to be the major cause of mild TBIs among children and youth.

Another way to examine the etiology of TBIs is to contrast unintentional and intentional injuries. Unintentional injuries are events such as motor vehicle accidents, sporting accidents, occupational injuries, and falls. Intentional injuries include those caused by street violence, violent crimes, child and domestic abuse, suicide attempts, and military actions. As Figure 2.2 reveals, the majority of injuries are unintentional. However, thousands of TBIs result year each from Shaken Baby Syndrome, handgun violence, and assaults. Risk factors associated with intentional TBI include male gender, minority race, young age, low income level, and drug and alcohol use (Wagner, Sasser, Hammond, Wiercisiewski, & Alexander, 2000).

Calendar Trends

The months from May through October might be considered "TBI season." Numerous researchers have confirmed that the majority of TBIs occur during this time (see Figure 2.3) (Cooper et al., 1983; Diamond, 1996; Klauber et al., 1981; Kraus, 1980; Whitman et al., 1984). The higher incidence of TBIs during these months is because greater numbers of people are outside, where most behaviors that place them at risk for sustaining TBIs occur.

Risk Factors

Certain behaviors and health factors place individuals at high risk for sustaining one or more TBIs during their life span.

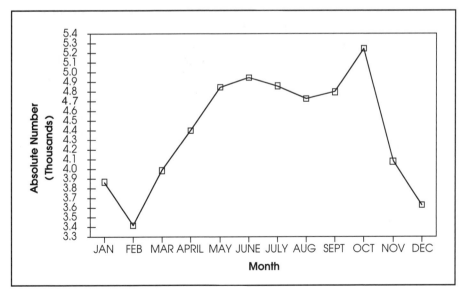

Figure 2.3. Head injury occurrence by month in the Commonwealth of Virginia, cumulative data for 1988–1993. *Note.* From "Brain Injury in the Commonwealth of Virginia: An Analysis of Central Registry Data 1988–1993," by P. T. Diamond, 1996, *Brain Injury, 10,* 413–419. Copyright 1996 by Taylor & Francis. Reprinted with permission.

Alcohol

One well-documented risk factor concerns alcohol use and abuse. Alcohol is often a contributing factor in motor vehicle accidents, pedestrian accidents, assaults, and falls; hence it contributes to the occurrence of TBI. According to the National Highway Traffic Safety Administration (n.d.), the drivers involved in more than one third of all traffic accidents that result in fatality have blood alcohol levels above the legal limit of 0.10 grams per deciliter.[1] Rimel (1981) reported that, among persons admitted for emergency room treatment because of TBIs sustained during motor vehicle accidents, blood alcohol levels of 0.10 g/dl or greater were present in 55% of cases. Furthermore, 17% of TBI survivors interviewed by Rimel and her colleagues (1982) reported having previously received some sort of treatment for alcohol abuse. Almost half of the 2,637 people included in a trauma registry because they sustained a TBI between January 1994 and September 1998 had alcohol in their bodies at the time of injury (Wagner, Sasser, et al., 2000).

Previous TBI

Another risk factor for TBI is having sustained a previous neurological injury. On average, the risk of sustaining a TBI at some point during the life span is 20% for men and 8% for women (Annegers et al., 1980). This risk rate increases by 3 times after one TBI has occurred and by 8 times after a second TBI (Annegers et al., 1980). Rimel and her colleagues (1982) reported that 42% of their sample of people with moderate TBIs and 31% of their sample of people with mild TBIs had histories of previous hospitalizations for head injury. Explanations for this phenomenon center around the existence of persistent cognitive and physical disabilities resulting from the first injury. In particular, cognitive deficits such as poor judgment, impulsivity, and decreased attention and concentration increase the likelihood of a person experiencing a second TBI. Physical impairments that affect motor control, coordination, strength, and speed are also potential contributors, especially when these impairments are mild enough not to limit participation in informal sports and recreational activities.

Preexisting Medical Conditions

In addition to prior head injury, certain other medical conditions are relatively common among the population of people with TBI. Specifically, Rimel (1981)

---

[1] On October 23, 2000, President Clinton signed into law a bill reducing the blood alcohol limit for drunkenness from 0.10 grams per deciliter to 0.08 grams per deciliter. States that do not implement the lower limit by 2004 will lose 2% of their federal highway money, with the penalty increasing to 8% by 2007.

found that 20% of patients admitted to an emergency room for treatment of TBI had histories of heart disease and high blood pressure. The co-occurrence of cardiac disorders and TBI probably relates to inadequacies in the blood supply to the brain and consequent lapses in consciousness or physical functioning.

Rimel (1981) also found that psychiatric illness was relatively common as a preexisting medical condition to TBI. Specifically, psychiatric illness occurred in 11% of the population sampled. The association between psychiatric illness and TBI probably relates to impairments in judgment, delusional thinking, and suicide attempts.

Severity of Injury

The medical classification of TBI often carries with it a specification of severity. However, the precise distribution of mild, moderate, and severe injuries is difficult to determine because epidemiology reports vary in the criteria used for classifying levels of severity. Also, many people with mild injuries do not seek medical attention, so the incidents remain unreported and are not tallied in epidemiology studies. Comparing data across multiple investigations reveals that mild TBIs account for 55% to 88% of all cases; moderate TBIs account for 9% to 34% of cases; and severe TBIs account for 5% to 21% of cases (Annegers et al., 1980; Caveness, 1979; Cohadon et al., 1991; Kraus et al., 1984; Kraus et al., 1994; Kraus & Nourjah, 1988; Miller & Jones, 1985; Rimel et al., 1982; Whitman et al., 1984). All reports are consistent in finding that mild TBIs are more common than either moderate or severe TBIs.

Another reason for confusion regarding the distribution of TBIs among the categories of mild, moderate, and severe is that the indication of a TBI as severe has distinctly different meanings for different professionals and at different points in the recovery process. The initial designation of an injury's severity typically refers solely to medical status. Hence, when a neurologist informs a family that their loved one has sustained a mild, moderate, or severe TBI, he or she is commenting primarily on the likelihood of the person surviving or dying. Only later, when survival is no longer in question, do severity judgments take into account quality-of-life issues. A person with a relatively mild injury may have persistent and profound impairments affecting success in academic, social, and vocational endeavors. In this case, the extent and impact of cognitive deficits will prompt rehabilitation professionals to refer to the TBI as severe, regardless of whether the initial injury was life threatening. Conversely, rehabilitation professionals may refer to the injury of a person who was initially near death but who experiences minimal long-term disability as a mild TBI. Readers of articles appearing in professional journals need to be particularly aware of differences in the use of severity terminology. Some people serving as research participants are categorized as severe because of the extent of their initial injury; others are categorized as severe because of their current level of functioning. This distinction becomes critical when researchers compare results across studies.

Prognosis for Recovery

Although many factors—such as age, educational background, psychosocial status, quality and extent of medical care and rehabilitation, family support, and personality characteristics—have the potential to affect TBI outcomes, two prognostic indicators are commonly used by medical professionals during the early stages of recovery: (a) the extent and location of brain damage and (b) the length of impaired consciousness, specifically regarding the duration of coma and posttraumatic amnesia. Recently, professionals have recognized a third prognostic indicator: the presence or absence of a specific gene.

Extent and Location of Brain Damage

An obvious factor in estimating the severity of a brain injury involves determining how much neural tissue has been damaged. Most people assume that the more brain matter damaged, the worse the potential outcome; however, some factors complicate this relation. First, much of the damage incurred during TBI is diffuse, occuring at cellular and microscopic levels, and may not be visible with currently available brain imaging techniques. This means that quantifying damage is not possible; instead, professionals rely on observing behaviors that suggest varying degrees of brain damage. Second, the *site* of damage often has more influence on a person's eventual outcome than the *amount* of damage. Destruction of neural tissue located in different regions of the brain will result in different functional impairments. For example, focal damage to the left perisylvian cortex typically results in aphasia, whereas an equal magnitude of focal damage to the occipital lobes may result in visual impairment or cortical blindness. Although both of these impairments cause obvious hardship and potential disability, they have quite distinct long-term implications.

Partially as a result of the complications associated with pairing injury severity with the amount and site of brain damage, behavioral observations that provide estimates of injury severity continue to be a primary prognostic indicator used by medical professionals. The Glasgow Coma Scale (Jennett & Teasdale, 1977; Teasdale & Jennett, 1974, 1976) is a tool frequently used for this purpose; initial Glasgow scores ranging from 3 to 8 correspond with severe brain damage, scores ranging from 9 to 12 correspond with moderate injury, and scores from 13 to 15 correspond with mild injuries. (Details about the Glasgow Coma Scale and its administration and scoring are provided in Chapter 5.)

Considerable research exists documenting the relation between patients' initial Glasgow scores and their eventual outcomes from TBI. Regarding mortality, Hill, Delaney, and Roncal (1997) found that two thirds of the individuals with initial Glasgow scores of 3 died; 18.13% of those with initial scores between 4 and 12 died; 7.81% of people with scores of 13 or 14 died; and only 3.91% of people with scores of 15 died. Miller and Jones (1985) found that only 20% of people with Glasgow scores below 8 had favorable outcomes (i.e., functioned independently despite some persistent cognitive or physical disabilities), whereas 80% of people with scores between 8 and 12 and 96% of people with scores above 12 experienced favorable recoveries. The work of Wagner and her colleagues (Wagner, Hammond, Sasser, Wiercisiewski, & Norton, 2000) confirmed these results through their finding that Glasgow scores of 8 or less were predictive of more disability and poorer community reintegration at 1 year postinjury than scores of 9 or higher.

Length of Impaired Consciousness

Professionals have long believed that injury severity and potential for recovery relate directly to the length of a patient's impaired consciousness. Over the years, two aspects of impaired consciousness have emerged as primary prognostic indicators—the length of coma and the length of posttraumatic amnesia. The term *coma* refers to a condition in which an individual lacks arousal and awareness of his or her surrounding (see Chapter 5). It corresponds with a Glasgow score of 8 or lower, with no eye opening response present. A person in coma does not follow commands and does not verbalize (Jennett & Teasdale, 1977, 1981). Posttraumatic amnesia (PTA) refers to the period during which an individual cannot store and recall ongoing events (Russell, 1932; Russell & Smith, 1961). It begins at the time of injury and extends until the survivor can recall information for a 24-hour period (including the period of coma).

Coma may last for less than 1 second or may persist indefinitely. In the former case, the person may not realize that he or she lost consciousness at all, and no report of coma may exist; in the latter case, the patient is said to be in a *persistent vegetative state* or to be *slow-to-recover* (see Chapter 5). Between these two extremes, levels of injury severity correspond with differing lengths of coma. According to Asikainen, Kaste, and Sarna (1998), approximately 50%

Why do physicians sometimes purposefully induce coma in TBI survivors?

People who sustain TBIs are sometimes combative and agitated, and they become more so when the external environment is highly stimulating—such as in an intensive care unit. Being in an agitated state tends to cause an increase in the level of intracranial pressure (ICP). Above a certain point, increases in ICP are life-threatening. To help control ICP, a physician may prescribe barbiturates that will keep a TBI survivor in a comatose state. When ICP stabilizes at an acceptable level, the drugs are slowly withdrawn while ICP monitoring continues. If ICP remains within certain limits, medical or rehabilitation professionals will assess the survivor's level of arousal and alertness to determine whether he or she is still in a state of impaired consciousness due to actual brain damage.

of children and young adults who were comatose for less than 30 minutes experienced a good recovery; in contrast, coma duration between 30 minutes and 1 week most often resulted in moderate disability, and coma duration longer than 1 week most frequently corresponded with severe disability. Of course, exceptions to these guidelines are not unusual, so length of coma should never serve as the sole prognostic indicator. In fact, many TBI professionals consider coma duration to be a rather crude measure of injury severity and believe that the duration of PTA is a better predictor of eventual outcome. Furthermore, sometimes medical professionals purposefully keep an individual in a comatose state through the administration of medications; clearly, coma duration is of little or no prognostic value in these incidences.

Researchers have estimated that, for most survivors, the duration of PTA is approximately 2 times that of coma duration or 4 times the period that it takes for a person to speak following injury (Jennett & Teasdale, 1981). Table 2.1 shows the guidelines established by Russell and Smith (1961) and Fortuny, Briggs, Newcombe, Ratcliff, and Thomas (1980) for equating PTA duration with injury severity. Table 2.2 shows the correlation established between the duration of PTA and three broad classifications of long-term recovery (Jennett & Teasdale, 1981).

Genetics: Apolipoprotein E

In recent years, researchers have attempted to determine whether differences exist among people in their genetic predisposition to respond favorably or unfavorably to nervous system injury. Research about Alzheimer's disease and TBI that targeted a gene responsible for production of apolipoprotein E (apoE) gave rise to the notion

Table 2.1
Association Between Duration of Posttraumatic Amnesia (PTA) and Injury Severity

Duration of PTA	Injury severity
Less than 10 minutes	Very mild injury
10 minutes to 60 minutes	Mild injury
1 hour to 24 hours	Moderate injury
1 day to 7 days	Severe injury
More than 7 days	Very severe injury

Table 2.2
Posttraumatic Amnesia and Outcome at 6 Months

PTA	n	Severely disabled (%)	Moderately disabled (%)	Good recovery (%)
<14 days	101	0	17	83
15–28 days	96	3	31	66
>28 days	289	30	43	27

Note. From *Management of Head Injuries,* by B. Jennett and G. Teasdale, 1981, New York: Oxford University Press. Copyright 1981 by Oxford University Press. Reprinted with permission.

that genetic differences may account for some of the variability in TBI recovery patterns.

The gene for apoE is located on chromosome 19 and has several different forms. The presence of a certain form (i.e., ε4) of the apoE gene is associated with the occurrence of substantial deposits of amyloid β-protein in the cerebral cortex—a prominent feature of Alzheimer's disease. Researchers have determined that people with the ε4 allele have a genetic predisposition to develop Alzheimer's disease (Corder et al., 1993; Poirer et al., 1993; Saunders et al., 1993) and to experience poor outcomes following neurological injuries (Alberts et al., 1995; Friedman et al., 1999; Mayeux et al., 1995; Sorbi et al., 1995; Teasdale, Nicoll, Murray, & Fiddes, 1997). Specifically, death following TBI is more than 3 times as likely among people with the ε4 allele than among those without it (Alberts et al., 1995), and less favorable outcome 6 months after injury is more likely among survivors with the ε4 allele than among those without that form of the gene (Friedman et al., 1999; Teasdale et al., 1997). Sorbi and her colleagues (1995) found a higher frequency of the apoE-ε4 allele among young adults who did not recover from prolonged coma following TBI than among young adults who did recover. They claimed that the presence or absence of the apoE-ε4 allele predicted outcome better than other prognostic indicators (e.g., age, duration of coma, and initial Glasgow Coma Scale score). In addition, Mayeux and colleagues (1995) reported that individuals with the apoE-ε4 allele and a history of head injury were 10 times more likely to develop Alzheimer's disease than TBI survivors without the ε4 allele.

Summary

Determining TBI frequency is difficult because of differences in definitions and tallying procedures. General consensus is that mild injuries are 2 to 3 times more common than moderate or severe injuries. Among children and young adults, the most common cause of severe TBI is motor vehicle crashes, and the most common cause of mild TBI is sporting accidents. Factors that increase a person's likelihood of sustaining a TBI include being male, being an adolescent or young adult, engaging in high-risk activities such as riding motorcycles or playing football, drinking alcohol excessively, having had a previous TBI, and having certain medical conditions such as cardiac disorder or psychiatric illness. The extent and location of brain damage, the duration of impaired consciousness, and the presence of a specific gene associated with poor recovery from neurological injury are the primary indicators professionals use to predict long-term outcome from TBI.

References

Alberts, M. J., Graffagnino, C., McClenny, C., DeLong, D., Strittmatter, W., Saunders, A. M., & Roses, A. D. (1995). ApoE genotype and survival from intracerebral haemorrhage. *Lancet, 346,* 575.

Alexander, R. C., & Smith, W. L. (1998). Shaken baby syndrome. *Infants and Young Children, 10*(3), 1–9.

Annegers, J. F., Grabow, J. D., Kurland, L. T., & Laws, E. R. (1980). The incidence, causes, and secular trends of head trauma in Olmstead County, Minnesota 1935–1974. *Neurology, 30,* 912–919.

Asikainen, I., Kaste, M., & Sarna, S. (1998). Predicting late outcome for patients with traumatic brain injury referred to a rehabilitation programme: A study of 508 Finnish patients 5 years or more after injury. *Brain Injury, 12,* 95–107.

Assistance to States for the Education of Children with Disabilities Program and Preschool Grants for Children with Disabilities, 57 Fed. Reg. 44794–44852 (September 29, 1992).

Caveness, W. F. (1979). Incidence of craniocerebral trauma in the United States in 1976 with trend from 1970 to 1975. *Advances in Neurology, 22,* 1–3.

Centers for Disease Control and Prevention. (1997). Traumatic brain injury—Colorado, Missouri, Oklahoma, and Utah, 1990–1993. *Morbidity and Mortality Weekly Report, 46*(1), 8–11.

Cohadon, F., Richer, E., & Castel, J. P. (1991). Head injuries: Incidence and outcome. *Journal of the Neurological Sciences, 103,* S27–S31.

Committee on Child Abuse and Neglect. (1993). Shaken baby syndrome: Inflicted cerebral trauma. *Pediatrics, 92,* 872–875.

Cooper, K. D., Tabaddor, K., Hauser, W. A., Shulman, K., Feiner, C., & Factor, P. R. (1983). The epidemiology of head injury in the Bronx. *Neuroepidemiology, 2,* 70–88.

Corder, E. H., Saunders, A. M., Strittmatter, W. J., Schmechel, D. E., Gaskell, P. C., Small, G. W., Roses, A. D., Haines, J. L., & Pericak-Vance, M. A. (1993). Gene dose of apolipoprotein E type 4 allele and the risk of Alzheimer's disease in late onset families. *Science, 261,* 921–923.

Diamond, P. T. (1996). Brain injury in the commonwealth of Virginia: An analysis of Central Registry data, 1988–1993. *Brain Injury, 10,* 413–419.

Fife, D., Faich, G., Hollinshead, W., & Boynton, W. (1986). Incidence and outcome of hospital-treated head injury in Rhode Island. *American Journal of Public Health, 76,* 773–778.

Fortuny, L. A., Briggs, M., Newcombe, F., Ratcliff, G., & Thomas, C. (1980). Measuring the duration of post-traumatic amnesia. *Journal of Neurology, Neurosurgery, and Psychiatry, 43,* 377–379.

Friedman, G., Froom, P., Sazbon, L., Grinblatt, I., Shochina, M., Tsenter, J., Babaey, S., Ben Yehuda, A., & Groswasser, Z. (1999). Apolipoprotein E-ε4 genotype predicts a poor outcome in survivors of traumatic brain injury. *Neurology, 52,* 244–248.

Hill, D. A., Delaney, L. M., & Roncal, S. (1997). A Chi-square automatic interaction detection (CHAID) analysis of factors determining trauma outcomes. *The Journal of Trauma: Injury, Infection, and Critical Care, 42,* 62–66.

Hux, K., Bond, V., Skinner, S., Belau, D., & Sanger, D. (1998). Parental report of occurrences and consequences of traumatic brain injury among delinquent and non-delinquent youth. *Brain Injury, 12,* 667–681.

Hux, K., Marquardt, J., Skinner, S., & Bond, V. (1999). Special education services provided to students with and without parental reports of traumatic brain injury. Brain Injury, 13, 447–455.

Individuals with Disabilities Education Act of 1990, 20 U.S.C. § 1400 *et seq.*

Individuals with Disabilities Education Act Amendments of 1991, 20 U.S.C. § 1400 *et seq.*

Jagger, J., Levine, J. I., Jane. J. A., & Rimel, R. W. (1984). Epidemiologic features of head injury in a predominantly rural population. *Journal of Trauma, 24,* 40–44.

Jennett, B., & MacMillan, R. (1981). Epidemiology of head injury. *British Medical Journal, 282,* 100–104.

Jennett, B., & Teasdale, G. (1977). Aspects of coma after severe head injury. *Lancet, 1,* 878–881.

Jennett, B., & Teasdale, G. (1981). *Management of head injuries.* New York: Oxford University Press.

Kalsbeek, W. D., McLaurin, R. L., Harris, B. S. H., & Miller, J. D. (1980). The national head and spinal cord injury survey: Major findings. *Journal of Neurosurgery, 53,* S19–S31.

Klauber, M. R., Barrett-Connor, E., Marshall, L. F., & Bowers, S. A. (1981). The epidemiology of head injury. *American Journal of Epidemiology, 113,* 500–509.

Kraus, J. F. (1980). A comparison of recent studies on the extent of the head and spinal cord injury problem in the United States. *Journal of Neurosurgery, 53*(Suppl.), S35–S43.

Kraus, J. F., Black, M. A., Hessol, N., Ley, P., Rokaw, W., Sullivan, C., Bowers, S., Knowlton, S., & Marshall, L. (1984). The incidence of acute brain injury and serious impairment in a defined population. *American Journal of Epidemiology, 119*, 186–201.

Kraus, J. F., McArthur, D. L., & Silberman, T. A. (1994). Epidemiology of mild brain injury. *Seminars in Neurology, 14*, 1–7.

Kraus, J. F., & Nourjah, P. (1988). The epidemiology of mild, uncomplicated brain injury. *The Journal of Trauma, 28*, 1637–1643.

Mayeux, R., Ottman, R., Maestre, G., Ngai, C., Tang, M.-X., Ginsberg, H., Chun, M., Tycko, B., & Shelanski, M. (1995). Synergistic effects of traumatic head injury and apolipoprotein-ε4 in patients with Alzheimer's disease. *Neurology, 45*, 555–557.

McAllister, T. W. (1992). Neuropsychiatric sequelae of head injuries. *Psychiatric Clinics of North America, 15*, 395–413.

Miller, J. D., & Jones, P. A. (1985). The work of a regional head injury service. *Lancet, 1*, 1141–1144.

National Highway Traffic Safety Administration. (n.d). *Traffic safety facts 2000: Alcohol.* Retrieved November 12, 2001, from www.nrd.nhtsa.dot.gov/pdf/nrd-30/ncsa/tsf2000/2001 2000alcfacts.pdf

NIH Consensus Development Panel on Rehabilitation of Persons with Traumatic Brain Injury. (1999). Rehabilitation of persons with traumatic brain injury. *Journal of the American Medical Association, 282*, 974–983.

Poirer, J., Davignon, J., Bouthillier, D., Kogan, S., Bertrand, P., & Gauthier, S. (1993). Apolipoprotein E polymorphism and Alzheimer's disease. *Lancet, 342*, 697–699.

Rimel, R. W. (1981). A prospective study of patients with central nervous system trauma. *Journal of Neurosurgical Nursing, 13*(3), 132–141.

Rimel, R. W., Giordani, B., Barth, J. T., Boll, T. J., & Jane, J. A. (1981). Disability caused by minor head injury. *Neurosurgery, 9*, 221–228.

Rimel, R. W., Giordani, B., Barth, J. T., & Jane, J. A. (1982). Moderate head injury: Completing the clinical spectrum of brain trauma. *Neurology, 11*, 344–351.

Russell, W. R. (1932). Cerebral involvement in head injury. *Brain, 55*, 549–603.

Russell, W. R., & Smith, A. (1961). Post-traumatic amnesia in closed head injury. *Archives of Neurology, 5*, 16–29.

Saunders, A. M., Strittmatter, W. J., Schmechel, D., St. George-Hyslop, P. H., Pericak-Vance, M. A., Joo, S. H., Rosi, B. L., Gusella, J. F., Crapper-MacLachlan, D. R., Alberts, M. J., Hulette, C., Crain, B., Goldgaber, D., & Roses, A. D. (1993). Association of apolipoprotein ε4 with late-onset familial and sporadic Alzheimer's disease. *Neurology, 43*, 1467–1472.

Sorbi, S., Nacmias, B., Piacentini, S., Repice, A., Latorraca, S., Forleo, P., & Amaducci, L. (1995). ApoE as a prognostic factor for post-traumatic coma. *Natural Medicine, 1*, 852.

Sosin, D. M., Sniezek, J. E., & Thurman, D. J. (1996). Incidence of mild and moderate brain injury in the United States, 1991. *Brain Injury, 10*, 47–54.

Starling, S. P., Holden, J. R., & Jenny, C. (1995). Abusive head trauma: The relationship of perpetrators to their victims. *Pediatrics, 95*, 259–262.

Teasdale, G., & Jennett, B. (1974). Assessment of coma and impaired consciousness. *Lancet, 2*, 81–84.

Teasdale, G., & Jennett, B. (1976). Assessment and prognosis of coma after head injury. *Acta Neurochirugia, 34*, 45–55.

Teasdale, G. M., Nicoll, J. A. R., Murray, G., & Fiddes, M. (1997). Association of apolipoprotein E polymorphism with outcome after head injury. *Lancet, 350,* 1069–1071.

Thurman, D., & Guerrero, J. (1999). Trends in hospitalization associated with traumatic brain injury. *Journal of the American Medical Association, 282,* 954–957.

Wagner, A. K., Hammond, F. M., Sasser, H. C., Wiercisiewski, D., & Norton, H. J. (2000). Use of injury severity variables in determining disability and community integration after traumatic brain injury. *The Journal of Trauma Injury, Infection, and Critical Care, 49,* 411–419.

Wagner, A. K., Sasser, H. C., Hammond, F. M., Wiercisiewski, D., & Alexander, J. (2000). Intentional traumatic brain injury: Epidemiology, risk factors, and associations with injury severity and mortality. *The Journal of Trauma Injury, Infection, and Critical Care, 49,* 404–410.

Whitman, S., Coonley-Hoganson, R., & Desai, B. T. (1984). Comparative head trauma experiences in two socioeconomically different Chicago-area communities: A population study. *American Journal of Epidemiology, 119,* 570–580.

Mild Traumatic Brain Injury

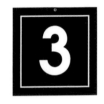

Karen Hux

> ❝ *I wish there had been blood and gore. Then, maybe people would believe that I really have a head injury.* ❞
>
> —*35-year-old survivor of mild TBI*

Many terms are used to refer to mild traumatic brain injury (TBI). In addition to *mild TBI*, current terminology includes *minor head injury, concussion,* and *postconcussive syndrome.* All of these terms are associated with a cluster of cognitive, physical, and behavioral symptoms that repeatedly appear in the complaints of people who have sustained what appear—at least initially—to be rather minor, insignificant injuries to the head.

In the past, additional terms have appeared in reference to mild TBI. Some of these terms—such as *ding amnestic syndrome* (referring to being "dinged" on the head; Yarnell & Lynch, 1973) and *accident neurosis* (Miller, 1961) or *compensation neurosis* (Noy, 1975), referring to fictitious problems that routinely disappear following the completion of litigation procedures—reflect the uncertainty that medical professionals and insurance company representatives have had concerning the legitimacy of mild TBI as a disabling condition. Indeed, one of the most pervasive debates in the mild TBI literature concerns distinguishing between people who have legitimate deficits following injury and those who are malingering (e.g., Binder & Willis, 1991; Ruff, Wylie, & Tennant, 1993; Stevens & Price, 1999).

No one doubts the existence of TBI when focal neurological deficits are evident upon physical examination or when structural changes can be observed on computerized tomography (CT) or magnetic resonance imaging (MRI) scans. Unfortunately, such evidence is not common among survivors of mild TBI; even brief losses of consciousness are not routine consequences of mild injury. Instead, professionals must make diagnostic decisions on the basis of clinical symptoms reported by survivors and observed during neuropsychological testing. However, the consistency with which people complain about specific and persistent cognitive, physical, and emotional challenges following mild injuries lends credence to the disorder and makes mild TBI an important area of consideration for medical, rehabilitation, and education professionals. The following sections provide information about defining mild TBI, describing its causes and frequency of occurrence, measuring its severity, describing prominent short-term and long-term characteristics, dealing with challenges of identification, and treating persistent problems. The final two sections address the phenomenon of second impact syndrome and provide guidelines for coaches and athletes about injury prevention and identification.

Definition

Professionals have struggled to define mild TBI. Because of the inherent anatomical and physiological variability among people, definitive statements cannot be made about the intensity or magnitude of neurological insult needed to cause brain damage. Instead, professionals must make judgments about the presence of brain damage based largely on anecdotal information provided by the survivor and behavioral observations. In an attempt to provide some standardization for claiming the occurrence of mild TBI, the Mild Traumatic Brain Injury Committee associated with the American Congress of Rehabilitation Medicine (1993) developed the following defining criteria:

> A person with mild traumatic brain injury is a person who has had a traumatically induced physiological disruption of brain function, as manifested by at least one of the following:
>
> 1. any period of loss of consciousness;
> 2. any loss of memory for events immediately before or after the accident;
> 3. any alteration in mental state at the time of the accident (e.g., feeling dazed, disoriented, or confused); and
> 4. focal neurological deficit(s) that may or may not be transient;
>
> but where the severity of the injury does not exceed the following:
>
> - loss of consciousness of approximately 30 minutes or less;
> - after 30 minutes, an initial Glasgow Coma Scale (GCS) of 13–15; and
> - posttraumatic amnesia (PTA) not greater than 24 hours. (p. 86)

Several features of these defining criteria are worthy of note. First, the criteria assume occurrence of an identifiable event originating outside the body as the cause of brain damage; events such as strokes, brain tumors, and infections are not included as potential causes of mild TBI. Second, the criteria do not require the substantiation of neurological damage through brain imaging procedures or routine neurological evaluations. Third, the person sustaining injury must experience at least one, but not necessarily more than one, of the previously listed symptoms. Hence, one individual sustaining a mild TBI may lose consciousness, but another may not; one individual may experience memory impairment, but another may not; one individual may display disorientation and confusion, but another may not.

Causes and Frequency

The causes of mild TBI differ somewhat from the causes of more severe TBI. In at least some reports, sporting accidents and falls replace motor vehicle accidents as the most common causes of injury (Guerrero, Thurman, & Sniezek, 2000; Hux, Bond, Skinner, Belau, & Sanger, 1998). Youth and young adults are most prone to acquiring mild TBI through sporting accidents, whereas toddlers and elderly adults most commonly sustain such injuries through falls.

Based on data from the Injury Supplement to the 1991 National Health Interview Survey, the estimated number of mild and moderate brain injuries sustained each year in the United States is 1.54 million (Sosin, Sniezek, & Thurman, 1996). For the purpose of this survey, mild and moderate head injuries were defined as blows to the head that resulted in a loss of consciousness but did not cause death or long-term hospitalization. Assuming that people who required hospitalization for more than 1 day represented those with moderate rather than mild injuries, the estimated number of mild TBIs is 1.29 million. However, because the data did not include people who sustained blows to the head not resulting in a loss of consciousness, 1.29 million must be regarded as an underestimate of the actual incidence of mild TBI. Among individuals reporting mild TBIs, 381,000 (29.5%) sought no medical care; 221,000 (17%) received treatment in clinics or doctors' offices; 543,000 (42%) received treatment in emergency departments; and 146,000 (11%) were hospitalized overnight.

Based on the same data set, the estimated number of sports-related concussions occurring every year in the United States is 308,000 (Sosin et al., 1996); over 150,000 of these result from bicycle accidents (Consumer Product Safety Commission, n.d.), and around 100,000 are from football (J. Powell, personal communication, as cited in Cantu, 1996). Bicycling and football are not the only sports associated with a high risk of mild TBI, however. In fact, some other sports—such as boxing, horseback riding, and race car driving—actually have higher frequencies of injury per participant, but, because fewer people engage in these sports, fewer injuries result from them. High-risk sports include boxing, football, ice hockey, martial arts, rugby, wrestling, soccer, auto racing, equestrian sports, gymnastics, motorcycle riding, diving, bicycling, snow skiing, basketball, baseball, softball, field hockey, pole vaulting, and volleyball. Figure 3.1 shows the percentage of mild brain injuries sustained by high school athletes in each of 10 sports (Powell & Barber-Foss, 1999); Table 3.1, based on data from the NCAA Injury Surveillance System, shows the frequency with which concussions occur among collegiate athletes involved in various sports.

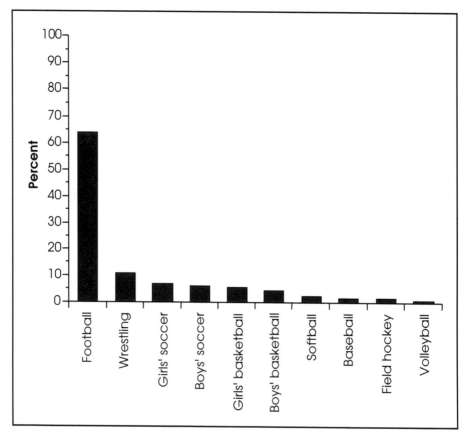

Figure 3.1. Percentage of high school students sustaining mild TBIs from each of 10 sports. *Note.* Based on data from Powell and Barber-Foss (1999).

Table 3.1
Frequency of Concussion Among College Athletes

Sport	Frequency per 100,000 athlete exposures[a]
Football	27
Ice hockey	25
Men's soccer	25
Women's soccer	24
Wrestling	20
Field hockey	20
Men's lacrosse	19
Women's lacrosse	16
Women's basketball	15
Men's basketball	12
Women's softball	11
Baseball	7

[a]Dick (1994) defined an athlete exposure as "one athlete participating in one practice or game where he or she is exposed to the possibility of athletic injury" (p. 15).

Note. Based on information from "A Summary of Head and Neck Injuries in Collegiate Athletics Using the NCAA Injury Surveillance System," by R. W. Dick, 1994, in *Head and Neck Injuries in Sports: ASTM Special Technical Publication 1229,* by E. F. Hoerner (Ed.), 1994, Philadelphia: American Society for Testing and Materials. Copyright 1994 by American Society for Testing and Materials. Adapted with permission.

Boxing is the only professional sport in which the objective is to inflict sufficient injury to render an opponent unconscious. The American Academy of Neurology (1983) and the American Academy of Pediatrics (1997) have both made formal statements opposing the sport of boxing and calling for its abolition.

Measuring Injury Severity

A concussion's severity is typically identified through a numeric label. Based on a consensus of experts in the field and a review of existing literature, the Quality Standards Subcommittee of the American Academy of Neurology (1997) recommended distinguishing three levels of concussion: Grade 1, Grade 2, and Grade 3. As shown in Table 3.2, the distinguishing feature

Table 3.2
Features Distinguishing Grade 1, 2, and 3 Concussions

Grade	Confusion	Loss of consciousness[a]	Duration of symptoms
1	Yes	No	<15 minutes
2	Yes	No	>15 minutes
3	Not applicable	Yes	Not applicable

[a] "Loss of consciousness" is said to be "brief" if it lasts a matter of seconds; it is said to be "prolonged" if it lasts a matter of minutes.

between Grade 1 and Grade 2 concussions is the duration of the symptoms; the distinguishing feature between Grade 2 and Grade 3 concussions is loss of consciousness.

An alternative method of identifying injury severity uses a combination of the duration of lost consciousness and the duration of posttraumatic amnesia (PTA)—that is, the period between the time of injury and the regaining of adequate memory to recall daily events (Russell, 1932; Russell & Smith, 1961; see Chapter 5 for additional information about PTA). This system, proposed by Ruff and Jurica (1999), classifies mild TBI into three types. Type I includes an altered state or transient loss of consciousness and a PTA duration of 1 to 60 seconds; Type II includes a definite loss of consciousness of unknown duration or less than 5 minutes and a PTA duration of 60 seconds to 12 hours; Type III includes a loss of consciousness between 5 and 30 minutes and a PTA duration of greater than 12 hours. Type I injuries roughly correspond with Grade 1 concussions; Type II and III injuries represent subdivisions of Grade 3 concussions.

Characteristics

Symptoms of mild TBI may be transient or may persist indefinitely. Table 3.3 lists many of the cognitive, physical, and behavioral symptoms that can appear in isolation or combination following mild TBI.

When a person sustains a mild TBI and complains of a cluster of symptoms from those listed in Table 3.3, the label *postconcussive syndrome* may be applied. The majority of people who sustain mild TBIs find that symptoms abate over time, and most recover fully within a few months; however, a subgroup of individuals experiences persistent cognitive, physical, and behavioral challenges (Alves, Macciocchi, & Barth, 1993; Binder, 1986, 1997; Cohadon, Richer, & Castel, 1991; Dikmen, Temkin, & Armsden, 1989; Jagoda & Riggio, 2000;

Table 3.3
Symptoms Associated with Mild TBI

Cognitive symptoms	Physical symptoms	Behavioral symptoms
Decreased attention	Headache	Irritability
Decreased concentration	Lethargy/lowered	Quickness to anger
Perceptual disturbances	stamina	Disinhibition
Memory impairment	Nausea	Emotional lability
Speech–language	Vomiting	Increased anxiety
problems	Dizziness	Depression
Poor executive functioning	Blurred vision	
Disorientation	Double vision	
	Hypersensitivity to light	
	Tinnitus	
	Sleep disturbance	
	Fatigue	

McLean, Temkin, Dikmen, & Wyler, 1983; Radanov, Di Stefano, Schnidrig, Sturzenegger, & Augustiny, 1993; Rimel, Giordani, Barth, Boll, & Jane, 1981; Rutherford, Merrett, & McDonald, 1978). Alves et al. (1993) documented that up to 40% of people admitted to a hospital with a diagnosis of uncomplicated mild TBI continued to display one or more postconcussive symptoms 1 year later. Other researchers have proposed a more moderate incidence rate of around 15% (Rutherford et al., 1978). Agreement exists, however, that the most common persistent complaint is chronic pain, usually in the form of headaches, followed by memory impairment, depression, and dizziness.

Some researchers have attempted to identify factors distinguishing individuals who do have from those who do not have persistent postconcussive symptoms. Through an examination of children with mild TBIs at 3 months postinjury, Ponsford and her colleagues (1999) found that those with persistent problems differed from those without residual complaints in their likelihood of having four premorbid factors: a previous head injury, neurological or psychiatric problems, learning difficulties, and stressors such as family breakdown. Among adults, multiple researchers have found that older age at the time of injury, preexisting psychosocial stressors, and lower levels of educational achievement are associated with persistent symptoms of postconcussive syndrome (Barth et al., 1983; Bohnen, Twijnstra, & Jolles, 1992;

Cohadon et al., 1991; Fenton, McClelland, Montgomery, MacFlynn, & Rutherford, 1993; Radanov et al., 1993; Rimel et al., 1981). What remains unknown is whether these preexisting conditions make people more vulnerable to postconcussive syndrome for organic reasons or psychological reasons. In other words, do postconcussive symptoms persist in a subset of people who sustain mild TBIs because, prior to injury, their brains are neurologically different from the brains of other people, or do the symptoms persist because, either prior to or as a result of injury, the people have psychosocial stressors (e.g., depression, family problems, litigation issues, etc.) that render them less able to recover fully?

Challenges with Identification

A major problem associated with mild TBI is identifying when it has occurred and conveying this information to the appropriate people. One factor contributing to this problem is that many people do not seek medical attention following a concussion because of its presumed triviality; hence, a medical record documenting the event may not exist. Although this is only problematic when postconcussive symptoms do not abate relatively quickly, researchers have estimated that this scenario occurs in up to 40% of cases of mild TBI (Alves et al., 1993).

Another factor contributing to the problem of identification occurs when individuals with mild TBIs receive medical attention but are not informed of the possible long-term consequences associated with their injury. Physicians are in a difficult position regarding this issue: They do not want to worry people unnecessarily, yet they need to alert them to possible problems. Some research suggests that the appearance and magnitude of postconcussive symptoms following mild TBIs match symptom expectations (Ferguson, Mittenberg, Barone, & Schneider, 1999). Hence, physicians may be reluctant to instill fears in people about the possible occurrence of changes in cognitive, emotional, or behavioral status. On the other hand, anger and frustration about postconcussive changes result when symptoms persist and individuals have not been informed of this possibility.

Another factor complicating identification concerns when and where most mild TBIs occur. Few injuries happen during school or work hours; most occur during recreational or sporting events that take place after hours or on weekends. Hence, school or work personnel may not be aware that a student or employee has sustained a mild TBI. Without this information, the symptoms of postconcussive syndrome may mistakenly be attributed to a lack of motivation or change in attitude. This is particularly likely with adolescents who, as they struggle with identity, adjustment, and maturation issues, often experience periods of variable academic performance. Distinguishing between a student who lacks motivation because of the challenges associated with adolescence and one who struggles academically, socially, or emotionally because of postconcussive symptoms is almost impossible when information about an injury has not been made available. To combat this problem, educators must be highly sensitive to changes in academic and psychosocial behaviors and seek out information about possible injuries that coincide in time with observed changes.

Treatment

As physicians and rehabilitation professionals have become increasingly aware of the potential for persistent problems following mild TBI and better able to identify individuals with postconcussive syndrome, efforts to develop and implement effective treatment strategies have increased. Neuropsychologists and speech–language pathologists have taken the lead in providing treatment for cognition problems (Harrington, Malec, Cicerone, & Katz, 1993). Treatment strategies run the gamut from educating survivors and family members about the consequences of mild TBI to providing formal cognitive rehabilitation.

In general, the role of speech–language pathologists working with survivors of mild TBI parallels that assumed when working with survivors of more severe injuries; the primary differences are in the intensity and duration of treatment. Whereas clinicians may work with survivors of severe TBI on a daily basis over a period of several months, the treatment for survivors of mild TBI may be required on a less frequent basis and last for only a few weeks (Harrington et al., 1993).

Second Impact Syndrome

Second impact syndrome, sometimes referred to as *malignant cerebral edema*, occurs when an individual sustains a second head injury before the symptoms of an earlier injury have resolved. Both the first and second injuries are typically mild; the first may or may not have resulted in a loss of consciousness. The two injuries together, however, have a compounding effect and catastrophic consequences. The second injury, despite its mildness, causes vasomotor paralysis, diffuse cerebral swelling, and a rapid increase in intracranial pressure. This leads to herniation of the brain stem and death, usually within a few minutes or hours. Most people who suffer second impact syndrome die (McCrory & Berkovic, 1998); virtually all who survive sustain massive brain damage (Cantu, 1998). Children and adolescents appear to be particularly susceptible to second impact syndrome (McCrory & Berkovic, 1998).

Prevention of second impact syndrome is the only real treatment. Changes in game rules, equipment, conditioning, and on-field medical care have greatly reduced the number of serious head injuries sustained during sporting events. However, because second impact syndrome typically results from mild TBIs that may or may not involve a loss of consciousness, its incidence has not been affected by these changes. Only when players, coaches, and medical personnel recognize all grades of concussion and insist that players refrain from practice or competition until they are completely asymptomatic will decreases in the incidence of second impact syndrome occur.

Attempts to reduce or limit the effects of second impact syndrome after a person collapses are only minimally successful. Rapid intubation, hyperventilation, and intravenous administration of diuretic medication may limit increases in intracranial pressure sufficiently to save some lives, but these measures rarely prevent extensive brain damage. Although second impact syndrome is an uncommon event, it is catastrophic when it does occur.

Information for Coaches and Athletes

Because mild TBI is so commonly associated with sporting accidents, coaches and athletes need information about when an injury warrants attention. The most basic question concerns when an athlete can safely return to play following a mild TBI. Coaches can use a screening tool such as the *Standardized Assessment of Concussion* (SAC; McCrea, Kelly, Kluge, Ackley, & Randolph, 1997) to determine the presence and severity of concussion. This tool includes a brief neurological screening and an assessment of orientation, immediate memory, concentration, and delayed recall after engaging in physical exertion. Using information such as that obtained through administration of the SAC or a similar tool, the Quality Standards Subcommittee of the American Academy of Neurology (1997) issued guidelines for managing concussions sustained during sporting events. The Quality Standards Subcommittee recommends that athletes wait 15 minutes to 1 month before returning to play. Specific guidelines relating to single and multiple incidents of Grade 1, 2, and 3 concussions are presented in Table 3.4.

Table 3.4

Return-to-Play Guidelines for Single and Multiple Grade 1, 2, and 3 Concussions

Grade	Immediate disposition	Sideline examination	Neurologic evaluation	CT or MRI scan	Return-to-play
1					
First instance	Remove to sideline	Every 5 minutes	No	No	Same game if symptom-free
Second instance	Remove to sideline	Every 5 minutes	No	No	After 1 week symptom-free at rest and with exertion
2					
First instance	Remove to sideline	Every 10 to 15 minutes	Yes	Yes, if headache or other symptoms worsen or persist longer than 1 week	After 1 week symptom-free at rest and with exertion
Second instance	Remove to sideline	Every 10 to 15 minutes	Yes	Yes, if headache or other symptoms worsen or persist longer than 1 week	After 2 weeks symptom-free at rest and with exertion
3					
First instance	Transport to hospital	Not applicable	Yes	Yes, as deemed appropriate by medical personnel	Brief loss of consciousness: After 1 week symptom-free at rest and with exertion. Prolonged loss of consciousness: After 2 weeks symptom-free at rest and with exertion
Second instance	Transport to hospital	Not applicable	Yes	Yes, as deemed appropriate by medical personnel	After 1 month symptom-free at rest and with exertion

Decisions about returning to play following a concussion should never be left to an athlete. While in the midst of competition, athletes, coaches, and fans can easily lose perspective about the balance between competitiveness and safety. Because of the dangers associated with second impact syndrome, athletes must never be permitted to return to practice or competition before they are asymptomatic. Youth, adolescents, and young adults often dread not being allowed to participate in sporting events; therefore, adults who are knowledgeable about the potential for catastrophic consequences must assume responsibility for enforcing return-to-play restrictions.

> **❝** These are kids, and they shouldn't have to risk their lives to play high school football. **❞**
> —Guynes, 1998

What is dementia pugilistica?

Dementia pugilistica is a condition sometimes referred to as the punch-drunk syndrome. It refers to the chronic brain damage sustained by boxers who receive repeated mild concussions. Between 9% and 55% of professional boxers eventually display dementia pugilistica (Jedlinski, Gatarski, & Szymusik, 1970; Roberts, 1969; Sercl & Jaros, 1962). Its first symptoms typically include incoordination and changes in affect and the control of emotions. As the syndrome progresses, dysarthria, tremors, and psychiatric disturbances emerge. Eventually, the person displays increasingly severe tremors and coordination problems as well as hearing and memory problems, difficulty with problem solving, poor social skills, changes in personality, and Parkinsonian symptoms.

References

Alves, W., Macciocchi, S. N., & Barth, J. T. (1993). Postconcussive symptoms after uncomplicated mild head injury. *Journal of Head Trauma Rehabilitation*, 8(3), 48–59.

American Academy of Neurology. (1983, May). *The American Board of Neurology opposes the practice of boxing* [Policy statement]. Executive Board Meeting, American Academy of Neurology.

American Academy of Pediatrics Committee on Sports Medicine and Fitness. (1997). Participation in boxing by children, adolescents, and young adults. *Pediatrics*, 99(1), 134–135.

Barth, J., Macciocchi, S., Giordani, B., Rimel, R., Jane, J. A., & Boll, T. J. (1983). Neuropsychological sequelae of minor head injury. *Neurosurgery*, 13, 529–533.

Binder, L. M. (1986). Persisting symptoms after mild head injury: A review of the postconcussive syndrome. *Journal of Clinical and Experimental Neuropsychology*, 8, 323–346.

Binder, L. M. (1997). A review of mild head trauma. Part II: Clinical implications. *Journal of Clinical and Experimental Neuropsychology*, 19, 432–457.

Binder, L. M., & Willis, S. C. (1991). Assessment of motivation after financially compensable minor head trauma. *Psychological Assessment*, 3, 175–181.

Bohnen, N., Twijnstra, A., & Jolles, J. (1992). Post-traumatic and emotional symptoms in different subgroups of patients with mild head injury. *Brain Injury*, 6, 481–487.

Cantu, R. C. (1996). Head injuries in sport. *British Journal of Sports Medicine*, 30, 289–296.

Cantu, R. C. (1998). Second-impact syndrome. *Clinics in Sports Medicine*, 17, 37–44.

Cohadon, R., Richer, E., & Castel, J. P. (1991). Head injuries: Incidence and outcome. *Journal of the Neurological Sciences*, 103, S27–S31.

Consumer Product Safety Commission. (n.d.). *Wear helmets to prevent sports related head injuries* (CPSC Document No. 5044). Retrieved November 12, 2001, from http://www.cpsc.gov/cpscpub/pubs/5044.html

Dick, R. W. (1994). A summary of head and neck injuries in collegiate athletics using the NCAA Injury Surveillance System. In E. F. Hoerner (Ed.), *Head and neck injuries in sports: ASTM special technical publication 1229* (pp. 13–19). Philadelphia: American Society for Testing and Materials.

Dikmen, S., Temkin, N., & Armsden, G. (1989). Neuropsychological recovery: Relationship to psychosocial functioning and postconcussional complaints. In H. S. Levin, H. M. Eisenberg, & A. L. Benton (Eds.), *Mild head injury* (pp. 229–241). New York: Oxford University Press.

Fenton, G., McClelland, R., Montgomery, A., MacFlynn, G., & Rutherford, W. (1993). The postconcussional syndrome: Social antecedents and psychological sequelae. *British Journal of Psychiatry*, 162, 493–497.

Ferguson, R. J., Mittenberg, W., Barone, D. F., & Schneider, B. (1999). Postconcussion syndrome following sports-related head injury: Expectation as etiology. *Neuropsychology*, 13, 582–589.

Guerrero, J. L., Thurman, D. J., & Sniezek, J. E. (2000). Emergency department visits associated with traumatic brain injury: United States, 1995–1996. *Brain Injury*, 14, 181–186.

Guynes, K. (1998, July). *Concussion in youth sports: Guidelines for evaluation and management of concussion in youth and prevention of secondary impact brain injury.* Conference presented by the Brain Injury Association of Nebraska, Lincoln.

Harrington, D. E., Malec, J., Cicerone, K., & Katz, H. T. (1993). Current perceptions of rehabilitation professionals towards mild traumatic brain injury. *Archives of Physical Medicine and Rehabilitation*, 74, 579–586.

Hux, K., Bond, V., Skinner, S., Belau, D., & Sanger, D. (1998). Parental report of occurrences and consequences of traumatic brain injury among delinquent and non-delinquent youth. *Brain Injury, 12*, 667–681.

Jagoda, A., & Riggio, S. (2000). Mild traumatic brain injury and the postconcussive syndrome. *Emergency Medicine Clinics of North America, 18*, 355–363.

Jedlinski, J., Gatarski, J., & Szymusik, A. (1970). Chronic posttraumatic changes in the central nervous system in pugilists. *Polish Medical Journal, 9*, 743–752.

McCrea, M., Kelly, J. P., Kluge, J., Ackley, B., & Randolph, C. (1997). Standardized assessment of concussion in football players. *Neurology, 48*, 586–588.

McCrory, P. R., & Berkovic, S. F. (1998). Second impact syndrome. *Neurology, 50*, 677–683.

McLean, A., Temkin, N. R., Dikmen, S., & Wyler, A. R. (1983). The behavioral sequelae of head injury. *Journal of Clinical Neuropsychology, 5*, 361–376.

Mild Traumatic Brain Injury Committee of the Head Injury Interdisciplinary Special Interest Group of the American Congress of Rehabilitation Medicine. (1993). Definition of mild traumatic brain injury. *Journal of Head Trauma Rehabilitation, 8*, 86–87.

Miller, H. (1961). Accident neurosis. *British Medical Journal, 1*, 919–925.

Noy, P. (1975). New views of the psychotherapy of compensation neurosis: A clinical study. In S. Arieti (Ed.), *New dimensions in psychiatry: A world view* (pp. 162–168). New York: Wiley.

Ponsford, J., Willmott, C., Rothwell, A., Cameron, P., Ayton, G., Nelms, R., Curran, C., & Ng, K. (1999). Cognitive and behavioral outcome following mild traumatic head injury in children. *Journal of Head Trauma Rehabilitation, 14*, 360–372.

Powell, J. W., & Barber-Foss, K. D. (1999). Traumatic brain injury in high school athletes. *Journal of the American Medical Association, 282*, 958–963.

Quality Standards Subcommittee of the American Academy of Neurology. (1997). Practice parameter: The management of concussion in sports (summary statement). *Neurology, 48*, 581–585.

Radanov, B. P., Di Stefano, G., Schnidrig, A., Sturzenegger, M., & Augustiny, K. F. (1993). Cognitive functioning after common whiplash: A controlled follow-up study. *Archives of Neurology, 50*, 87–91.

Rimel, R. W., Giordani, B., Barth, J. T., Boll, T. J., & Jane, J. A. (1981). Disability caused by minor head injury. *Neurosurgery, 9*, 221–228.

Roberts, A. H. (1969). *Brain damage in boxers: A study of prevalence of traumatic encephalopathy among ex-professional boxers.* London: Pitman.

Ruff, R. M., & Jurica, P. (1999). In search of a unified definition for mild traumatic brain injury. *Brain Injury, 13*, 943–952.

Ruff, R. M., Wylie, T., & Tennant, W. (1993). Malingering and malingering-like aspects of mild closed head injury. *Journal of Head Trauma Rehabilitation, 8*(3), 60–73.

Russell, W. R. (1932). Cerebral involvement in head injury. *Brain, 55*, 549–603.

Russell, W. R., & Smith, A. (1961). Post-traumatic amnesia in closed head injury. *Archives of Neurology, 5*, 16–29.

Rutherford, W. H., Merrett, J. D., & McDonald, J. R. (1978). Symptoms at one year following concussion from minor head injuries. *Injury: The British Journal of Accident Surgery, 10*, 225–230.

Sercl, M., & Jaros, O. (1962). The mechanisms of cerebral concussion in boxing and their consequences. *World Neurology, 3*, 351–357.

Sosin, D. M., Sniezek, J. E., & Thurman, D. J. (1996). Incidence of mild and moderate brain injury in the United States, 1991. *Brain Injury, 10*, 47–54.

Stevens, K. B., & Price, J. R. (1999). Social and legal impact of malingered mild traumatic brain injury. In M. J. Raymond, T. L. Bennett, L. C. Hartlage, & C. M. Cullum (Eds.), *Mild traumatic brain injury: A clinician's guide* (pp. 187–200). Austin, TX: PRO-ED.

Yarnell, P. R., & Lynch, S. (1973). The "ding:" Amnestic states in football trauma. *Neurology, 23,* 196–197.

Mechanisms of Severe Injury
Damage to the Central Nervous System

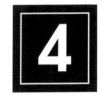

Karen Hux

U nderstanding the effect that TBI has on neural structures requires knowledge about the anatomy and physiology of the head. This chapter provides a review of pertinent anatomy and physiology, then provides explanations of the mechanisms of injury when acceleration–deceleration forces act upon the skull and brain.

Anatomy and Physiology of the Head

Cranial Bones

The brain is one of the best protected structures of the human body. Its first form of protection is encasement in a bony vault called the cranium. The *cranium* consists of eight bones fused together to form a structure that is roughly ovoid in shape. Table 4.1 lists the bones of the cranium and their location; Figures 4.1, 4.2, and 4.3 show the location of the bones of the cranium when the skull is viewed from various directions.

The outer surface of the cranium is generally smooth. In contrast, the inner surface varies in topography from region to region. Multiple bony protuberances that extend inward from the ethmoid, sphenoid, and right and left temporal bones make the portion of the cranium surrounding the lower part of the frontal and temporal lobes of the brain rough and jagged. In particular, the crista galli of the ethmoid bone, the lesser wings and sella turcica of the sphenoid bone, and the petrous portion of the temporal bones form ridges and spikes on the inner surface of the cranium. The inner surface of the cranium surrounding the occipital and parietal lobes is relatively smooth and free from jagged edges and bony protuberances.

The cranium serves to protect the brain from exposure to the external world. It is a barrier against infection as well as a hard shield to absorb the impact of blows to the head. Sometimes a blow to the head causes one or more bones of the skull to break. The bones most susceptible to fracture are the cribiform plate of the ethmoid bone, the orbital plates of the frontal bone, and the portions of the

Table 4.1
Bones of the Cranium and Their Location

Bone	Location
Frontal	Forms the forehead—the anterior portion of the cranium
Left and right parietal	Form the center portion of the top of the head
Occipital	Forms the back portion and part of the underneath portion of the cranium; contains the foramen magnum
Left and right temporal	Form the sides of the cranium and contain within them the middle and inner ear structures
Ethmoid	Forms a small portion of the anterior floor of the cranium
Sphenoid	Forms a major portion of the floor of the cranium

sphenoid and temporal bones that surround the sphenoidal sinuses and middle ear cavities. Symptoms of fractures to these bones include bulging of the eyes and blood, and cerebrospinal fluid leakage from the nose and ears.

Skull fractures present an interesting scenario in terms of TBI. A simple fracture of a cranial bone may actually protect the brain somewhat by dispersing the force of the impact. However, a depressed skull fracture—in which a cranial bone breaks in such a way that it projects inward—may expose the central nervous system to the external environment and allow infection. This is particularly true of depressed skull fractures that penetrate one or more of the meningeal layers.

Skull fractures occur in approximately one fourth of all TBIs, with simple fractures being about 4 times more common than depressed ones (Rimel, 1981). Based on examination of over 1,000 consecutive cases of skull fractures, Rimel documented breaks to the frontal region in 39% of cases, basilar region in 21% of cases, parietal region in 19% of cases, occipital region in 14% of cases, and temporal region in 7% of cases.

Meninges

A second layer of brain protection comes from the *meninges*, the three layers of coverings that separate the central nervous system from the cranial and spinal bones. The three layers of meninges are the dura mater, the arachnoid mater, and the pia mater. The *dura mater*—literally "hard mother"—is a tough mem-

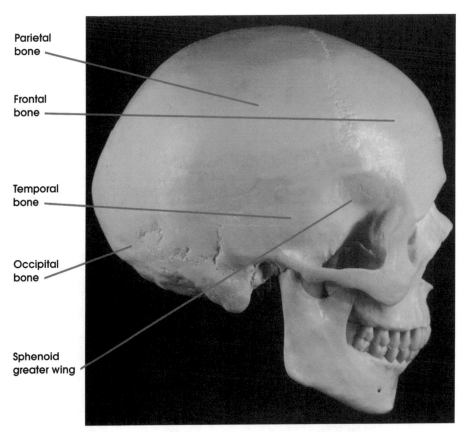

Figure 4.1. Lateral view of the skull.

brane that adheres tightly to the interior surface of the cranium. The cranial nerves pass through the dura mater as they exit the central nervous system, and the dura mater also encases sinuses into which the veins carrying blood away from the cerebral hemispheres drain. Directly below and tightly attached to the dura mater is the second layer of meninges, the *arachnoid mater*; similar in appearance to the cobwebs of arachnid spiders, the arachnoid is a delicate, fibrous membrane. Underneath it is a space, the *subarachnoid space*, that contains cerebrospinal fluid. The final meningeal layer, the *pia mater*—literally "little mother"—is the thinnest of the three meninges and adheres tightly to the outer surface of the brain.

Together, the three layers of meninges and the fluid-filled subarachnoid space absorb shock and protect the brain. Because the dura mater adheres tightly to the interior surface of the skull, a blow that causes movement of the skull will also cause the dura mater and the arachnoid mater to move. However,

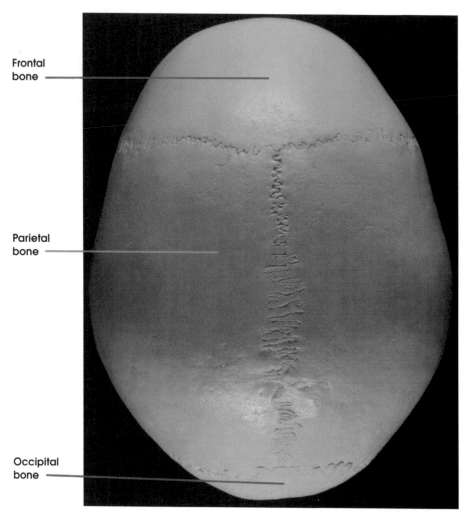

Frontal
bone

Parietal
bone

Occipital
bone

Figure 4.2. Superior view of the skull.

the fluid in the subarachnoid space allows for a slipping action such that the pia mater does not move as much as the outer meningeal layers. This eases the effect on the brain caused by sudden skull movement.

Ventricular System

Another mechanism that serves to protect the brain from TBI is the ventricular system. The ventricular system includes four ventricles (or cavities)—the right and left lateral ventricles, the third ventricle, and the fourth ventricle—

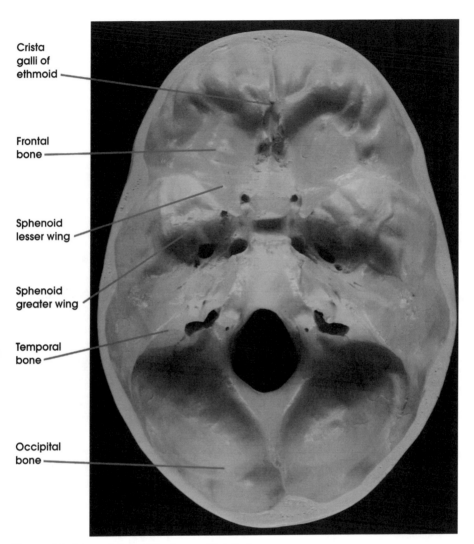

Crista galli of ethmoid

Frontal bone

Sphenoid lesser wing

Sphenoid greater wing

Temporal bone

Occipital bone

Figure 4.3. Internal view of the base of the skull.

the subarachnoid space, and the cerebrospinal fluid. The two lateral ventricles are relatively large structures within the cerebral hemispheres. They join the centrally located third ventricle as it enters the diencephalon. In turn, the third ventricle joins the fourth ventricle at the level of the pons. The fourth ventricle continues descending the spinal cord as the central canal and has three openings connecting it to the subarachnoid space.

A primary purpose of the ventricles is production of *cerebrospinal fluid*, a clear, colorless fluid that acts as a cushion and spatial buffer for the brain

Why is it important to remain stationary, in bed, for at least 24 hours following a spinal tap? A spinal tap (also called a lumbar puncture) is a procedure in which a physician inserts a needle into the lower portion of the spinal cord. A small amount of cerebrospinal fluid is withdrawn and sent to a laboratory for analysis. During the next several hours, the brain produces additional cerebrospinal fluid to replace that which was removed. Until a sufficient amount of new cerebrospinal fluid is produced, the subarachnoid space provides less than normal cushioning between the brain and skull. When the person raises his or her head, gravity and the lack of adequate cerebrospinal fluid allow the brain to rub against the bottom of the cranial vault causing an excruciating headache. A similar situation occurs if an individual has an undetected skull fracture that causes a leaking of cerebrospinal fluid; indeed, the revealing symptom of such an injury is often a severe headache that worsens when the person is upright and lessens when he or she lies down.

and spinal cord. Because rigid bones encase the brain, the only way something within the cranium can enlarge and not cause neurological damage is for something else of equal size to leave the cranial vault. The cerebrospinal fluid in the ventricles and subarachnoid space serves this role; whenever events related to TBI—such as brain swelling or the pooling of spilled blood—create an increased need for space within the cranium, cerebrospinal fluid is pushed out of the ventricles and subarachnoid space surrounding the brain.

Mechanisms of Injury

The neurological effects of TBI occur in two stages, referred to as primary and secondary mechanisms of injury. *Primary mechanisms of injury* occur at the actual time of a traumatic event. They relate to the instantaneous effects of acceleration–deceleration forces on the skull and brain. *Secondary mechanisms of injury* are consequences of the primary injuries and do not occur at the actual time of trauma. They are a chain of events that occur a few minutes to several weeks later. For interested readers, Graham (1999) provides a detailed review of the damage associated with various primary and secondary mechanisms of injury.

Primary Mechanisms of Injury

Acceleration–deceleration forces are major contributors to brain damage incurred at the actual time of most injuries. These forces exist whenever the head undergoes a sudden change in its rate of movement. This occurs any time a moving head stops abruptly because of contact with a hard object (e.g., falling from a height and landing on a hard surface), a stationary head accelerates quickly because of impact of another object (e.g., being struck on the head with a blunt object), or a rapid and uncontrolled back-and-forth movement of the head causes repeated changes in acceleration and deceleration (e.g., sustaining a whiplash injury). Only in rare instances is a head immobilized at the time that it makes contact with another object. In these situations, primary brain injury results from fragments of crushed skull bones penetrating the brain rather than from the impact of acceleration–deceleration forces. The amount of damage caused by a moderate blow to a mobile head is often extreme, whereas the amount of damage caused by a blow —even one that is 20 times more intense—is minimal when a head is immobilized (Denny-Brown & Russell, 1941).

   Two types of acceleration–deceleration forces —translational and rotational—can cause damage to the brain. *Translational forces* occur when a force travels through a head's center of gravity. The effect of a translational force is linear acceleration—a pushing of the head in one direction (Figure 4.4a). *Rotational forces* occur when a force passes through the head in a place other than its center of gravity. The effect of a rotational force is to rotate the head in horizontal, vertical, or simultaneous horizontal and vertical directions (Figure 4.4b). In virtually all instances of acceleration–deceleration dependent injuries, both translational and rotational forces are present.

Translational Forces

A blow through a head's center of gravity causes an abrupt change in movement of the skull. Because of inertia and the brain's separation from the skull by the meninges and subarachnoid space, the corresponding change in the brain's movement lags behind until the skull actually begins pushing against it. When this contact involves a part of the skull that has rough inner

Emergency medical technicians often refer to the first 60 minutes following an injury as the "golden hour." A person is much more likely to survive a severe TBI if he or she makes it to the hospital within 1 hour, because physicians have a better chance to controlling and minimizing the effects of secondary mechanisms of injury.

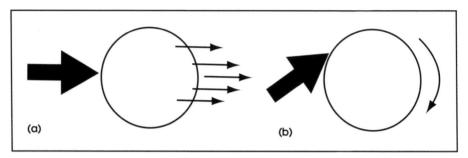

Figure 4.4. (a) Translational acceleration; (b) Rotational acceleration.

surfaces, severe lacerations of the underlying cortex and veins occur. As the skull decelerates to a still position, the brain repeatedly scrapes against the inner surface of the skull. This accounts for many of the cortical contusions evident in the frontal and temporal lobes (Lindenberg & Freytag, 1960). When the damage is at the site of impact, the injury is a *coup injury*. (*Coup* is a French word meaning "blow" or "stroke.") When the damage is at the point opposite the site of impact, it is a *contrecoup injury*, meaning an injury "counter to (or opposite) the blow."

In addition to causing differential movement of the skull and brain, translational acceleration causes a region of positive pressure at the site of impact and a region of negative pressure—equal in magnitude to that of the positive pressure—at the site directly opposite the point of impact (Figure 4.5). No pressure change occurs at the center of the brain. Because all of the particles of the brain are traveling at the same speed and in the same direction, no intermolecular stress within the brain accompanies the application of a translational force. Furthermore, the brain can tolerate a lot of positive pressure without sustaining damage (Unterharnscheidt & Sellier, 1966). However, brain tissue is quite susceptible to damage from negative pressure, and brain damage is often present in the region opposite the site of impact.

Negative pressure causes brain damage because of cavitation effects. *Cavitation effects* occur when the translational force is sufficient to cause the negative pressure at the point opposite impact to drop below the vapor pressure level of the liquid contents of the brain. *Vapor pressure level* is the point at which a liquid changes to a gas. When pressure drops below vapor pressure level, the intracellular and extracellular fluid within the brain converts to a gaseous state, resulting in the formation of gas bubbles. Within a few milliseconds, the negative pressure rises and returns to a level above vapor pressure level. The gas bubbles burst as they return to a liquid state, much like bubbles

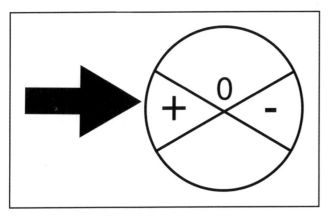

Figure 4.5. Pressure changes with application of translational force.

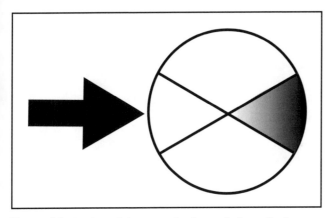

Figure 4.6. Region of damage due to cavitation effects.

burst when water boils. This bursting is similar in effect to multiple small explosions that destroy brain cells by ripping them apart. A wedge-shaped region of damage (in the area where pressure drops below vapor pressure level) results at the point opposite the impact (Figure 4.6).

Rotational Forces

A blow that does not pass through a head's center of gravity will cause a rotating movement. Because of the structure of the meninges, rotational forces make a skull move slightly ahead of the underlying brain. As the skull begins to move, bony protuberances on its inner surface catch the brain and drag it along. The resultant *shearing strain* causes lacerations to the cortex of the brain. Particularly severe injury occurs in the frontal and temporal regions, because these are the parts of the brain into which the majority of bony prominences extend.

Shearing strain is also thought to be responsible for damage deep within the brain. In contrast to translational acceleration—in which all particles move in the same direction and at the same speed—rotational acceleration causes adjacent structures to move along slightly different paths, at slightly different speeds. Thus, rotational forces pull adjacent structures in two directions at once and, if the structures are not tightly bound to one another, rip them apart. Resulting disruptions to synaptic connections between neurons and separations between cell bodies and their axons cause diffuse white matter lesions throughout the deep structures of the brain.

Shearing strain is most common between neural structures of differing densities; places where gray and white matter meet are particularly susceptible. Hence, the basal ganglia, the cerebellar peduncles, the corpus callosum, and the fiber tracts within the brain stem are likely to sustain damage from shearing strain. Other differences in density between adjacent structures occur between neural tissue and blood vessels and between neural tissue and the cerebrospinal fluid contained in the ventricles and subarachnoid space.

Secondary Mechanisms of Injury

Primary damage leads to secondary mechanisms of brain injury. For example, shearing strain may tear blood vessels which, in turn, may lead to hematoma formation—a relatively common secondary mechanism of injury. Secondary damage can also promote further mechanisms of injury. For example, hematomas cause increased intracranial pressure. The secondary mechanisms of injury most frequently observed following TBI include hematomas, acute cerebral swelling, cerebral edema, and increased intracranial pressure.

Hematomas

Hematomas are localized pools of blood found outside the circulatory system. With respect to TBI, epidural, subdural, subarachnoid, and intracranial hematomas are most serious.

Epidural hematomas (also called extradural hematomas) form between the skull and the outermost meningeal covering of the brain (i.e., the dura mater) and occur in 6% to 10% of TBI survivors (Foulkes et al., 1991; Graham, Adams, Nicoll, Maxwell, & Gennarelli, 1995). Their most common cause is a tearing of one of the arteries supplying blood to the meninges; less frequently, they result from a rupture to one of the dural sinuses. In 85% of

adult cases of epidural hematoma, a skull fracture also occurs. As an epidural hematoma expands, it pushes on the underlying brain tissue.
If identified quickly, epidural hematomas are the
least dangerous of the various types of hematomas because they do not invade neural tissue
and are not difficult to surgically drain. However, epidural hematomas are likely to be fatal if
not treated quickly.

Subdural hematomas form between the dura
mater and the arachnoid mater. Although a
space does not typically exist between these
meningeal layers, the tearing of a cerebral vein as
it enters a dural sinus and the subsequent spilling
of blood can force an opening. This often happens in TBI because application of rotational
forces causes the dural sinuses to move with the
skull, but the cerebral veins extending into the
brain lag behind and can tear.

Subdural hematomas are more common and
more serious than epidural hematomas; they occur in 24% of survivors of severe TBI (Foulkes
et al., 1991). Although still separated from the
brain by the arachnoid and pia mater, the subdural hematoma can push inward and cause compression and shift of brain tissue. Surgeons can
drain these hematomas in much the same way
that they drain epidural hematomas or, if the
progression is sufficiently slow, the body can reabsorb the spilled blood. However, the reabsorp-
tion process is quite slow; it can take up to a year
for the body to reabsorb the spilled blood completely.

Another disorder similar to a subdural hematoma is called a subdural hygroma (sometimes
called a subdural hydroma). A subdural hygroma
results from a tear in the arachnoid that allows
cerebral spinal fluid to collect between the dura
mater and arachnoid. It has the same effect as a
subdural hematoma and is equally slow to be re-
absorbed.

Any surgical procedure in which the skull is opened is a craniotomy. Hence, any-time surgery occurs to treat a hematoma, the patient undergoes a craniotomy. Draining a hematoma is called evacuating a clot.

Subarachnoid hematomas form in the subarachnoid space. They most often result from the tearing of a cerebral artery or vein. Whenever subarachnoid hematomas are present, performance of a spinal tap will reveal considerable amounts of blood mixed with cerebrospinal fluid.

Intracranial hematomas (also called intracerebral hematomas) are the most serious type of brain hematoma and are also the most difficult to treat. They occur within the brain itself, thus having an immediate impact on surrounding neural tissue. The onset of intracranial hematomas may be delayed several hours, days, or even weeks because brain swelling initially controls the bleeding. As the swelling reduces, bleeding can occur or recur resulting in the formation of new hematomas. Delayed intracranial hematomas occur in 5% to 10% of survivors of severe TBI (Foulkes et al., 1991).

Acute Cerebral Swelling

The body's response to many injuries is to increase blood flow to the affected part. When a disruption occurs in the system regulating the amount of blood flow to the brain, acute cerebral swelling may result. Either an elevation in blood pressure or a change in the dilation of vessels supplying blood to the brain can cause an increase in blood volume within the cranium. If this increase is excessive and accompanies other secondary mechanisms of injury, pressure will rise within the cranium, and damage will result when structures press against one another. Acute cerebral swelling is more common among pediatric survivors of traumatic brain injury than among adult survivors.

Cerebral Edema

Cerebral edema reflects an increase in water content within the brain. Two forms of cerebral edema exist: vasogenic edema and cytotoxic edema. *Vasogenic edema* is the most common form of edema following TBI. It results from a breakdown in the blood–brain barrier such that capillary walls become more permeable than usual and allow fluid from the bloodstream to pass into the extracellular spaces of the brain. *Cytotoxic edema* occurs when damage to brain cells causes their membranes to have increased permeability. An excess of accumulating intracelluar fluid causes neurons to become engorged with liquid.

Increased Intracranial Pressure

The most common cause of death in neurosurgical intensive care units is increased intracranial pressure. Seventy-five percent of people who die from TBI have increased intracranial pressure (Graham et al., 1995; Graham, Lawrence,

Adams, Doyle, & McLellan, 1987). Occurrence of any of the other secondary mechanisms of injury can also cause an increase in the pressure within the brain. For example, hematomas, cerebral swelling, or cerebral edema all cause increased volume within the brain, resulting in a corresponding increase in pressure. Although the brain's ventricular system combats fluctuations in intracranial pressure, rapid and uncontrolled pressure rises can quickly destroy brain tissue and lead to death. The actual cause of death is typically compression of brain stem structures as they are pushed downward by the increasing volume within the cranium.

Intracranial pressure in a normal adult ranges from 5 to 13 mmHg (millimeters of mercury). The initial increase from a normal intracranial pressure reading to one around 20 mmHg may occur relatively slowly because the ventricular system prompts the removal of cerebrospinal fluid from within the cranial vault. However, after all of the cerebrospinal fluid has been removed, any further increase in volume will cause a rapid rise in intracranial pressure. A pressure reading above 20 mmHg is abnormal, and brain damage invariably occurs when intracranial pressure exceeds 40 mmHg. Persons with intracranial pressure above 60 mmHg almost always die.

Treatment of increased intracranial pressure typically begins when pressure readings reach 20 to 25 mmHg. The first step in treatment is elevation of the individual's head to approximately 30°. This helps by increasing venous drainage while only minimally decreasing arterial blood flow to the brain. Next, physicians can administer diuretic medications to draw fluids out of brain cells thus decreasing intracranial pressure. If intracranial pressure still remains dangerously high, hyperventilation can reduce it further. Finally, as a last resort, a physician may administer high doses of barbiturates to control intracranial pressure; however, such treatment has a high risk of significant complications.

Summary

TBI can result in damage to multiple cortical and subcortical regions. Primary mechanisms of injury cause diffuse damage as the rough interior surface of the skull scrapes against the brain and as shearing strains tear adjacent structures from one another. Focal regions of damage may also result—particularly at the point of impact and at the point opposite impact. Secondary mechanisms of injury occur in reaction to primary injuries. Mechanisms such as acute cerebral swelling, cerebral edema, and increased intracranial pressure result in additional diffuse damage; hematomas can cause both focal and diffuse damage.

References

Denny-Brown, D. E., & Russell, W. R. (1941). Experimental cerebral concussion. *Brain, 64,* 93–164.

Foulkes, M. A., Eisenberg, H. M., Jane, J. A., Marmarou, A., Marshall, L. F., & The Traumatic Coma Data Bank Research Group. (1991). The traumatic coma data bank: Design, methods, and baseline characteristics. *Journal of Neurosurgery, 75,* S8–S13.

Graham, D. I. (1999). Pathophysiological aspects of injury and mechanisms of recovery. In M. Rosenthal, E. R. Griffith, J. S. Kreutzer, & B. Pentland (Eds.), *Rehabilitation of the adult and child with traumatic brain injury* (3rd ed., pp. 19–41). Philadelphia: Davis.

Graham, D. I., Adams, J. H., Nicoll, J. A. R., Maxwell, W. L., & Gennarelli, T. A. (1995). The nature, distribution, and causes of traumatic brain injury. *Brain Pathology, 4,* 397–406.

Graham, D. I., Lawrence, A. E., Adams, J. H., Doyle, D., & McLellan, R. (1987). Brain damage in non-missile head injury secondary to high intracranial pressure. *Neuropathology and Applied Neurobiology, 13,* 209–217.

Lindenberg, R., & Freytag, E. (1960). The mechanisms of cerebral contusions. *Archives of Pathology, 69,* 440–469.

Rimel, R. W. (1981). A prospective study of patients with central nervous system trauma. *Journal of Neurosurgical Nursing, 13*(3), 132–141.

Unterharnscheidt, F., & Sellier, K. (1966). Mechanics and pathomorphology of closed brain injuries. In W. F. Caveness & A. E. Walker (Eds.), *Head injury* (pp. 321–341). Philadelphia: Lippincott.

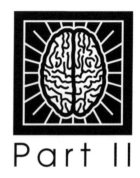

Part II

Understanding the Role of Speech–Language Pathologists

Assessment and Treatment of Impaired Consciousness
Coma, Vegetative State, Minimal Responsiveness, and Posttraumatic Amnesia

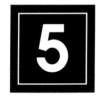

Karen Hux and Rebecca Burke

Coma, Vegetative State, and Minimal Responsiveness

Terminology

The term *coma* comes from the Greek word *koma*, meaning "deep sleep." A comatose individual is one who demonstrates no arousal or awareness of the environment, does not open his or her eyes, and does not have apparent sleep–wake cycles (American Congress of Rehabilitation Medicine, 1995; American Neurological Association, 1993; Berrol, 1990; Jennett, 1997). Coma may be very brief or may persist for the first few weeks following injury. After 2 to 3 weeks, eye opening usually happens spontaneously and sleep–wake cycles begin to appear. The appearance of these behaviors marks the end of coma.

A person who continues to not respond to or show awareness of the environment but who demonstrates spontaneous eye opening and sleep–wake cycles is in a *vegetative state* (American Congress of Rehabilitation Medicine, 1995; American Neurological Association, 1993; Berrol, 1986, 1990; Jennett & Plum, 1972). This condition may be termed a *persistent vegetative state* if it lasts longer than 1 month, although there is no universal agreement regarding the length of time needed to classify the condition as persistent (American Congress of Rehabilitation Medicine, 1995). Furthermore, use of the term *persistent* does not imply that neurological improvement will never occur; many people in persistent vegetative states remain severely impaired on a permanent basis, but some progress to the point of having relatively good functional outcomes (Giacino et al., 1997; Jennett, 1997).

After 1 year in a vegetative state, the term *permanent vegetative state* is sometimes applied. However, some professionals argue strongly against use of this term because this diagnosis has at times been used as a rationale for withdrawing or witholding care, denying rehabilitation services, or providing less

When is hope of recovery from a persistent vegetative state no longer realistic?

Most professionals agree that the prognosis for regaining consciousness is very poor after a person has remained in a vegetative state for more than 12 months following a traumatic injury (Multi-Society Task Force on PVS, 1994). Even when consciousness is regained after this length of time, the survivor typically remains severely disabled.

Are sleep disorders following TBI related to the reticular activating system?

Sleep disorders are not unusual following TBI. At least some instances of sleep disorder are due to damage to the reticular activating system. In these cases, the injury to the reticular activating system keeps the individual in a state of over-arousal rather than the state of underarousal associated with coma. The condition of overarousal may or may not follow a period of coma or minimal responsiveness.

aggressive management of coexisting medical problems (American Congress of Rehabilitation Medicine, 1995; Giacino et al., 1997; Jennett, 1997).

Once individuals begin to respond—even minimally—to environmental stimuli, they enter a state of minimal responsiveness. *Minimally responsive* (sometimes "minimally conscious") individuals demonstrate inconsistent control of voluntary movements or behaviors (American Congress of Rehabilitation Medicine, 1995; Giacino et al., 1997). Such individuals may sporadically perform meaningful behaviors such as grasping an object or moving a body part in response to a command or environmental trigger. Professionals may refer to survivors of TBI who remain at this stage of recovery for an extended period of time as *slow to recover*. This includes as many as 5% to 20% of the survivors of severe TBI (Jennett et al., 1979; Levin et al., 1990).

Considerable confusion exists about use of the terms *coma*, *vegetative state*, and *minimally responsive*. Because of negative connotations associated with referring to a person as vegetative (literally, "like a vegetable"; Committee for Pro-Life Activities–National Conference of Catholic Bishops, 1992), some professionals avoid use of the terms vegetative state and persistent vegetative state altogether and continue to use the term comatose even after eye opening and sleep–wake cycles appear. In a similar misuse of diagnostic terminology, some professionals persist in using the term vegetative state beyond the time when a person begins responding to environmental stimuli. Sometimes, the term comatose or vegetative state is used right up to the time a person can respond consistently to commands. Figure 5.1 shows the contrast in terminology between professionals who use only a single label (i.e., coma) and those who use multiple labels (i.e.,

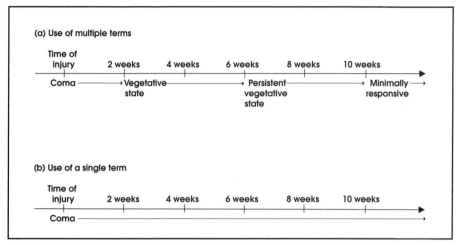

Figure 5.1. Example timeline for coma, vegetative state, and minimal responsiveness.

coma, vegetative state, persistent vegetative state, and minimally responsive) to describe various stages of impaired consciousness. Specific terminology—terminology that uses narrowly defined diagnoses—can be very helpful when information is passed from one professional (or one facility) to another. Because of the misuse of terms, over one third of individuals in acute brain injury rehabilitation programs may have inaccurate diagnostic labels at the time of admission (Childs, Mercer, & Childs, 1993).

Physiological Correlates on the Continuum of Consciousness

Coma from traumatically induced brain damage is associated with severe, diffuse lesions to both cerebral hemispheres and with brain stem injury (Plum & Posner, 1983). Coma resulting from injuries involving only the brain stem reflects a change in the functioning of the *reticular activating system*. This system—also called the *reticular formation*—is located in the upper two thirds of the brain stem and has projections to and from multiple cortical regions. Its primary purpose is to maintain consciousness and arousal. When a temporary disruption occurs as a result of trauma, a person enters a comatose state. In contrast to the brain stem damage evident in many people who experience coma for a time following traumatic injury, survivors who remain in minimally responsive states for extended periods postinjury typically have widespread and pervasive cortical damage (Ingvar, Brun, Johansson, & Samuelsson, 1978).

Do people who are in coma-tose, vegetative, or minimally responsive states understand things that are said or done to them?

Although a survivor of TBI may have a few isolated memories (e.g., arriving at the emergency room or hearing a family member's voice), most people do not recall many events relating to their injury or the period of impaired consciousness. Because of this general lack of recall, little is to be gained by questioning people about what they understood when in a state of impaired consciousness. Such questioning does not provide a conclusive answer to the question of what a person understands when in a comatose, vegetative, or minimally responsive state. Without evidence about the adequacy or inadequacy of comprehension, professionals and family members should always assume that survivors of TBI understand everything that is said and done around them. Negative comments about medical status or potential for recovery should never be made in a survivor's presence.

A second type of coma associated with TBI is a barbiturate coma. This is a drug-induced coma that physicians use to reduce dangerously high intracranial pressure when other methods—such as administration of other medications, controlled hyperventilation, moderate hypothermia, and removal of small amounts of cerebrospinal fluid—have not been sufficient. A barbiturate coma serves to protect the brain by slowing bodily functions and decreasing the brain's need for oxygen and nutrients.

Measuring Depth and Duration of Impaired Consciousness

Defining Behaviors

Professionals often use the duration of impaired consciousness as a prognostic indicator of long-term outcome following TBI. One of the challenges associated with doing this is determining precisely when a survivor moves from one state (coma, vegetative, and minimally responsive) to another. Regaining full consciousness is typically a gradual, erratic process that does not have a clear stopping point; the level of arousal and awareness (i.e., the level of consciousness) observed in survivors of TBI often fluctuates considerably from hour to hour and from day to day. In an attempt to regulate diagnosis terminology, professionals have defined behaviors that indicate the end of each of the various states of impaired consciousness. The termination of coma is the point at which spontaneous eye opening and sleep–wake cycles occur; the termination of a vegetative state is the point at which an individual begins to follow simple commands, manipulate objects, utter recognizable words, or gesture or verbalize yes and no responses; the termination of a minimally responsive state is the point at which a person demonstrates reliable and consistent interactive communication or functional use of objects (Giacino et al., 1997).

This progression through several types of responses is typical during recovery from a state of impaired consciousness. In the deepest stage of coma, a person is totally unresponsive to any stimuli—even painful or aversive ones. The next response type typical of emergence from coma or vegetative state is production of unconscious, subcortical *reflexive behaviors* (see Appendix 5.A), such as extensor posturing to pain and the production of primitive reflexes following specific stimulation. *Generalized responses* are said to occur when stimulation triggers movement of a body part not associated directly with the actual stimulus presented; for example, a noise in the environment might prompt a chewing response. The precise location and extent of brain damage determines which stimuli are likely to cause an individual survivor to respond; for example, a person whose injury severed the right and left olfactory nerves will not respond to smells but may respond to tactile stimuli. The next stage of recovery involves production of more specific and *localized responses*; when a noise occurs in the environment, the survivor might turn to face the source of the stimulus. Gradually, as the specificity of responses increases, the survivor begins to vocalize and to follow simple commands such as, "Squeeze my hand." Continued improvement toward full consciousness is indicated by increased specificity, consistency, and complexity of responses.

In addition to making simple observations, professionals can measure various physiological responses to determine whether a person in coma or vegetative state is aware of environmental events. Changes in body temperature, breathing rate, heart rate, oxygen saturation level, blood pressure, and pupil dilation or constriction are examples of physiological responses that may change in reaction to various stimuli.

Rating Levels of Consciousness and Cognitive Functioning

Several scales exist to measure the depth and duration of impairments to consciousness. The most commonly used scales include the Glasgow Coma Scale (Teasdale & Jennett, 1974), the Rappaport Coma/Near Coma Scale (Rappaport, Dougherty, & Kelting, 1992), the Western Neuro Sensory Stimulation Profile (Ansell & Keenan, 1989), and the Rancho Los Amigos Levels of Cognitive Functioning (Hagen, 1982, 2000).

Glasgow Coma Scale. The Glasgow Coma Scale was developed by Teasdale and Jennett (1974) as a means of using behavioral observations to judge the depth and duration of impaired consciousness following injury to the brain. Administration of the Glasgow Coma Scale requires observation of survivors'

What are primitive reflexes?

Primitive reflexes are behaviors that are present at birth but are normally suppressed within the first several months of life. TBI sometimes causes a recurrence of primitive reflexes suppressed since infancy. Other types of reflexes persist throughout life and serve as protective mechanisms. TBI can also cause the suppression of reflexes that are normally present throughout life. Appendix 5.A lists and describes several primitive reflexes affected by TBI and several normal reflexes that TBI may suppress.

eye opening, motor, and verbal responses during conversation and stimulation specifically geared to elicit responses. A score ranging from 3 to 15 points is obtained by summing points assigned for eye opening, best motor response, and best verbal response. Table 5.1 outlines the examiner's role, survivor's response, and assignment of points within each area of observation. Glasgow Coma Scale scores of 8 or less are generally considered indicative of coma or vegetative state; scores between 9 and 14 reflect less severe impairments to consciousness (American Congress of Rehabilitation Medicine, 1995; Binder, 1997); and a score of 15 indicates normal consciousness.

Although it is used extensively as a prognostic indicator of long-term outcome, several features of the Glasgow Coma Scale limit its fit for this purpose. First, much research correlating the Glasgow Coma Scale with long-term outcome uses scores obtained at the time a person arrives at an emergency room. This initial score fails to consider the length of time it takes to rescue and transport an individual to the hospital. Hence, a lack of uniformity exists in the time postinjury that the Glasgow Coma Scale is administered. Second, a person who has been administered medications at the scene of an accident or has alcohol or street drugs in his or her system at the time of injury may receive an artificially low Glasgow Coma Scale score because of drug-induced depression of central nervous system functioning. Third, a person with focal brain damage or a spinal cord injury may experience aphasia or motor impairment that will affect performance on the verbal or motor aspects of the assessment; again, an artificially low Glasgow Coma Scale score will result.

Rappaport Coma/Near Coma Scale. Rappaport et al. (1992) developed the Rappaport Coma/Near Coma Scale to assist professionals

Table 5.1
Glasgow Coma Scale Administration and Scoring

Behavior	Examiner's test	Survivor's response	Score
Eye opening	Enter room	Open eyes spontaneously	4
	Call patient's name	Open eyes when spoken to	3
	Apply a painful stimulus	Open eyes when pressure is applied	2
	Apply a painful stimulus	Do not open eyes	1
Best motor response	Tell patient to raise hand	Follow simple commands	6
	Apply stimulation to head, neck, or trunk of body	Use arm or leg to push examiner's hand away—localizing response	5
	Apply pressure to nail bed	Pull away from examiner—withdrawing response	4
	Apply pressure to nail bed	Flex arm or hand abnormally—flexor response	3
	Apply pressure to nail bed	Extend elbow in rigid position—extensor posturing	2
	Apply pressure to nail bed	No motor response	1
Best verbal response	Converse with patient	Engage in conversation and be oriented to person, time, and place	5
	Converse with patient	Display confusion or disorientation	4
	Converse with patient	Use words to speak but do not engage in conversational exchange	3
	Converse with patient	Make sounds that are not intelligible	2
	Converse with patient	Make no vocalizations	1

Note. Adapted from "Assessment of Coma and Impaired Consciousness: A Practical Scale," by G. Teasdale and B. Jennett, 1974, *Lancet, 2,* 81–84.

in measuring small changes in the responsiveness and awareness of people in vegetative and minimally responsive states. By administering up to 10 sensory stimuli and monitoring for spontaneous vocalizations, a professional determines a score that corresponds to one of five levels describing the severity of a person's deficits in sensory, perceptual, and primitive responses. Table 5.2

Table 5.2

Levels of the Rappaport Coma/Near Coma Scale

Level	Description
No coma	Person responds consistently and without delay to at least 3 of 10 stimulus modalities and responds consistently to simple commands
Near coma	Person responds consistently to 2 of 10 stimulus modalities and responds inconsistently or incompletely to simple commands
Moderate coma	Person responds inconsistently to 2 or 3 of 10 stimulus modalities but does not respond to simple commands; person may vocalize but does not produce recognizable words
Marked coma	Person responds inconsistently to 1 of 10 stimulus modalities and does not respond to simple commands; person does not vocalize
Extreme coma	Person does not respond to any sensory stimuli or simple commands; person does not vocalize

Note. Adapted from "Evaluation of Coma and Vegetative States," by M. Rappaport, A. M. Dougherty, and D. L. Kelting, 1992, *Archives of Physical Medicine and Rehabilitation, 73*, 628–634.

lists and describes each of the five levels of responsiveness; Table 5.3 lists each stimulus type, frequency, and response for the tested sensory modalities. Additional instructions for administration and scoring are provided on the protocol form for the scale.

Western Neuro Sensory Stimulation Profile. The purpose of the Western Neuro Sensory Stimulation Profile (Ansell & Keenan, 1989) is similar to that of the Rappaport Coma/Near Coma Scale: It provides a means of objectively measuring the small changes in cognitive status that minimally responsive survivors of TBI demonstrate during the early stages of recovery. The scale includes 32 items addressing arousal and attention; expressive communication; and auditory, visual, tactile, and olfactory responsiveness. Individual profile items are scored on an item-specific point scale (scales range from 0 to 1 points to 0 to 5 points) with higher point values corresponding with greater cognitive ability. Subscale scores can be obtained by summing the points scored in each of six subscales (i.e., Arousal/Attention, Auditory Comprehension, Visual Comprehension, Visual Tracking, Object Manipulation, and Tactile/Olfactory Response).

Rancho Los Amigos Levels of Cognitive Functioning. The Rancho scale (Hagen, 1982, 2000) differs from the Glasgow Coma Scale, Rappaport Coma/Near

Table 5.3
Modalities Tested, Type and Number of Stimulus Presentations, and Response Possibilities for the Rappaport Coma/Near Coma Scale

Modality	Stimulus	Maximum number of trials	Response
Auditory	1. Ring a bell for 5 seconds; repeat at 10-second intervals	3	Eye opening or orientation toward sound
	2. Request person to open or close eyes, mouth, or move finger, hand, or leg	3	Follows or attempts to follow command
Visual	3. Flash a light 1 time per second for 5 seconds	5	Fixation or avoidance
	4. Tell person, "Look at me," while moving your face from side to side	5	Fixation and tracking
	5. Quickly move hand forward to within 1 to 3 inches of eyes	3	Eye blink
Olfactory	6. Hold ammonia capsule or bottle 1 inch under person's nose for about 2 seconds	3	Withdrawal or other response linked to stimulus
Tactile	7. Briskly tap person's shoulder 3 times without speaking; test each side	3	Head or eye orientation or shoulder movement
	8. Place nasal swab at entrance of nostril; test each side	3	Withdrawal, eye blink, or mouth twitch
Pain	9. Pinch person's fingertip firmly or press wooden part of a pencil on fingernail; test each side	3	Withdrawal or other response linked to stimulus
	10. Pinch or pull person's ear 3 times; test each side	3	Withdrawal or other response linked to stimulus
Vocalization	11. None	—	Spontaneous production of words or nonverbal vocalizations

Note. Adapted from "Evaluation of Coma and Vegetative States," by M. Rappaport, A. M. Dougherty, and D. L. Kelting, 1992, *Archives of Physical Medicine and Rehabilitation, 73,* 628–634.

Coma Scale, and Western Neuro Sensory Stimulation Profile in that it provides a way to describe cognitive functioning in both the early and late stages of recovery from TBI. The original version of the scale (Hagen, 1982) included eight levels of cognitive functioning based on general descriptions of behaviors. The updated version (Hagen, 2000) includes Levels I through VII from the original scale with Level VIII expanded into Levels VIII, IX, and X to provide greater identification and recognition of persistent challenges in high-level cognitive processes, independent functioning, and social behaviors. To date, no research exists establishing the reliability and validity of the 10-level version of the Rancho scale. However, the expanded scale has considerable appeal to rehabilitation professionals because of its increased attention to late stages of recovery. Appendix 5.B provides the revised version of the Rancho Los Amigos Levels of Cognitive Functioning.

Behaviors observed when determining a Rancho Level for a survivor of TBI include responsiveness to stimuli, level of agitation and confusion, awareness of deficits, dependence on others to maintain attention to tasks, response delays, and the need for supervision when performing academic, vocational, and daily living activities. Levels I, II, and III deal with emergence from coma, persistent vegetative state, and minimal responsiveness; Levels IV, V, and VI describe individuals who are in the process of regaining the orientation and memory skills needed for full consciousness. Levels VII through X address persistent cognitive, social, and emotional challenges and are pertinent to discussions provided in later chapters of this book.

Sensory Stimulation

The terms *sensory stimulation*, *multisensory stimulation*, and *coma stimulation* are often used interchangeably. Technically, because coma rarely extends beyond a few weeks, *coma stimulation* is probably not an appropriate term to use with survivors of TBI who are minimally responsive for an extended period of time. Because of this, sensory stimulation is the term used in the remainder of this chapter to refer to programs aimed at increasing the arousal, awareness, and responsiveness of slow-to-recover individuals. When sensory stimulation occurs through several modalities (i.e., visual, auditory, tactile, gustatory, olfactory, and kinesthetic), the term multisensory stimulation can be correctly applied.

Designing and Implementing a Program

Typically, service providers from a variety of professions participate in the development and provision of sensory stimulation programs. Traditionally, speech–language pathologists or occupational therapists have assumed roles as team leaders to establish and implement sensory stimulation programs; however, anyone actively involved in a survivor's care can and should play a role. This includes family members, friends, nurses, aides, recreational therapists, physicians, psychologists, neuropsychologists, and physical therapists.

Using input from all team members, the team leader determines what type of stimuli to present and how often to present it to a survivor. Table 5.4 lists examples of stimulation appropriate for inclusion in a multisensory stimulation program. The team leader also establishes a system for tracking responses to various types of stimuli and for monitoring the overall success of the program. Figure 5.2 provides a sample form for recording stimuli presented, responses elicited, current cognitive status, and the date and time of sensory stimulation sessions.

Controversies Associated with Sensory Stimulation Programs

Several controversies surround the use of sensory stimulation for individuals emerging from states of impaired consciousness: the potential for misuse of health care funds, the potential for abuse of survivors, the appropriateness of various stimuli and activities, the frequency with which stimulation should be provided, and the poorly documented value of sensory stimulation programs.

Misuse of Funds. By definition, a person in a state of minimal consciousness is not fully aware of his or her surroundings. Because of this, the survivor cannot report or complain about services received. This creates a scenario with the potential for inappropriate service provision and overbilling.

Inappropriate services occur when a professional claims to be providing sensory stimulation but does not use materials appropriate to the individual's level of responsiveness or does not monitor and record responses to the stimuli presented. For example, a service provider who enters a room, starts an audiotape, and then leaves without monitoring the survivor's responses has not performed sensory stimulation. Billing for provision of such services is unethical.

Abuse. Another potential problem that arises from a survivor's inability to report inappropriate services is the possibility for physical maltreatment. People in comatose, vegetative, or minimally responsive states are at risk both for intentional and unintentional physical abuse because of their medically fragile condition and their inability to respond verbally to pain. Intentional abuse usually stems from staff or family members' frustration relating to survivors' inconsistent pattern of responsiveness. Unintentional abuse can occur with overzealous applications of sensory stimulation procedures that include painful or aversive stimuli. Although occasionally inflicting pain in a controlled manner may be necessary to determine a person's level of responsiveness, to administer

(*text continues on page 74*)

Table 5.4
Stimulation Ideas for Multisensory Stimulation Programs

Modality	Stimuli
Visual	Visits from family and friends Photographs of family, friends, and familiar places Various levels of lighting (avoid flashing lights due to risk of seizure) Colored balloons Streamers Soap bubbles Get-well cards Printed words
Auditory	Tapes of preferred music Voices of family and friends (taped or live) Tapes of soothing, environmental sounds Preferred television or radio shows Spoken commands
Tactile	Stroking or gently rubbing face or limbs with materials of varying textures: feather, Q-tip, satin, lotion, burlap, cotton ball Holding hands Stroking or gently rubbing face or limbs with cool or warm washcloth
Olfactory	Familiar cologne/perfume Baked goods Spices, herbs, and extracts Fruits Freshly ground coffee Chocolate Air fresheners Dryer sheets/freshly laundered clothing Flowers
Gustatory[a]	Lemon glycerin swab Ice chips/lemon ice/popsicles Mint-flavored toothette Cotton swab or gauze-covered tongue blade dipped in juice
Kinesthetic	Elevating and lowering the bed to various positions Positioning individual on his or her back, side, or stomach Moving the person in a rocking chair Performing passive range-of-motion exercises

[a] Only introduce items orally if the person does not have swallowing problems.

SENSORY STIMULATION RESPONSE FORM

Patient's name: _____ Session date: _____

Rancho Level: I   II   III   IV   V   VI   VII   VIII   IX   X

Level of arousal:
1. no arousal
2. opens eyes with tactile stimulation
3. opens eyes with auditory stimulation
4. opens eyes spontaneously

Length of arousal:
1 minute or less (0–1)
2 to 5 minutes (2–5)
6 to 15 minutes (6–15)
16 to 30 minutes (16–30)
intermittent (int)

Responses:

No response	Facial grimace	Head movement	Withdrawal
Chewing response	Smile	Eye opening	Flexion
Biting response	Hand/arm movement	Visual tracking	Agitation
Swallow response	Foot/leg movement	Eye contact	Startle response

Session number	1	2	3	4	5
Beginning and ending time					
Staff name and discipline					
Level and length of arousal					
Auditory					
Visual					
Olfactory					
Tactile					
Gustatory					
Kinesthetic					

Figure 5.2. Sensory Stimulation Response Form.
© 2002 by PRO-ED, Inc.

a medically necessary procedure, or to stretch muscles to avoid contractures, painful stimuli should not be a routine part of sensory stimulation programs. Similarly, professionals should avoid the use of aversive stimuli such as unpleasant odors and excessively loud or irritating noises. As often as possible, the stimuli selected should reflect survivor preferences. Optimally, the presentation of sensory stimuli should be a pleasant experience for the survivor.

Appropriateness of Stimuli and Activities. Another controversy about sensory stimulation programs concerns the type of stimuli presented to survivors. Some professionals advocate presenting stimuli in a sequential manner progressing from phylogenetically primitive subcortical sensory systems (including touch, smell, and movement) to more cortically controlled systems (including hearing and vision) (Smith & Ylvisaker, 1985). Other professionals advocate introducing stimuli to all sensory modalities from the start (Wilson, Powell, Brock, & Thwaites, 1996). The rationale for targeting phylogenetically older sensory systems first is that they have a greater number of multisensory connections, greater redundancy and bilateral central nervous system representation, and, in many cases, more resiliency in terms of recovery from acquired injury. In contrast, the rationale for targeting all sensory modalities at the initiation of treatment relates to the uncertainty that professionals have about the integrity of various sensory systems within individual survivors. For a given survivor, subcortical functions may be impaired to a greater extent than cortically controlled functions. If so, devoting large amounts of therapy time to subcortical modalities may be of little value.

Yet another important issue is the personal relevance of stimuli used in sensory stimulation programs. In a case study with a minimally responsive adolescent, Jones, Hux, Morton-Anderson, and Knepper (1994) found that playing audiotapes of friends and family members talking to the survivor was more effective in increasing arousal than playing tapes of other types of auditory stimuli. Similarly, Hall, MacDonald, and Young (1992) found that a combination of general sensory stimulation and personally relevant sensory stimulation (e.g., presenting family photographs and favorite music) elicited more frequent eye movements and motor responses among survivors of TBI with impaired consciousness than stimulation involving only the oral reading (i.e., single sensory) of a generic passage. Ansell (1995) found that survivors achieved significantly higher scores on a visual tracking procedure when they observed their own faces in a mirror rather than other visual stimuli in the environment. Typically, survivors of TBI are more likely to respond to stimuli that are familiar and relevant to them.

Frequency of Intervention. Professionals disagree about the optimal amount of stimulation to provide individuals who are comatose or who are in vegetative or minimally responsive states. At one extreme is the notion that the person needs virtually constant stimulation throughout each day to facilitate recovery, with caretakers and assistants working in shifts and adhering to a strict schedule of treatment activities. At the other extreme is the notion that a minimally responsive person needs rest in an environment that is as quiet and as free from stimulation as possible.

An approach falling between these two extremes is probably appropriate for most survivors. Providing constant stimulation may lead a survivor to ignore all environmental stimuli—exactly the opposite of the intended effect of sensory stimulation. Conversely, providing minimally responsive individuals with no stimulation creates sensory deprivation that may hinder cognitive recovery. Furthermore, if no stimulation is provided, families and professionals have no way to assess changes in responsiveness or monitor improvement. A compromise—short periods of stimulation several times throughout the day interspersed with rest periods—is probably appropriate for the majority of people in minimally responsive states (Wood, 1991).

Effectiveness of Sensory Stimulation Programs. Little research has been done to document the effectiveness of sensory stimulation programs. The research that does exist is open to criticism because of small sample sizes, variations across participants in the time between injury and intervention, lack of control groups (ethical questions surround withholding care), selection biases, and methodological problems (Andrews, 1996; Giacino, 1996), especially the challenge of differentiating treatment effects from spontaneous recovery (Wilson, Powell, Elliott, & Thwaites, 1991).

Despite these challenges, a number of researchers have documented positive outcomes associated with sensory stimulation based on Rancho Level several months posttreatment, increased eye opening and body movements, and changes in pulse rate, EEG readings, and heart rate (Hall et al., 1992; Jones et al., 1994; Kater, 1989; Pfurtschuller, Schwarz, & List, 1986; Wilson, Powell, et al., 1991; Wilson, Brock, Powell, Thwaites, & Elliott, 1996). In contrast, some researchers have reported that sensory stimulation programs yield mixed outcomes (Wilson, Brock, Powell, Thwaites, & Elliott, 1996) or inconclusive outcomes (Johnson, Roethig-Johnston, & Richards, 1993), or have no significant impact on the recovery of full consciousness (Pierce et al., 1990).

Posttraumatic Amnesia

As individuals emerge from minimal responsiveness, they often experience a period of posttraumatic amnesia (PTA). Actually, PTA is present during the period of coma, vegetative state, and minimal responsiveness, but it does not become readily apparent until the survivor is engaging regularly in communicative interactions with others. As defined by Russell (1932) and Russell and Smith (1961), posttraumatic amnesia refers to the period between the time of injury and the return of adequate memory to recall daily events. It is characterized by disorientation and anterograde and retrograde memory impairment. A person experiencing PTA is not likely to have consistent recall of activities, visitors, or meals on any given day.

Measuring PTA Duration

As with the duration of impaired consciousness, the duration of PTA often serves as a prognostic indicator of long-term outcome. Using PTA for this purpose requires a consistent and reliable way to determine its end. To address this problem, Levin, O'Donnell, and Grossman (1975) developed the Galveston Orientation and Amnesia Test (GOAT; see Figure 5.3). Ewing-Cobbs and her colleagues (Ewing-Cobbs, Levin, Fletcher, Miner, & Eisenberg, 1990) developed a version to use with survivors between 3 and 15 years of age called the Children's Orientation and Amnesia Test (COAT). The GOAT or COAT is administered daily until a survivor achieves a score within the normal range (i.e., 75 points or more for the GOAT; less than two standard deviations below the mean for a child's age for the COAT) for 2 consecutive days. That accomplishment marks the end of PTA.

Researchers have correlated the duration of PTA with the quality of long-term outcome (Fortuny, Briggs, Newcombe, Ratcliff, & Thomas, 1980; Jennett & Teasdale, 1981; Russell & Smith, 1961). A PTA duration of less than 1 hour is indicative of a mild injury and is typically associated with good recovery. A PTA duration between 1 hour and 1 day corresponds with moderate injury; again, good physical recovery with functional independence is typical. When PTA persists for longer than 1 day, the injury is severe, and the quality of recovery is less certain. (See Chapter 2 for more information on PTA.)

Treatment

Transitioning from Passive to Active Participation

When survivors of TBI progress from vegetative states to minimally responsive states, and again when they progress from being minimally responsive to displaying characteristics of posttraumatic amnesia, substantial changes occur in treatment participation and orientation. In essence, rehabilitation professionals impose sensory stimulation treatment on survivors of TBI during the early stages of recovery; the role of the survivor is a passive one. However, once a

Name _____   **Date of Test** |__|__|__|
                                                             mo day yr

Age _____   **Sex**   M   F   **Day of the week** s m t w t f s

Date of birth |__|__|__| **Time**   AM   PM
                 mo day yr

Diagnosis _____   **Date of injury** |__|__|__|
                                                                mo day yr

GALVESTON ORIENTATION AND AMNESIA TEST (GOAT)   **Error Points**
                                                                    |__|__|
 1. What is your name? (2) _____
    When were you born? (4) _____
    Where do you live? (4) _____

 2. Where are you now? (5) city _____ |__|__|
    hospital (5) _____
    (unnecessary to state name of hospital)

 3. On what date were you admitted to this hospital? (5) _____ |__|__|
    How did you get here? (5) _____

 4. What is the first event you can remember <u>after</u> the injury? (5) ___ |__|__|

    _____

    Can you describe in detail (e.g., date, time, companions) the first
    event you can recall after injury? (5) _____

    _____

 5. Can you describe the last event you recall <u>before</u> the accident? |__|__|
    (5) _____

    _____

    Can you describe in detail (e.g., date, time, companions) the first
    event you can recall <u>before</u> the injury? (5) _____

    _____

 6. What time is it now? _____ (−1 for each ½ hour |__|__|
    removed from correct time to maximum of −5)

 7. What day of the week is it? _____ (−1 for each day |__|__|
    removed from the correct one)

 8. What day of the month is it? _____ (−1 for each day |__|__|
    removed from correct date to maximum of −5)

 9. What is the month? _____ (−5 for each month removed |__|__|
    from correct one to maximum of −15)

10. What is the year? _____ (−10 for each year removed |__|__|
    from correct one to maximum of −30)

                                          Total Error Points |__|__|

             Total Goat Score (100 − total error points) |__|__|

Figure 5.3. The Galveston Orientation and Amnesia Test form. *Note.* From "The Galveston Orientation and Amnesia Test: A Practical Scale To Assess Cognition After Head Injury," by H. S. Levin, V. M. O'Donnell, and R. G. Grossman, 1975, *Journal of Nervous and Mental Disorders, 167,* 675–684. Copyright 1975 by Lippincott, Williams & Wilkins. Reprinted with permission.

survivor begins responding consistently to environmental stimuli, passive participation in treatment changes to active participation. Rehabilitation professionals can facilitate the shift to active participation by presenting minimally responsive survivors with tasks that allow choice making via switch activation. Switch activation requires identification of a body part over which a survivor has some (usually inconsistent) control. Placing the switch in proximity to the selected body part and connecting it to an electronic device that controls either an environmental feature (e.g., changing the lights or adjusting the bed) or the presentation of stimulation (e.g., turning on music or television) encourages and assists survivors to activate the switch, thus reclaiming some control over the events that occur around them. In addition to empowering survivors to perform tasks independently, switch activation educates clients about the concept of using switches to control equipment—a skill survivors may need later to implement assistive technology or augmentative and alternative communication systems (see Chapter 8).

As a survivor gains skill and consistency in switch activation or the use of natural or augmented communication, the introduction of choice-making activities is appropriate. Here, switch activation, eye gaze, eye blink, gestural responses, or verbalizations can indicate a preference for one activity or item over another. For example, a survivor might use eye gaze to indicate which of two audiotape recordings he or she would like to hear. Again, the goals are to allow the survivor as much control over events as possible, to encourage communicative interaction with others, and to facilitate active participation in therapy. Choice-making activities also serve as a bridge to the more formal and traditional forms of therapy that are typically used to assist individuals who display the attention, memory, and orientation problems characteristic of PTA.

Treatment Focus

Cognitive treatment during PTA primarily focuses on improving attention, orientation, and memory. Although interrelated, each of these cognitive functions has unique features that warrant separate discussion.

Attention. Paying attention to environmental events and stimuli is a fundamental underlying process of learning and memory. Three kinds of attention—sustained attention, focused attention, and divided attention—can be negatively affected by TBI. *Sustained attention* refers to maintaining focus on a given task for a protracted period of time. Sustained attention tasks for a survivor of TBI might involve looking at family pictures, listening to music, or answering biographical questions. *Focused attention* involves attending to one task despite the presence of distracting stimuli in the immediate environment. The same types of activities used to foster sustained attention can also foster focused attention, but additional distractors must be present. *Divided attention* requires a shift between two or more activities occurring simultaneously. When working on divided attention, a therapist might request that a survivor of TBI alternately read sentences on one piece of paper and write key words on another.

As attention improves, additional environmental distractors can be added so that therapy situations become less sterile and more like vocational and academic settings. However, inconsistent attention is a hallmark of TBI, especially when a survivor is experiencing agitation. Because of this, professionals should expect survivors to vary considerably in their attending behavior based on level of fatigue, changes in medication, and overall emotional and cognitive status.

Orientation. Typically, people possess orientation in relation to four factors: person (i.e., who a person is), place (i.e., where a person is), time (i.e., the day, date, and time), and situation (i.e., what has happened to bring the person to the current situation). In hospitals and rehabilitation facilities, a person's orientation status is typically reported as "oriented × 1," "oriented × 2," "oriented × 3," or "oriented × 4"; the numbers refer to person, place, time, and situation, respectively. Hence, a person who is "oriented × 2" knows who he or she is and where he or she is but does not know the day, date, time, or reasons surrounding his or her present situation. This numbering system reflects the typical order in which orientation skills are regained following neurological injury.

As people progress through PTA, they become increasingly aware of their environment and those around them. Although this awareness serves as a major contributor to the reestablishment of orientation, family members and rehabilitation staff can also provide verbal reminders and environmental cues to foster further the reacquisition process. Appropriate environmental cues include calendars, signs stating the facility name and location, labels providing the names of specific rooms within the facility (e.g., physical therapy, cafeteria, nursing station), written schedules of daily activities, maps of the facility, directional cues (e.g., arrows or color-coded lines) for navigating from one place to another, and simple memory logs to record daily events. (See Chapter 8 for additional information on the use of memory logs.) The case example ("Regaining Orientation") documents the typical progression of recovery of orientation.

Memory. The predominant memory impairments associated with PTA are retrograde and anterograde amnesia. As shown in Figure 5.4, retrograde amnesia

Case Example: Regaining Orientation

Regaining orientation to person, time, place, and situation is sometimes a very rapid process and sometimes never occurs fully. A typical progression is evident in the example of John, a 25-year-old man who sustained a moderate TBI in a car accident. During the period of PTA, John displayed orientation to person but not to time, place, or situation. One example of his disorientation occurred during occupational therapy, while he was performing a ring throwing task to improve upper extremity strength and range of motion. The ring targets were pegs mounted on a wall, with each peg surrounded by numbers. John interpreted the ring target to be the control panel of an airplane cockpit and reported this to his therapist. However, within 1 week of beginning treatment to work on regaining orientation skills, John no longer displayed this confusion and consistently knew where he was and the time of day. His reacquisition of orientation to date and situation required additional time and intervention, but he also reacquired these skills given cues to consult his memory log or a newspaper or calendar.

refers to memory loss extending backward in time from the moment of injury. For many survivors, the time period of retrograde amnesia is initially quite large, spanning several weeks, months, or even years; however, with recovery, this time period often decreases to a few days or hours. Anterograde amnesia refers to memory loss for events occurring after the time of trauma (see Figure 5.4). This includes the period of coma, vegetative state, and minimal responsiveness. The end of PTA typically coincides with the end of anterograde amnesia, although some survivors who have specific and severe deficits in forming new memories may experience persistent anterograde amnesia despite the resolution of other characteristics of PTA.

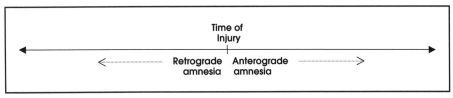

Figure 5.4. Retrograde and anterograde amnesia.

Formal treatment of retrograde amnesia occurs primarily during the period of PTA and involves exposing a survivor to artifacts from or descriptions of major life events in the hopes of stimulating recall. This can be done through review of photo albums and mementos supplied by family members or through construction of an autobiographical notebook featuring a chronology of major life events (e.g., birth, graduation from high school, first job, marriage).

Treatment for anterograde amnesia begins during PTA but may extend into later stages of recovery based on the particular constellation of memory problems displayed by an individual survivor. Initial treatment strategies are similar to those used to facilitate recovery of orientation—provision of verbal prompts and environmental cues. One of the most frequently used techniques is to record daily events in a memory log or journal. Initially, family members and rehabilitation staff record journal information; later, as survivors regain written language skills, they can assume responsibility for writing brief synopses of events and activities as they occur throughout the day. Chapters 6 and 8 provide additional details about the use of memory logs and the implementation of compensatory strategies by survivors of TBI whose pervasive memory impairments persist beyond the period of PTA.

Appendix 5.A
Reflexive Behaviors

Reflex	Elicitation	Description	Associated central or peripheral nervous system component
Primitive Reflexes Affected by TBI			
Asymmetrical tonic neck reflex	In supine position, turn head to side for 5 seconds	Extension of extremities on side to which head is facing and flexion of extremities on other side	Cerebral cortex and peripheral nervous system
Symmetrical tonic neck reflex	In midline position, flex and extend neck 5 times	Extension of arms and flexion of legs when head is extended	Cerebral cortex and peripheral nervous system
		Flexion of arms and extension of legs when head is flexed	
Grasp reflex	Press object on the palm of the hand	Closure of the hand around object	Cerebral cortex and peripheral nervous system
Babinski reflex	Scratch the sole of the foot along its lateral margin from heel to toe	Extension and flaring of toes	Cerebral peduncle or pyramid of the corticospinal tract and peripheral nervous system
Clasp knife reflex	Rapidly stretch and bend arm	Brief "catch" in limb movement	Golgi tendon organs of the peripheral nervous system
Moro (startle) reflex	In supine position, raise head 3 cm from padded surface and allow it to drop suddenly OR Make a sudden loud noise	Rapid and symmetrical spread of the arms, with fingers extended, followed by flexion of the arms	Cerebral cortex and peripheral nervous system
Oral Reflexes			
Jaw thrust reflex	Present food	Forceful downward extension of mandible	Cranial nerves V (trigeminal) and VII (facial)
Rooting reflex	Touch face around the mouth or gently tap corners of mouth	Turning of the head toward the side touched and suckling	Cranial nerves V (trigeminal), VII (facial), XI (spinal accessory), and XII (hypoglossal)

Reflex	Stimulus	Response	Cranial Nerves
Tongue thrust reflex	Present liquid	Forceful movement of the tongue between or against the upper teeth during swallow	Cranial nerve XII (hypoglossal)
Tonic bite reflex	Apply moderate pressure to the gums	Closure of the jaws in a biting movement	Cranial nerves V (trigeminal) and VII (facial)
Chewing reflex	Rub anterior and lateral surfaces of the teeth	Rhythmic chewing movements without jaw closure	Cranial nerves V (facial) and VII (facial)
Suckling/sucking reflex	Place finger in mouth or on lips and move in a rotary pattern	Grasping of stimulus object with lips and forward, upward, and inward movement of tongue; may be followed by a swallow	Cranial nerves V (trigeminal), VII (facial), IX (glossopharyngeal), X (vagus), and XII (hypoglossal)

Normal Reflexes Affected by TBI

Reflex	Stimulus	Response	Cranial Nerves
Corneal blink	Touch the cornea of one eye	Immediate blinking of *both* eyes	Cranial nerves V (trigeminal), VII (facial)
Flexor reflex	Apply painful stimulus (e.g., pinch)	Quick withdrawal of extremity	Peripheral nervous system
Pupillary light reflex	Shine light in eyes	Constriction of both pupils	Cranial nerves II (optic) and III (oculomotor)
Pendular muscle stretch reflex (knee jerk reflex)	Strike patellar leg tendon with a reflex hammer when leg can swing freely	Forward movement of lower leg	Peripheral nervous system
Oral Reflexes Swallowing	Present liquid or solid food to posterior part of oral cavity	Completed swallow within approximately 1 second	Cranial nerves V (trigeminal), VII (facial), IX (glossopharyngeal), X (vagus), and XII (hypoglossal)
Gag reflex	Stimulus (e.g., toothbrush or tongue blade) placed on back half of tongue or side wall of the pharynx	Rapid velopharyngeal closure, symmetrical pharyngeal closure, mouth opening, head extension	Cranial nerves IX (glossopharyngeal) and X (vagus)

Appendix 5.B

Rancho Los Amigos Levels of Cognitive Functioning (I to X)

I. NO RESPONSE—Total assistance

- Complete absence of observable change in behavior when presented visual, auditory, tactile, proprioceptive, vestibular, or painful stimuli.

II. GENERALIZED RESPONSE—Total assistance

- Demonstrates generalized reflex response to painful stimuli.
- Responds to repeated auditory stimuli with increased or decreased activity.
- Responds to external stimuli with physiological changes, generalized, gross body movement, and/or not purposeful vocalization.
- Responses noted above may be same regardless of type and location of stimulation.
- Responses may be significantly delayed.

III. LOCALIZED RESPONSE—Total assistance

- Demonstrates withdrawal or vocalization to painful stimuli.
- Turns toward or away from auditory stimuli.
- Blinks when strong light crosses visual field.
- Follows moving object passed within visual field.
- Responds to discomfort by pulling tubes or restraints.
- Responds inconsistently to simple commands.
- Responses directly related to type of stimulus.
- May respond to some persons (especially family and friends) but not to others.

Note. Adapted from *Rancho Los Amigos Levels of Cognitive Functioning–Revised,* by C. Hagen, 2000, February, Presentation at TBI Rehabilitation in a Managed Care Environment: An Interdisciplinary Approach to Rehabilitation, Continuing Education Programs of America, San Antonio, TX. Copyright 2000 by C. Hagen. Adapted with permission.

IV. CONFUSED–AGITATED—Maximal assistance

- Alert and in heightened state of activity.

- Purposeful attempts to remove restraints or tubes or crawl out of bed.

- May perform motor activities such as sitting, reaching, and walking but without any apparent purpose or upon another's request.

- Very brief and usually nonpurposeful moments of sustained attention and divided attention.

- Absent short-term memory.

- Absent goal-directed, problem-solving, self-monitoring behavior.

- May cry out or scream out of proportion to stimulus even after its removal.

- May exhibit aggressive or flight behavior.

- Mood may swing from euphoric to hostile with no apparent relationship to environmental events.

- Unable to cooperate with treatment efforts.

- Verbalizations are frequently incoherent and/or inappropriate to activity or environment.

V. CONFUSED–INAPPROPRIATE–NONAGITATED— Maximal assistance

- Alert, not agitated but may wander randomly or with a vague intention of going home.

- May become agitated in response to external stimulation and/or lack of environmental structure.

- Not oriented to person, place, or time.

- Frequent brief periods of nonpurposeful sustained attention.

- Severely impaired recent memory, with confusion of past and present in reaction to ongoing activity.

- Absent goal-directed, problem-solving, self-monitoring behavior.

- Often demonstrates inappropriate use of objects without external direction.

- May be able to perform previously learned tasks when structure and cues provided.

- Unable to learn new information.

- Able to respond appropriately to simple commands fairly consistently with external structure and cues.

- Responses to simple commands without external structure are random and nonpurposeful in relation to the command.

- Able to converse on a social, automatic level for brief periods of time when provided external structure and cues.

- Verbalizations about present event become inappropriate and confabulatory when external structure and cues are not provided.

VI. CONFUSED–APPROPRIATE—Moderate assistance

- Inconsistently oriented to person and place.

- Able to attend to highly familiar tasks in nondistracting environment for 30 minutes with moderate redirection.

- Remote memory has more depth and detail than recent memory.

- Vague recognition of some staff.

- Able to use assistive memory aid with maximum assistance.

- Emerging awareness of appropriate response to self, family, and basic needs.

- Emerging goal-directed behavior related to meeting basic personal needs.

- Moderate assist to problem solve barriers to task completion.

- Supervised for old learning (e.g., self care).

- Shows carryover for relearned familiar tasks (e.g., self care).

- Maximum assistance for new learning, with little or no carryover.

- Unaware of impairments, disabilities, and safety risks.

- Consistently follows simple directions.

- Verbal expressions are appropriate in highly familiar and structured situations.

VII. AUTOMATIC–APPROPRIATE—Minimal assistance for routine daily living skills

- Consistently oriented to person and place within highly familiar environments. Moderate assistance for orientation to time.

- Able to attend to highly familiar tasks in a nondistracting environment for at least 30 minutes with minimal assistance to complete tasks.

- Able to use assistive memory devices with minimal assistance.

- Minimal supervision for new learning.

- Demonstrates carryover of new learning.

- Initiates and carries out steps to complete familiar personal and household routines but has shallow recall of what he or she has been doing.

- Able to monitor accuracy and completeness of each step in routine personal and household activities of daily living (ADLs) and modify plan with minimum assistance.

- Superficial awareness of his or her condition but unaware of specific impairments and disabilities and the limits they place on his or her ability to safely, accurately, and completely carry out his or her household, community, work, and leisure ADLs.

- Minimal supervision for safety in routine home and community activities.

- Unrealistic planning for the future.

- Unable to think about consequences of a decision or action.

- Overestimates abilities.

- Unaware of others' needs and feelings.

- Oppositional/uncooperative.

- Unable to recognize inappropriate social interaction behavior.

VIII. PURPOSEFUL AND APPROPRIATE—Standby assistance

- Consistently oriented to person, place, and time.

- Independently attends to and completes familiar tasks for 1 hour in a distracting environment.

- Able to recall and integrate past and recent events.

- Uses assistive memory devices to recall daily schedule, "to do" lists, and record critical information for later use with standby assistance.

- Initiates and carries out steps to complete familiar personal, household, community, work, and leisure routines with standby assistance and can modify the plan when needed with minimal assistance.

- Requires no assistance once new tasks/activities are learned.

- Aware of and acknowledges impairments and disabilities when they interfere with task completion but requires standby assistance to take appropriate corrective action.

- Thinks about consequences of a decision or an action with minimal assistance.

- Overestimates or underestimates abilities.

- Acknowledges others' needs and feelings and responds appropriately with minimal assistance.

- Depressed.

- Irritable.

- Low frustration tolerance/easily angered.

- Argumentative.

- Self centered.

- Uncharacteristically dependent/independent.

- Able to recognize and acknowledge inappropriate social interaction behavior while it is occurring and takes corrective action with minimal assistance.

IX. PURPOSEFUL AND APPROPRIATE—Standby assistance on request

- Independently shifts back and forth between tasks and completes them accurately for at least 2 consecutive hours.

- Uses assistive memory devices to recall daily schedule and "to do" lists, and to record critical information for later use with assistance when requested.

- Initiates and carries out steps to complete familiar personal, household, work, and leisure tasks independently and unfamiliar personal, household, work, and leisure tasks with assistance when requested.

- Aware of and acknowledges impairments and disabilities when they interfere with task completion and takes appropriate corrective action but requires standby assistance to anticipate a problem before it occurs and take action to avoid it.

- Able to think about consequences of decisions or actions with assistance when requested.

- Accurately estimates abilities but requires standby assistance to adjust to task demands.

- Acknowledges others' needs and feelings and responds appropriately with standby assistance.

- Depression may continue.

- May be easily irritable.

- May have low frustration tolerance.

- Able to self-monitor appropriateness of social interaction with standby assistance.

X. PURPOSEFUL AND APPROPRIATE—Modified independent

- Able to handle multiple tasks simultaneously in all environments but may require periodic breaks.

- Able to independently procure, create, and maintain own assistive memory devices.

- Independently initiates and carries out steps to complete familiarand unfamiliar personal, household, community, work, and leisure tasks but may require more than the usual amount of time and/or compensatory strategies to complete them.

- Anticipates impact of impairments and disabilities on ability to complete daily living tasks and takes action to avoid problems before they occur but may require more than the usual amount of time and/or compensatory strategies.

- Able to think independently about consequences of decisions or action but may require more than the usual amount of time and/or compensatory strategies to select the appropriate decision or action.

- Accurately estimates abilities and independently adjusts to task demands.

- Able to recognize the needs and feelings of others and automatically respond in appropriate manner.

- Periodic periods of depression may occur.

- Irritability and low frustration tolerance when sick, fatigued, and/or under emotional stress.

- Social interaction behavior is consistently appropriate.

References

American Congress of Rehabilitation Medicine. (1995). Recommendations for use of uniform nomenclature pertinent to patients with severe alterations in consciousness. *Archives of Physical Medicine and Rehabilitation, 76*, 205–209.

American Neurological Association. (1993). Persistent vegetative state: Report of the American Neurological Association Committee on Ethical Affairs. *Annals of Neurology, 33*, 386–390.

Andrews, K. (1996). International working party on the management of the vegetative state: Summary report. *Brain Injury, 10*, 797–806.

Ansell, B. (1995). Visual tracking behavior in low functioning head-injured adults. *Archives of Physical Medicine and Rehabilitation, 76*, 726–731.

Ansell, B. J., & Keenan, J. E. (1989). The Western Neuro Sensory Stimulation Profile: A tool for assessing slow-to-recover head-injured patients. *Archives of Physical Medicine and Rehabilitation, 70*, 104–108.

Berrol, S. (1986). Considerations for the management of the persistent vegetative state. *Archives of Physical Medicine and Rehabilitation, 67*, 283–285.

Berrol, S. (1990). Persistent vegetative state. *Physical Medicine and Rehabilitation: State of the Art Reviews, 4*, 559–567.

Binder, L. M. (1997). A review of mild head trauma: Part II. Clinical implications. *Journal of Clinical and Experimental Neuropsychology, 19*, 432–457.

Childs, N. L., Mercer, W. N., & Childs, H. W. (1993). Accuracy of diagnosis of persistent vegetative state. *Neurology, 43*, 1465–1467.

Committee for Pro-Life Activities–National Conference of Catholic Bishops. (1992). Nutrition and hydration: Moral and pastoral reflections. *Issues in Law and Medicine, 8*, 387–406.

Ewing-Cobbs, L., Levin, H. S., Fletcher, J. M., Miner, M. E., & Eisenberg, H. M. (1990). The Children's Orientation and Amnesia Test: Relationship to severity of acute head injury and to recovery of memory. *Neurosurgery, 27*, 683–691.

Fortuny, L. A., Briggs, M., Newcombe, F., Ratcliff, G., & Thomas, C. (1980). Measuring the duration of post-traumatic amnesia. *Journal of Neurology, Neurosurgery, and Psychiatry, 43,* 377–379.

Giacino, J. T. (1996). Sensory stimulation: Theoretical perspectives and the evidence for effectiveness. *NeuroRehabilitation, 6,* 69–78.

Giacino, J. T., Zasler, N. D., Katz, D. I., Kelly, J. P., Rosenberg, J. H., & Filley, C. M. (1997). Development of practice guidelines for assessment and management of the vegetative and minimally conscious states. *Journal of Head Trauma Rehabilitation, 12*(4), 79–89.

Hagen, C. (1982). Language–cognitive disorganization following closed head injury: A conceptualization. In L. E. Trexler (Ed.), *Cognitive rehabilitation: Conceptualization and intervention* (pp. 131–151). New York: Plenum.

Hagen, C. (2000, February). *Rancho Los Amigos Levels of Cognitive Functioning–Revised.* Presentation at TBI Rehabilitation in a Managed Care Environment: An Interdisciplinary Approach to Rehabilitation. Continuing Education Programs of America, San Antonio, TX.

Hall, M. E., MacDonald, S., & Young, G. C. (1992). The effectiveness of directed multisensory stimulation versus non-directed stimulation in comatose CHI patients: Pilot study of a single subject design. *Brain Injury, 6,* 435–445.

Ingvar, D. H., Brun, A., Johansson, L., & Samuelsson, S. M. (1978). Survival after severe cerebral anoxia with destruction of cerebral cortex: Apallic syndrome. *Annals of the New York Academy of Science, 315,* 184–214.

Jennett, B. (1997). A quarter century of the vegetative state: An international perspective. *Journal of Head Trauma Rehabilitation, 12*(4), 1–12.

Jennett, B., & Plum, F. (1972). Persistent vegetative state after brain damage. *Lancet, 1,* 734–737.

Jennett, B., & Teasdale, G. (1981). *Management of head injuries.* New York: Oxford University Press.

Jennett, B., Teasdale, G., Braakman, R., Minderhoud, J., Heldon, J., & Kurze, T. (1979). Prognosis of patients with severe head injury. *Neurosurgery, 4,* 283–289.

Johnson, D., Roethig-Johnston, K., & Richards, D. (1993). Biochemical and physiological parameters of recovery in acute severe head injury: Responses to multisensory stimulation. *Brain Injury, 7,* 491–499.

Jones, R., Hux, K., Morton-Anderson, A., & Knepper, L. (1994). Auditory stimulation effect on a comatose survivor of traumatic brain injury. *Archives of Physical Medicine and Rehabilitation, 75,* 164–171.

Kater, K. M. (1989). Response of head-injury patients to sensory stimulation. *Western Journal of Nursing Research, 11*(1), 20–33.

Levin, H. S., Gary, H. E., Eisenberg, H. M., Ruff, R. M., Barth, J. T., Kreutzer, J., High, W. M., Portman, S., Foulkes, M. A., Jane, J. A., Marmarou, A., & Marshall, L. F. (1990). Neurobehavioral outcome 1 year after severe head injury. *Journal of Neurosurgery, 73,* 699–709.

Levin, H. S., O'Donnell, V. M., & Grossman, R. G. (1975). The Galveston Orientation and Amnesia Test: A practical scale to assess cognition after head injury. *Journal of Nervous and Mental Disorders, 167,* 675–684.

Multi-Society Task Force on PVS. (1994). Medical aspects of the persistent vegetative state (Part 2). *New England Journal of Medicine, 330,* 1572–1579.

Pfurtscheller, G., Schwarz, G., & List, W. (1986). Long-lasting EEG reactions in comatose patients after repetitive stimulation. *Electroencephalography and Clinical Neurophysiology, 64,* 402–410.

Pierce, J. P., Lyle, D. M., Quine, S., Evans, N. J., Morris, J., & Fearnside, M. R. (1990). The effectiveness of coma arousal intervention. *Brain Injury, 4*, 191–197.

Plum, R., & Posner, J. B. (1983). *The diagnosis of stupor and coma* (3rd ed.). Philadelphia: Davis.

Rappaport, M., Dougherty, A. M., & Kelting, D. L. (1992). Evaluation of coma and vegetative states. *Archives of Physical Medicine and Rehabilitation, 73*, 628–634.

Russell, W. R. (1932). Cerebral involvement in head injury. *Brain, 55*, 549–603.

Russell, W. R., & Smith, A. (1961). Post-traumatic amnesia in closed head injury. *Archives of Neurology, 5*, 16–29.

Smith, G. J., & Ylvisaker, M. (1985). Cognitive rehabilitation therapy: Early stages of recovery. In M. Ylvisaker (Ed.), *Head injury rehabilitation: Children and adolescents* (pp. 275–286). San Diego: College-Hill Press.

Teasdale, G., & Jennett, B. (1974). Assessment of coma and impaired consciousness: A practical scale. *Lancet, 2*, 81–84.

Wilson, S. L., Brock, D., Powell, G. E., Thwaites, H., & Elliott, K. (1996). Constructing arousal profiles for vegetative state patients—A preliminary report. *Brain Injury, 10*, 105–113.

Wilson, S. L., Powell, G. E., Brock, D., & Thwaites, H. (1996). Vegetative state and responses to sensory stimulation: An analysis of 24 cases. *Brain Injury, 10*, 807–818.

Wilson, S. L., Powell, G. E., Elliott, K., & Thwaites, H. (1991). Sensory stimulation in prolonged coma: Four single case studies. *Brain Injury, 5*, 393–400.

Wood, R. L. (1991). Critical analysis of the concept of sensory stimulation for patients in vegetative states. *Brain Injury, 5*, 401–409.

Assessment and Treatment of Cognitive–Communication Impairments

Karen Hux and Nancy Manasse

Communication Problems Associated with TBI: A Syndrome in Search of a Name

Speech–language pathologists have struggled to identify and label the language-related communication challenges of survivors of TBI. During the past 70 years, professionals have progressed through a succession of previously existing and newly coined names to classify and describe the communication behaviors displayed by survivors of TBI. Terms such as *aphasia, language of confusion,* and *subclinical aphasia* preceded use of the label most commonly used today—that is, *cognitive–communication impairment*. All of these terms, however, have valid associations with TBI and have contributed to the current understanding of the language-related and cognition-related communication challenges of people with TBI.

When Aphasia Is Not Aphasia

During the early years of diagnosing and treating survivors of TBI, aphasia was the only known language disorder to result from acquired brain damage; hence, clinicians referred to the communication challenges of all survivors of TBI as aphasia. For some survivors, *aphasia* may be an appropriate diagnostic label; for others, it definitely is not.

Aphasia is defined as a chronic, acquired impairment in the comprehension and formulation of language caused by a focal lesion to a part of the brain concerned specifically with language processing—typically the perisylvian region of the left cortical hemisphere (Dirckx, 1997; Rosenbek, LaPointe, & Wertz, 1989). The language-related communication challenges typical in people with TBI do not match all of the qualifying criteria contained in this definition of aphasia. First, TBI usually causes diffuse damage to multiple

Perhaps in no other realm of recovery from TBI is there greater discrepancy than occurs when discussing cognition. People who have escaped obvious physical impairment are often described as having made "remarkable" or even "excellent" recoveries. These descriptions ignore the tremendous impact of cognitive deficits on long-term outcome and overall life quality. The fact that cognitive deficits are, in fact, hidden inside the person's brain makes them much more difficult to identify, quantify, and treat than some other types of impairments.

cortical and subcortical regions; focal damage to language processing areas of the brain may or may not occur. When such focal damage does exist and, consequently, the individual displays language processing behaviors consistent with aphasia symptomology, *aphasia* is probably an appropriate label. However, when clinicians observe communication challenges with characteristics that do not correspond with traditional aphasia and that are not associated with focal lesions, they need to use another diagnostic label.

Second, some survivors of TBI display aphasia-like symptoms during early stages of recovery. However, the aphasia-like language challenges of people with TBI differ from the traditional disorder in terms of their chronicity. Some people with aphasia from strokes recover functional language skills, but most never regain their prior facility with language processing. Even with treatment, most stroke survivors with aphasia have language challenges that persist throughout the remainder of their lives. On the other hand, most survivors of TBI do not display language-based impairments that persist in the same manner as aphasia; aphasia-like symptoms often appear during the early stages of recovery, but the linguistic impairments of survivors of TBI tend to be transient rather than permanent. Within a few days or weeks of regaining speech, most survivors of TBI have minimal difficulty with structural aspects of language, although problems may persist in their word retrieval ability or their ability to maintain sufficient attention and concentration to engage fully in conversations.

The presence of a temporary or transient form of aphasia may seem puzzling. Why do symptoms of aphasia appear during the early stage of TBI recovery despite a lack of focal damage to the perisylvian region of the language-dominant hemisphere? The explanation for this phenomenon lies in the brain's physiological recovery. Early in the recovery process, a great deal of cerebral swelling and edema typically occurs. This swelling and edema increases pressure on neural structures and can cause temporary symptoms of many disorders. As swelling reduces, many symptoms of language, cognitive, physical, and neurological disorders dissipate. Only then do the persistent effects of brain trauma become visible.

A problem arises when speech–language pathologists or medical professionals use the term *aphasia* to describe the transient, aphasia-like symptoms that survivors of TBI often display during the early stage of recovery. Although aphasia in its traditional form rarely extends past Rancho Level V (see Appendix 5.B in Chapter 5), the label may stay with an individual for years. Of greater concern is the possibility that the incorrect diagnosis will limit exploration and treatment of the actual cognitive deficits contributing to ineffective or inefficient communication.

Despite the preceding warnings about misdiagnosing aphasia, the disorder in its traditional and chronic form sometimes results from TBI. In about one third of cases of severe TBI, the acquired brain damage results in true aphasia (Sarno, 1980; Sarno, Buonaguro, & Levita, 1986). When this occurs, the language impairment matches that caused by strokes. However, an important difference still exists between survivors of TBI with aphasia and survivors of strokes with aphasia. Specifically, the survivor of TBI with aphasia almost invariably has other language-related and cognition-related communication problems as well; a survivor of stroke, on the other hand, is more likely than the TBI survivor to have aphasia in isolation.

The Confusion of *Language of Confusion*

In the 1970s and 1980s, researchers and clinicians began to realize that the communication challenges of people with TBI differed from those of people with strokes; as a result, the search for an alternative diagnostic label began. One option was to use the label *language of confusion* to identify the communication challenges associated with the impaired mental functioning that neurologists term *confusion* (Darley, 1982; Halpern, Darley, & Brown, 1973). Clinical confusion typically results from multiple or diffuse brain lesions and is associated with disorientation, reduced comprehension or awareness of surroundings, and memory deficits. The expressive language of confused individuals often contains confabulation and irrelevant or peculiar responses despite relatively preserved syntax, morphology, and phonology.

Normally, a confused mental state and the associated language behaviors are temporary. Once the confusion dissipates, the language of survivors of TBI becomes more appropriate and less bizarre and confabulatory; as a result clinicians attempting to describe and treat the *chronic* communication challenges of survivors of TBI find language of confusion an inadequate term. Recognition that some TBI survivors had continuing communication challenges even after the resolution of confusion prompted clinicians to explore further the persistent language challenges associated with TBI and to continue the search for an appropriate term for the chronic condition.

Subclinical Aphasia

By the 1980s, professionals began realizing that persistent communication challenges affected the ability of survivors of TBI to perform academic and vocational endeavors despite their having recovered from language of confusion or aphasia. Across two research studies, Sarno (1980) and her colleagues (Sarno et al., 1986) administered a battery of aphasia tests to survivors of TBI and determined that, although most did not score low enough to qualify as having aphasia, all performed at a level lower than that of neurologically intact adults. Sarno coined the term *subclinical aphasia* to describe communication impairments of this population of survivors. However, as with similar terms such as *latent aphasia* (Boller & Vignolo, 1966) and *nonaphasic naming disorders* (Geschwind, 1964, 1967), subclinical aphasia never gained widespread use in clinical settings. This may have reflected a reluctance on the part of professionals to add another adjective to the long list used to describe variations in aphasic syndromes (e.g., Broca's aphasia, conduction aphasia, global aphasia, sensory aphasia, receptive aphasia), or it may have reflected a growing awareness of the role of cognitive deficits in the communication challenges of people with TBI—that is, scientists may have wanted the name to reflect the actual source of the condition.

Cognitive–Communication Impairments

In the late 1980s, professionals from fields such as neurology, linguistics, and psychology began raising questions about brain–language relations, specifically wanting to know how a normal brain processes and represents language and how an injury to the brain can disrupt those processes and representations. Because of its rule-based nature, professionals began conceptualizing language as separate and unique from other aspects of cognition. As depicted in Figure 6.1, communicative competence requires both knowledge of rule-based aspects of language and intact cognitive functioning. An impairment to communicative performance occurs when a disruption to either the language rule system or cognitive functioning occurs. The effect of focal brain damage to the perisylvian region of the language-dominant hemisphere—as occurs with some strokes—causes aphasia because of a disruption in the efficiency with which an individual can access and use one or more of the language rule systems: relational semantics, morphology, syntax, or phonology (see Figure 6.2). In contrast, individuals with diffuse brain damage from TBIs may have intact language rule systems but have decreases in one or more aspects of cognition that cause them to be inefficient and ineffective in their communicative performance (see Figure 6.3). Professionals have labeled the resulting disorder a *cognitive–communication impairment* and have defined it as a decreased ability to perform language-based activities because of a deficit in one or more of the cognitive functions that underlie communication (e.g., attention, perception, memory) (American Speech-Language-Hearing Association, 1991).

In some cases, TBI affects language functioning and cognitive functioning; in other cases, it affects only one of the two. Figure 6.4 depicts the interaction of language and cognition and shows how impairment to one or both processes can affect communicative performance. As shown in Figure 6.5, the most common language-related disorder to result from TBI is cognitive–communication impairment. This occurs whenever a disruption in one or more aspects of cognitive functioning has a negative impact on communicative performance. In contrast, the most common disorder to result from stroke damage to the language-dominant hemisphere is aphasia. True aphasia can be caused by TBI, but it is rare because damage typically is not restricted to the cortical regions responsible for language processing. Usually when TBI causes focal damage to language processing centers of the brain, damage to other cortical regions accompanies it, causing a combination of cognitive–communication impairment and aphasia.

Because cognitive–communication impairment is pervasive among survivors of TBI, can have substantial negative effects on academic, social, and vocational functioning, and constitutes a relatively new diagnostic category within the profession of speech–language pathology, the remainder of this chapter focuses solely on this disorder. A description of the characteristics and behaviors associated with cognitive–communication impairments, guidelines for performing assessments, and suggestions concerning intervention strategies and techniques are included.

(*text continues on page 100*)

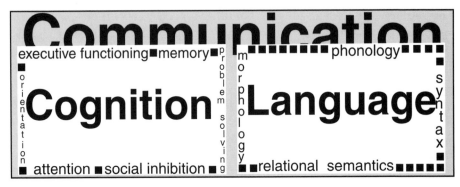

Figure 6.1. Communicative competence.

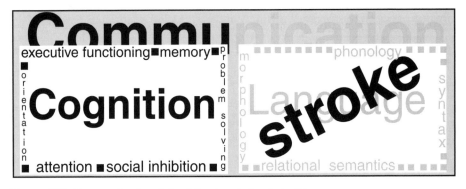

Figure 6.2. Communicative status following stroke: Aphasia.

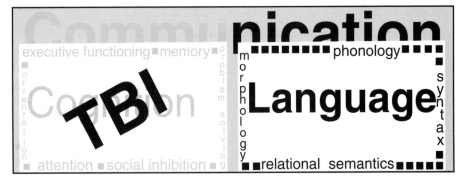

Figure 6.3. Communicative status following TBI: Cognitive–communication impairment.

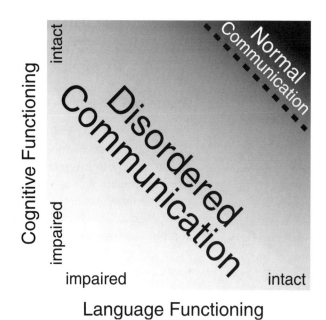

Figure 6.4. Effects of language and cognitive impairments on communication.

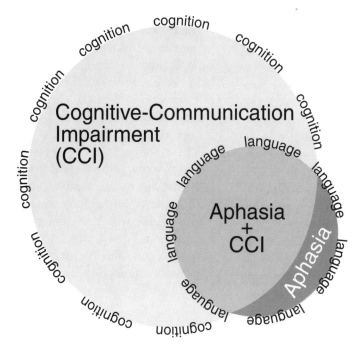

Figure 6.5. Occurrence of language-related disorders following TBI.

How do physiological changes within an individual contribute to variations in cognitive functioning?

The autonomic nervous system regulates the environment within the human body. It controls basic sensations such as the level of alertness, feelings of hunger and thirst, and temperature regulation, and it controls the involuntary muscles regulating functions such as heart rate, blood pressure, and respiratory rate. Fluctuations in the internal environment occur on a constant basis. Typically, these fluctuations do not interfere with cognitive status or performance; however, when a person ignores a basic need (such as the need for food) for an extended period of time, the resulting discomfort may interfere with performance of other tasks.

Among survivors of TBI, abnormal functioning of the nervous system may cause a phenomenon called internal distractibility. A survivor with internal distractibility is more sensitive to changes in the internal environment than neurologically intact individuals; cognitive resources become directed toward bodily sensations rather than toward performance or awareness of external activities and events. Survivors of TBI susceptible to internal distractibility show decreases in cognitive functioning whenever they cannot divert their attention away from internal sensations.

Characteristics of Cognitive–Communication Impairments

Areas of Cognitive Challenge

Several aspects of cognition—such as orientation, attention, memory, problem solving, executive functioning, critical thinking, and psychosocial responses—underlie communicative performance and, when impaired, have the potential to contribute to cognitive–communication impairments. Table 6.1 provides definitions of many communication-related aspects of cognition that TBI can affect.

A decrease in a single aspect of cognition is enough to create a negative effect on communicative competence, and survivors of TBI typically experience multiple cognitive disruptions simultaneously. Furthermore, the extent of cognitive impairment tends to fluctuate on a daily (sometimes hourly) basis, depending on changes in the individual or in the environment. The numerous possible variations and combinations of cognitive deficits following TBI and the variability in cognitive performance that is a hallmark of TBI complicate the process of identifying and describing the factors that contribute to cognitive–communication impairments. The situation is further complicated by overlap and interdependence among some aspects of cognition. For example, a problem with attention can affect cognitive processes such as memory, orientation, executive functioning, and problem solving.

Table 6.1
Aspects of Cognition Associated
with Cognitive–Communication Impairments

Cognitive Component	Definition
Orientation	
Person	Knowing name, birth date, and age
Place	Knowing location (city, state, and type of facility)
Time	Knowing the date, month, year, day of week, and approximate time of day
Purpose	Knowing what happened and why therapy is necessary
Attention	
Sustained	Maintaining attention to single tasks in quiet environments
Selective	Focusing on one task in the presence of distractions
Alternating	Switching between two tasks while maintaining speed and accuracy
Divided	Switching between visual and verbal information while performing two or more tasks
Memory	
Short term	Immediate recall of newly learned verbal and visual information
Recent	Delayed recall (approximately 30 minutes) of newly learned information
Long term	Recall of previously known information—including general knowledge information, content-specific information, and personal and biographical information
Procedural	Recall of an acquired pattern or process (e.g., riding a bike)
Prospective	Recall of information needed in the near future (e.g., remembering to call a doctor to obtain test results)
Episodic	Recall of temporally dated events and the temporal–spatial relation between events (e.g., remembering the first day of school)
Problem Solving	
Identifying problems	Identifying and acknowledging the existence of actual or potential problems
Generating solutions	Formulating appropriate and effective solutions

(continues)

Table 6.1 *Continued.*

Cognitive Component	Definition
Problem Solving *Continued.*	
Organizing	Collecting and arranging any materials needed
Sequencing	Determining the order in which events should occur
Implementing solutions	Actively putting a solution to work
Managing time	Knowing how long each step of the process should take and actively maintaining prospective time frames
Self-monitoring	Checking progress toward goals
Maintaining safety	Identifying potential dangers to oneself or others and taking appropriate actions to minimize dangers
Executive Functioning	
Insight	Accurately perceiving strengths and weaknesses
Goal setting	Choosing realistic goals based on personal ability
Planning and organizing	Determining what approach to take and the order of steps needed to attain a goal
Self-initiation	Having an active desire and motivation to pursue goals
Implementation	Carrying out a plan
Self-evaluation	Making judgments about performance in relation to a goal
Problem solving	Strategically modifying plans if confronted with obstacles prohibiting goal attainment
Carryover	Transferring new skills to a variety of environments and situations
Critical Thinking	
Drawing inferences	Making a connection between two otherwise unrelated facts
Deductive reasoning	Drawing a specific conclusion from given information
Inductive reasoning	Drawing a general conclusion from inferred information
Abstract reasoning	Drawing conclusions based on notions, ideas, and concepts that are not tangible
Flexibility of thought	Shifting from one idea to another with relative ease
Psychosocial Responses	
Inhibition	Suppressing instinctual or unconscious tendencies, especially those that conflict with societal norms
Emotional stability	Displaying emotional responses proportionate to external stimuli

Areas of Communication Challenge

Cognitive–communication impairments affect overall communicative competence. Typically, survivors of TBI with cognitive–communication impairments have intact grammar, syntax, and vocabulary knowledge, but they can not participate efficiently and effectively in communicative exchanges. In other words, they talk better than they communicate (Milton, Prutting, & Binder, 1984; Sohlberg & Mateer, 1989a). Because the language production of people with cognitive–communication impairment is generally fluent and free of grammatical errors, the communication problem may not be readily apparent to untrained listeners during informal conversation. Nevertheless, cognitive–communication impairments can substantially affect the social, academic, behavioral, and vocational lives of survivors.

Table 6.2 lists and defines specific behaviors associated with cognitive–communication impairments. A large number of these behaviors fall under the broad category of *pragmatics*: the functional use of verbal and nonverbal modes of communication to convey and interpret intended messages. The specific constellation of behaviors associated with an individual survivor's cognitive–communication impairment depends on his or her particular set of cognitive strengths and challenges.

Many of the symptoms of cognitive–communication impairments are readily apparent in the discourse of people with TBI. The following sample from a 56-year-old male survivor of severe TBI is representative. The sample was from an initial meeting between the survivor (G) and a clinician (C) during which the survivor initiated a conversation about his neighbor. Characteristics of cognitive–communication impairments are identified in parentheses immediately following the behavior. In particular, note the rambling nature of the text and the inclusion of many irrelevant details. Syntactic and morphologic structures that deviate from Standard American English were assumed to reflect dialectal variation rather than language impairment and, hence, were not marked as errors.

G: He was, he was (verbal dysfluency) married before, and his first wife died. Then he married his second wife, and that didn't go off so good. So this girl (lack of cohesion) that was working for him. . . . And he started up this pizza place on the corner (lack of saliency). She (lack of cohesion) was working for him. He got to know her pretty good, so he took her out a couple of times. Then he got married. You see, he's got a daughter, 27 years old from his second wife, er, from the first wife (revision). And, uh, (verbal dysfluency) this woman he married

(*text continues on page 106*)

Table 6.2

Communication Behaviors Associated
with Cognitive–Communication Impairments

Behavior	Definition
Semantics	
Word retrieval deficits	Difficulty recalling specific words to refer to objects, people, concepts, or ideas; may lead to word choice errors or delays, verbal dysfluency, circumlocution, use of nonspecific vocabulary, or frequent revision behaviors
Lexical rigidity	Difficulty recognizing multiple meanings of words or expressions
Lack of cohesion	Limited use of cohesive ties involving personal, possessive, and demonstrative pronouns, ellipses, conjunctions, and lexical substitutions
Concrete language	Failure to recognize abstract interpretations of expressions and concepts (e.g., humor, proverbs, and idioms)
Decreased integration	Difficulty associating and connecting new information with previous knowledge
Decreased synthesis	Difficulty assembling multiple pieces of spoken or written information to make a cohesive whole
Rigidity of thought	Lack of flexibility in interpreting or generating language
Confabulation	Lack of truthfulness in expressive language due to memory, attention, or orientation impairments
Decreased recognition of saliency	Difficulty discriminating between salient and irrelevant pieces of information
Slowed speed of processing	Difficulty processing verbal and/or nonverbal information as rapidly as average people without neurological damage; as task complexity increases, speed of processing typically decreases disproportionately
Verbal Pragmatics	
Tangential speech	Sudden shifts in conversational topic without appropriate signaling to a listener; person often requires redirection to task to reestablish original topic

(*continues*)

Table 6.2 *Continued.*

Behavior	Definition
Verbal Pragmatics *Continued.*	
Topic shading	Subtle shifts in topic that gradually cause a change in conversational focus
Decreased organization	Failure to recognize or adhere to the sequential or hierarchical nature of information; failure to identify or follow spatial or temporal sequences
Decreased communication	Limited initiation and maintenance of conversational interactions with others
Decreased topic maintenance	Difficulty generating novel messages associated with an established topic of conversation
Inappropriate topic selection	Failure to recognize or adhere to societal norms dictating the appropriateness of various conversational topics; often associated with disinhibition
Inadequate relevance	Difficulty determining the relevancy of information regarding a particular topic or goal
Poor presupposition skills	Difficulty assuming a listener's perspective when distinguishing new and old information
Nonverbal Pragmatics	
Dysprosody	Limited variation in vocal inflection or inappropriate selection of speech registers when conversing
Poor eye contact	Limited or excessive establishment of eye contact with communication partners
Flat affect	Limited use of facial expressions to convey emotions
Lability	Display of emotions (e.g., laughing, crying) in excess to the surrounding conditions
Decreased use of gestures	Failure to supplement verbal messages with appropriate limb or body movements
Inappropriate proxemics	Failure to recognize or adhere to societal norms dictating the distance between conversational partners
Inappropriate physical contact	Failure to recognize or adhere to societal norms dictating the use of touch during conversational interactions
Decreased understanding of nonverbal cues	Failure to recognize or interpret correctly the nonverbal communication attempts of others

is 27 years old, too. They've got a little boy. He's 2 years old. He always calls, "George, George!" (lack of saliency). And, uh, now they're expecting their second boy . . .

G: Oh, they're happy though.

C: Are they?

G: The only thing is, he, since he's (revision) had this business, he hasn't bought a home (tangential speech). He lives in an apartment there. It's out on the ground floor, but it's on the corner of—Oh, you don't know Westin. Where are you from (topic shading)?

C: Eagle Rock.

G: Eagle Rock, yeah?

C: So, he's living in an apartment (redirection to task)?

G: Yeah. He's on the ground floor. And uh, (verbal dysfluency) he got a lot of room there, too. The only thing, he had a Lincoln Towncar (tangential speech). And, he had trouble with it. So he bought it, he went on himself, he bought himself (revision) a Pontiac, uh, Bonneville. Oh, he likes that very much. Oh, and I clean up around there for him, too, after they close (tangential speech) . . .

C: Sounds like you're pretty handy.

G: Oh, oh, I can do anything you want.

C: Really?

G: Work on automobiles, anything.

C: Oh? Where'd you learn that?

G: Oh, from my father. I had 2 years of autoshop at high school in Springfield, Illinois. My father was the chief motor machinist for the Coast Guards (lack of cohesion) [starts crying] (lability). Oh, we were, uh, in the peninsula first (tangential speech). And then, mmm, I'd say about 2 years later we moved to uh—No, he was, no, (revision) they transferred and he was out, out (verbal dysfluency) East Coast. . . . Yeah. So, when he was over there, we's, I was (revision) about 13 years old, and I was going to high school. And this woman in there was telling me, she says, "Boy, you know a lot about, uh, (verbal dysfluency) motors, don't ya?" (topic shading). I says, "Yes." She goes, "Would you take my uh, motor, my generator motor (revision)"—where she makes electricity—"Would you take that motor out of there and fix it up for me?" So, I says, "Sure." So I went home and we had a truck and it was made out of an old '27 Studabaker (lack of saliency). Put a box on it. I put it (lack of cohesion) in there and brought it home. And we had an old trailer we used as a, as a, uh, (verbal dysfluency) mechanic shop. So, I put it (lack of cohesion) in there, and I started taking it apart. And my dad come home. "Where'd ya get this from?" I says, "Mrs. Paine. Uh, lights, lights, (verbal dysfluency) where she makes her lights (word finding)." "What'd you do that for?" "I told her I could fix it." He says, "That'll be the day." So I looked at a book, and I just followed everything in the book. And I ordered the parts and put new rings in there and new bearings and everything else. And, a new wrist pit in there. And, uh, my dad says, "How ya gonna get that going?" I says, "Watch." So after I got done I put it on there (lack of cohesion). Went down there, turned the switch on. The battery was charged. Turned it on and away it went. He says, well, he knows better now!

C: Hmm. That's pretty good . . .

G: Yeah. Oh, one time I was going down to see Dave (tangential speech; poor presupposition). I was going down the back streets and I come to the top of a hill. I was, I was gonna, er, (verbal dysfluency) top of a hill, and I started going down. And the car started sliding. I put on the brakes. And here was another car going east. Went right across in front of me. I went right in, I hit him (revision), and I hit the snow bank, too. Oh, they (lack of cohesion) fixed the car up. I brought it to the Chevrolet garage, and they fixed it up real good, yeah.

C: So I guess you've had a lot of experience fixing things up.

G: Yes. Deer hunting, everything (irrelevant information).

C: That's a good skill to have.

Assessment of Cognitive-Communication Impairments

Dramatic changes in cognitive and physical functioning may occur during early stages of recovery from TBI. During this period, many individuals do not have adequate attention or stamina to participate fully in assessment or treatment activities. Obviously, this lack of full engagement can affect test performance, and speech–language pathologists should not confuse initial evaluations with comprehensive evaluations.

During the initial recovery period, informal assessment should occur on a daily basis as part of intervention sessions. Later, when an individual has emerged from posttraumatic amnesia and can participate actively in a variety of activities, a speech–language pathologist should perform a comprehensive evaluation of the functional impact of cognitive–communication impairments on a survivor's life. Periodic reevaluations may be necessary for an extended time period postinjury—often for several years.

The complex relation between cognitive processes and communication processes makes multidisciplinary assessment beneficial. Speech–language pathologists, occupational therapists, psychologists, and neuropsychologists may share responsibility for assessing various aspects of cognitive and communication functioning. Typically, trends develop within hospital and rehabilitation settings to distribute the assessment responsibilities and avoid duplication.

Goals and Procedures of Early Assessments

Early assessments of communicative functioning often involve one or more scales designed to describe overall cognitive and physical status. Three such scales are common: (a) the World Health Organization's Model of Disablements found in *The International Classification of Functioning, Disability and Health* (ICIDH–2; World Health Organzation [WHO], 1999), (b) the Functional Independence Measures (FIM; State University of New York [SUNY] at Buffalo, 1997), and (c) the Rancho Los Amigos Levels of Cognitive Functioning (I to X) (Hagen, 2000). These scales identify an individual's status in a variety of health care domains. Professionals from multiple fields are familiar with the scales and the corresponding terminology, and many hospitals and rehabilitation centers nationwide use the scales to indicate recovery status and to compare progress across survivors. As a result, the scales are excellent supplements to formal, domain-specific assessment procedures. Administration of these assessments typically begins during the early stages of recovery and continues throughout the entire rehabilitation process.

World Health Organization Model

The World Health Organization Model in the ICIDH–2 delineates three main concepts characterizing current functioning level: impairment, activity, and participation (WHO, 1999). *Impairment* refers to a "loss or abnormality in cognitive, communicative, physical, emotional, physiological, or anatomical structure or function" (Rogers, Alarcon, & Olswang, 1999, p. 910). TBI can affect any or all of these areas, although the level of impairment across areas varies within and across persons. *Activity* (previously identified as *disability*) refers to one's ability to perform customary tasks or activities. Limitations in this area arise from current impairments. For example, impaired memory and attention can lead to difficulty engaging in conversations, watching television or movies, or taking notes in class. *Participation* (previously identified as *handicap*) refers to "an individual's involvement in life situations in relation to Health Conditions, Body Functions and Structures, Activities, and Contextual Factors" (WHO, 1999, p. 14). Participation restrictions are problems an individual may have in the manner or extent of involvement in life situations. For example, participation limitations related to impaired memory and attention may include reduced engagement in recreational, self-care, educational, and occupational activities. While similarities exist among the population of survivors of TBI as a whole, the extent of involvement across the levels of functioning varies depending on a survivor's usual and customary activities of daily living.

Functional Independence Measures

The FIM scale (SUNY at Buffalo, 1997) includes seven levels for assessing independent functioning across multiple areas and disciplines. Areas pertaining to cognitive–communication abilities include comprehension, expression, social interaction, problem solving, and memory (see Table 6.3). Although variations exist for each area of functioning, in general, the seven scoring levels include Complete Independence (7), Modified Independence (6), Standby Prompting (5), Minimal Prompting (4), Moderate Prompting (3), Maximal Prompting (2), and Total Assistance (1). A speech–language pathologist or another trained professional assigns the number that best corresponds to the individual's current level of performance.

A unique characteristic of the FIM scale is that it has multiple uses beyond assessment. The seven levels enable speech–language pathologists to identify one level of functioning as representative of current performance, a second level as a short-term goal, and yet another level as a long-term goal. Professionals also use the scale to describe outcome levels attained by individuals at the time of discharge. Hence, the scale can serve as an assessment measure, a progress measure, and an outcome measure.

Rancho Los Amigos Levels of Cognitive Functioning (I to X)

The Rancho Levels were developed by Hagen and Malkmus (1979) and recently revised by Hagen (2000). This 10-level scale focuses on numerous behavioral characteristics displayed by people with TBI throughout the recovery process.

Table 6.3
FIM Areas Related to Cognitive–Communication Functioning

Subskill area	Definition
Comprehension	Understanding of auditory or visual communication, whichever is used most frequently
Expression	Using verbal or nonverbal means (e.g., speaking, writing, using a communication device) to express communicative intents clearly
Social Interaction	Getting along and participating with others in group situations to meet personal needs and the needs of others; includes behaviors such as controlling temper, accepting criticism, and being aware of how words and actions affect others
Problem Solving	Identifying, initiating, and executing steps in a reasonable, safe, and timely manner to solve problems pertaining to financial, social, and personal affairs
Memory	Remembering verbal and visual information necessary for the recognition of frequently encountered people, the recall of daily routines, and the independent execution of requests

The scale is presented in its entirety in Appendix 5.B of this text. Although the levels primarily address changes in cognitive functioning, they include behavioral characteristics associated with cognitive–communication impairments. For example, incoherent verbalizations that do not relate to the present activity or environment characterize Level IV; inappropriate verbalizations about present events (which may be accompanied by confabulation when external structure and cues are minimal) characterize Level V. Although somewhat subjective in nature, the Rancho Levels provide a systematic way to summarize initial status and progressive changes in cognitive–communicative abilities.

As a person emerges from coma or a state of minimal consciousness and progresses through the first three Rancho Levels, pervasive medical and cognitive problems mask language functioning. Systematic assessment of cognitive–communication deficits is not possible at this time, and the lack of functional communication does not indicate future cognitive–communication abilities. Assessment of communicative functioning focuses primarily on language comprehension—specifically, the individual's ability to follow one-step commands. Only about 50% of survivors of severe TBI follow simple commands—an initial sign of emergence from coma or vegetative state—within the first 3 months of recovery (Bricolo, Turazzi, & Feriotti, 1980).

Goals and Procedures of Comprehensive Assessments

Hoogeveen (1993) outlined several general principles that relate specifically to performing comprehensive assessments of the cognitive and communication status of people with TBI. After a description of each principle, procedures are provided for performing functional evaluations of cognitive–communication impairments.

General Assessment Principles

Rely on Clinical Judgment. Over the years, clinical practitioners from a variety of disciplines have been encouraged to rely on objective scores rather than subjective observations and clinical judgment. Unfortunately, much important information is lost when speech–language pathologists ignore their "gut-level" reactions. When assessing the communication skills of people with TBI, clinical judgment is paramount. Because many aspects of cognitive–communication impairments relate to pragmatic behaviors that are not easily quantified through standardized measures, speech–language pathologists must rely on clinical judgment. Anytime a clinician thinks or feels that interactions with a survivor are strange, uncomfortable, or unusual, he or she needs to pay attention to those observations and examine carefully the individual's communication behaviors. Many times, the discomfort stems from violations of verbal and nonverbal pragmatic conventions. In all likelihood, if a professional reacts negatively when interacting with a survivor of TBI, so will other people. Speech–language pathologists need to trust their clinical judgment: If something feels wrong, it probably is.

Observations Are More Important Than Scores. The lure of standardized assessment procedures is that they provide a score for comparison with normative data. However, normative data do not generally exist for survivors of TBI, and, because of the tremendous variability among survivors, such data are never likely to exist in a worthwhile form. Instead, the value of assessment procedures is in the opportunity to observe how an individual approaches the problems presented. Tests with which a speech–language pathologist is highly familiar and that he or she has given to many other people are helpful. By using familiar tests, the clinician knows what to expect from people of a given age and background and will more readily recognize deviations from normal performance.

Perform Real-World Observations. Oftentimes, survivors of TBI perform better on standardized tests than they do in real life. This discrepancy reflects the benefit of the high degree of structure inherent in standardized tests and contributes an important piece of diagnostic information. However, determining how an individual performs in an actual classroom, social, or vocational situation is much more important than determining his or her score on a standardized test. Although performing real-world observations is more difficult than administering standardized measures, such observations are imperative when assessing and developing rehabilitation and reintegration programs for people with cognitive–communication impairments.

Recognize the Importance of Personal History and Life Scripts. As noted in Chapter 2, the TBI population does not represent a random sampling of the general population. As a group, survivors of TBI are more likely to have histories of speech and language challenges, learning disabilities, risk-taking behaviors, and underachievement than people who do not sustain TBIs. This does not imply that individuals are in some way responsible or to blame for their injuries; a substantial proportion of people who sustain TBIs are simply in the wrong place at the wrong time. However, the behaviors and cognitive characteristics that initially increase the likelihood of TBI are certainly not improved by brain damage. Hence, knowing the preinjury academic, social, and behavioral history of an individual is crucial and provides important information and clues about how that person is likely to perform following injury. Practitioners must avoid the temptation of trying to fix problems that were not amenable to change prior to injury.

Examine Family Dynamics and Social Stressors. TBI does not happen to individuals; it happens to families (see Chapter 13). How various family members cope with the ongoing trauma and recovery process will have a direct impact on a survivor's emotional status and recovery. If the family as a whole is in crisis, the survivor will be in crisis as well and will not perform at his or her optimum level.

Expect Variability. One of the hallmarks of TBI is variability. Expect day-to-day and even hour-to-hour fluctuations in performance due to attention problems and internal and external distractibility. Decreases in communication performance are particularly common when cognitive demands increase. Speech–language pathologists and other rehabilitation practitioners need to recognize that an individual with a cognitive–communication impairment may be a functional communicator in some situations but not in others.

Reject a "Standard Battery." Do not expect one assessment tool to work for all survivors of TBI with cognitive–communication impairments. Using subtests from multiple sources is appropriate, as are using informal measures and developing individualized assessment tools. Administration of the same test battery to all survivors of TBI signals a lack of understanding about the nature and variability of cognitive–communication impairments.

Functional Assessments

Several subtests from formal communication and cognitive evaluation batteries may be beneficial in helping professionals understand the nature and extent of cognitive–communication impairments and their impact on various aspects of everyday functioning. Table 6.4 lists several areas of assessment and formal measures or subtests that may assist in the evaluation process.

In conjunction with formal tests, clinicians should observe individuals with TBI in functional situations that are a part of daily routines. An assessment report documenting cognitive–communication status may include subtest scores from one or more standardized batteries, but it also must contain observational reports of a person in a variety of simulated or actual real-world situations and reports of interviews with the survivor and his or her family or caregivers. Combining formal and informal assessment strategies provides a comprehensive and accurate picture of an individual's communicative functioning.

Informal assessment does not require the use of any particular test protocol or standardized tool—that is what makes it informal. Some procedures result in numerical scores, while others provide strictly descriptive information. Interviews and discourse sample analyses are among the most common and useful ways to learn about a survivor's previous lifestyle and current communication abilities. Although some therapists are uncomfortable assessing communication informally, a variety of scales and guidelines exist to help them make accurate judgments about a survivor's cognitive–communication status. The following sections describe the Functional Living Scale (Hagen, 1999), the American Speech-Language-Hearing Association *Functional Assessment of Communication Skills for Adults* (ASHA-FACS) (Frattali, Thompson, Holland, Wohl, & Ferketic, 1995), and outline procedures for performing discourse analyses of TBI survivors.

Functional Living Scale. The Functional Living Scale is an informal assessment tool developed by Hagen (1999). Because entire rehabilitation teams use the Functional Living Scale, it targets physical and general cognitive abilities as well as those skills particular to cognitive–communication status. The first section of this scale—Individual Daily Living Skills—addresses a

(*text continues on page 117*)

Table 6.4

Formal Measures and Subtests for Assessing Various Aspects
of Cognitive–Communication Impairments

Assessment area	Formal measure	Subtests
Abstract language	*Mini Inventory of Right Brain Injury* (Pimental & Kingsbury 1989)	Higher Level Receptive and Expressive Language Skills
	Rehabilitation Institute of Chicago Evaluation of Communication Problems in Right Hemisphere Dysfunction (Burns, Halper, & Mogil, 1985)	Metaphorical Language Test
Auditory comprehension	*Brief Test of Head Injury* (Helm-Estabrooks & Hotz, 1991)	Items 8–13, 37–40
	Boston Diagnostic Aphasia Examination (Goodglass & Kaplan, 1983)	Complex Ideational Material
	Discourse Comprehension Test (Brookshire & Nicholas, 1993)	Listening Comprehension Version
	Scales of Cognitive Ability for Traumatic Brain Injury (Adamovich & Henderson, 1992)	Recall (Items 8 and 9)
	Woodcock-Johnson Psycho-Educational Battery–Revised: Tests of Cognitive Ability (Woodcock & Johnson, 1989)	Listening Comprehension
Integration and synthesis	*Woodcock–Johnson Psycho-Educational Battery–Revised: Tests of Cognitive Ability* (Woodcock & Johnson, 1989)	Analysis–Synthesis
Orientation, memory, and attention	*Brief Test of Head Injury* (Helm-Estabrooks & Hotz, 1991)	Items 1–7, 34–36, 48–49
	Rey Auditory Verbal Learning Test (Schmidt, 1996)	

(*continues*)

Table 6.4 *Continued.*

Assessment area	Formal measure	Subtests
	Ross Information Processing Assessment–Second Edition (Ross-Swain, 1996)	Immediate Memory
		Recent Memory
		Temporal Orientation (Recent Memory)
		Temporal Orientation (Remote Memory)
		Orientation to Environment
	Scales of Cognitive Ability for Traumatic Brain Injury (Adamovich & Henderson, 1992)	Perception and Discrimination
		Orientation
		Recall
	Selective Reminding Test (Buschke, 1973; Buschke & Fuld, 1974)	
	Wechsler Memory Scale–III (Russell, 1975; Stone, Girdner, & Albrecht, 1946; Wechsler, 1945, 1997b)	Associate Learning
		Digit Span
		Logical Memory
		Visual Reproduction
	Woodcock-Johnson Psycho-Educational Battery–Revised: Tests of Cognitive Ability (Woodcock & Johnson, 1989)	Memory for Names (Immediate and Delayed)
		Visual–Auditory Learning (Immediate and Delayed)
		Memory for Sentences
		Memory for Words
		Numbers Reversed
Reasoning	*Brief Test of Head Injury* (Helm-Estabrooks & Hotz, 1991)	Items 19–23
	Ross Information Processing Assessment–Second Edition (Ross-Swain, 1996)	Problem Solving/Reasoning
	Ross Test of Higher Cognitive Processes (Ross & Ross, 1976)	Deductive Reasoning
		Missing Premises
		Questioning Strategies
		Analysis of Relevant and Irrelevant Information

(*continues*)

Table 6.4 *Continued.*

Assessment area	Formal measure	Subtests
	Scales of Cognitive Ability for Traumatic Brain Injury (Adamovich & Henderson, 1992)	Organization Reasoning
	Stanford-Binet Intelligence Scale–Fourth Edition (Thorndike, Hagen, & Sattler, 1986)	Verbal Absurdities Pictured Absurdities
	Wechsler Adult Intelligence Scale–III (Wechsler, 1997a)	Similarities Comprehension Arithmetic Picture Arrangement
	Wisconsin Card Sorting Test (Heaton, 1981)	
	Woodcock-Johnson Psycho-Educational Battery–Revised: Tests of Cognitive Ability (Woodcock & Johnson, 1989)	Verbal Analogies Spatial Relations Concept Formation
Speed of processing	*Wechsler Adult Intelligence Scale–III* (Wechsler, 1997a)	Digit Symbol
	Woodcock-Johnson Psycho-Educational Battery–Revised: Tests of Cognitive Ability (Woodcock & Johnson, 1989)	Visual Matching Cross Out
Word finding	*Brief Test of Head Injury* (Helm-Estabrooks & Hotz, 1991)	Items 30–33, 41–42
	Boston Diagnostic Aphasia Examination (Goodglass & Kaplan, 1983)	Word Fluency
	Boston Naming Test (Kaplan, Goodglass, & Weintraub, 1983)	
	Neurosensory Center Comprehensive Examination for Aphasia (Spreen & Benton, 1977)	Word Fluency
	Scales of Cognitive Ability for Traumatic Brain Injury (Adamovich & Henderson, 1992)	Recall (Items 2 and 7)

person's ability to perform usual and customary activities in the areas of safety, health maintenance, personal care, household management, community access, productive activity, and leisure. Having team members rate the severity of impairment on multiple activities in each designated area provides a means of assessing the impact of cognitive–communication impairments on daily skills.

A speech–language pathologist administering the Individual Daily Living Skills portion of the Functional Living Scale performs role plays or interviews with a survivor or family member to determine the extent to which a cognitive–communication impairment affects various situations. For example, in the section concerning safety, the clinician must make a judgment about and assign a severity rating to a survivor's ability to dial a telephone to obtain emergency assistance if another person unexpectedly passed out. The clinician's belief about how successfully and independently a survivor could execute the task determines the severity rating assigned for the skills of "seeking help" and "handling emergencies." Ratings for each skill contribute to determination of the survivor's overall functional living level.

ASHA-FACS. Speech–language pathologists or family members perform direct observations to assess the four communication domains included in the ASHA-FACS: (a) social communication; (b) communication of basic needs; (c) reading, writing, and number concepts; and (d) daily planning. Within each domain, a scale of Qualitative Dimensions (i.e., adequacy, appropriateness, promptness, and communication sharing) is rated on a 5-point scale. ASHA-FACS yields mean scores, overall scores, and profiles of both Communication Independence and Qualitative Dimensions.

Discourse Analyses. The analysis of discourse is one of the most important diagnostic tools available for evaluating cognitive–communication impairments. Whenever possible, clinicians should obtain and analyze samples from multiple settings and with multiple communication partners. Discourse samples need to include opportunities for survivors to engage in informal conversation, language-based problem-solving activities, verbal sequencing, narrative tasks, divergent thinking, and abstract language usage. Cherney (1998) suggests including several varieties of discourse in a comprehensive sample. Table 6.5 provides definitions of various discourse genres and examples of elicitation tasks for each.

Videotaping discourse samples is essential to assess verbal and nonverbal behaviors. Conversely, transcription of discourse samples and performance of extensive syntactic or morphologic analyses are usually unnecessary because people with cognitive–communication impairments do not typically have

Table 6.5
Definitions and Elicitation Activities for Various Discourse Genres

Discourse genre	Definition	Elicitation activities
Descriptive	Relaying static concepts, attributes, and relations	Describe what is happening in this Norman Rockwell picture. Describe what your living room looks like.
Narrative	Relaying actions or events revealed over time	Listen to this story, and then tell it back to me. Look at these sequence cards, and tell me a story about them.
Procedural	Relaying a sequence of instructions or steps	How do you change a flat tire? How do you bake a cake?
Persuasive	Relaying facts or a rationale to support an opinion	Explain why you believe states should or should not adopt and enforce seat belt laws.
Expository	Relaying factual and interpretive information about a particular topic	Explain the advantages and disadvantages of home schooling versus public schooling for young children.
Conversational	Relaying information in a cooperative interaction with others	What would you like to talk about?

challenges with the structural aspects of language. Instead, a checklist of be-haviors such as the one presented in Figure 6.6 can help identify various communication behaviors affected by cognitive impairments. After identi-fying a behavior as being potentially problematic, the speech–language pathologist should use future interactions or formal measures to investigate it further. Figure 6.6 includes markings to indicate the appropriate and inap-propriate areas of performance for the discourse sample provided earlier in this chapter.

Behavior	Appropriate	Inappropriate
Nonverbal Pragmatics		
Physical contact with others	✓	
Proxemics—distance between conversation partners	✓	
Use of gestures and facial expressions		✓
Interpretation of nonverbal cues from others		✓
Establishment and maintenance of eye contact	✓	
Emotional lability		✓
Verbal Pragmatics		
Selection of appropriate speech registers	✓	
Prosody—use of vocal inflection	✓	
Appropriate topic selection		✓
Disinhibition	✓	
Initiation of communication	✓	
Semantics		
Use of nonspecific vocabulary/word retrieval deficits		✓
Provision of clear pronoun referents		✓
Word choice errors or delays		✓
Flexibility in word use	✓	
Verbal fluency (minimal use of mazes and revisions)		✓
Discourse Organization		
Topic maintenance		✓
Need for redirection to the task		✓
Use of cohesive ties		✓
Maintenance of spatial or temporal sequences	✓	
Discrimination of salient and irrelevant information		✓
Integration and synthesis of information	✓	
Flexibility of thought	✓	
Processing delays	✓	
Truthful and plausible content/lack of confabulation	✓	

Figure 6.6. Discourse Analysis Checklist.

Treatment

A two-stage pattern of cognitive and communication recovery typically occurs following TBI. First, as the brain heals itself, a certain amount of improved functioning occurs spontaneously. Several months after the resolution of post-traumatic amnesia, a second stage of recovery begins. At this time, persistent areas of impairment and their functional impact on an individual's participation in daily activities become evident.

Because of this pattern of recovery, rehabilitation professionals must provide two types of intervention: one that facilitates restoration of basic cognitive and communication processes and another that facilitates mastery, implementation, and generalization of compensatory strategies. During early stages of recovery, determining what changes are due to treatment effects and what changes are due to spontaneous recovery can be difficult. Researchers have performed several studies documenting improvements in basic cognitive processes such as attention and memory through the implementation of specific treatment programs (e.g., Ben-Yishay, Piasetsky, & Rattok, 1987; Malec & Questad, 1983; Ruff et al., 1994; Sohlberg & Mateer, 1987). A major concern with much of this work, however, is the questionable generalization of targeted skills to real-world situations (Glisky, Schacter, & Tulving, 1986; Lawson & Rice, 1989; Nieman, Ruff, & Baser, 1990; O'Connor & Cermak, 1987; Parente & Anderson-Parente, 1989). When recovery of basic processes appears to be maximized, intervention efforts should shift to teaching survivors compensatory and accommodation strategies. The remainder of this chapter provides (a) general guidelines for cognitive and cognitive–communication treatment and (b) treatment approaches for facilitating learning and mastery of compensatory and accommodation strategies in specific areas of impairment.

General Guidelines

Several considerations guide the development of appropriate cognitive–communication treatment plans for survivors. First and foremost, program plans must be individualized. Multiple survivors may have apparently similar deficits in a particular area of functioning; however, because each survivor differed prior to injury, the effect on each person's life will be unique. As a result, a clinician must consider the individual effect of an impairment when developing a treatment plan. That is, the clinician must determine how underlying impairments in cognition and communication (e.g., deficits in memory, problem solving, attention, reasoning) contribute to current disabilities (e.g., the inability to work, attend school, participate in community and leisure activities). When targeting these impairments and disabilities, clinicians should use personally relevant materials and should implement activities in settings consistent with preinjury lifestyles. Such materials provide a means of increasing the functionality of treatment and facilitate awareness of how deficits negatively affect daily life.

A second consideration is the need for multidisciplinary input when developing a treatment plan. Because cognitive and communication impairments may prohibit survivors from accurately conveying information, professionals need to consult with family members and survivors to determine current disabilities. As a team, professionals, family members, and survivors identify activities that were important prior to injury and activities that continue to be important postinjury. Communication with other rehabilitation professionals (e.g., physical therapist, occupational therapist, recreational therapist) prevents duplication of effort and services. This comprehensive communication allows for the formation of a treatment plan aimed at increasing independence in specified areas.

Additional guiding principles of cognitive–communication rehabilitation concern the implementation of treatment programs. First, task analysis is an important factor in identifying component parts of activities. Initially, worksheets may be helpful in providing a survivor with cues to identify and locate materials, sequence the steps involved, estimate the time needed, and document the execution and success of each step involved in an activity. Once such steps are mastered by survivors, clinicians should help survivors transition from reliance on external supports to use of self-monitoring or self-quizzing (Yorkston & Kennedy, 1999). Second, structured repetition across multiple trials, settings, and people is essential for successful generalization. Additionally, researchers have recently promoted the use of "errorless learning"—a technique in which the production of incorrect responses is minimized during the early stages of learning (Baddeley & Wilson, 1994; Glisky & Delaney, 1996; Hunkin, Squires, Aldrich, & Parkin, 1998; Hunkin, Squires, Parkin, & Tidy, 1998).

Treatment plans include both long-term and short-term goals. Long-term goals directly and functionally address a survivor's usual and customary day-to-day living skills. For example, a long-term goal might be for a person to seek and obtain routine health care services with minimal assistance from others. Short-term goals address underlying impairments that negatively affect a survivor's independent performance of activities identified in long-term goals. For the above goal of seeking health care, underlying impairments might include decreased memory, poor problem solving, limited executive functioning, word retrieval deficits, decreased synthesis and integration of information, and inappropriate verbal or nonverbal pragmatic behaviors. Short-term goals might include locating a phone number from a directory to develop problem-solving skills; calling and scheduling a doctor's appointment to develop executive functioning; and independently writing down the appointment time, doctor's name, and office location to compensate for memory problems.

Initial treatment for underlying impairments or cognitive subskills is usually provided in individual or small group settings; as a survivor masters compensatory techniques, treatment should more closely simulate realistic and natural settings. The following sections provide suggestions for treating various subskill areas that typically affect survivors' activity level and participation in daily living.

Treatment of Cognitive Subskills

Orientation

Orientation refers to a person's conscious awareness of self, time, place, and situation. As described in Chapter 5, the restoration of orientation skills often coincides with the end of posttraumatic amnesia. Rehabilitation staff and family members can assist in the restoration of orientation by providing verbal cues and access to external aids such as calendars and schedule cards. Depending on the severity of orientation impairment, survivors may use external aids for a short period of time or depend on them indefinitely. Controversy exists about the value of external aids because of concerns about whether survivors use them independently once discharged from therapy (Sohlberg & Mateer, 1989b).

Memory

In addition to memory logs (see Chapters 5 and 8), many other external aids can assist people with memory impairments. Watches with alarms, alarm clocks, or timers can help survivors recall tasks needing attention at a later time. For example, a survivor can set a watch alarm to ring when it is time to take medicine or make a phone call. Another alternative is posting sticky notes with written reminders in highly visible places. Posting a note on the front door or by the car keys can serve as a reminder to take something to work in the morning.

Learning and implementing *mnemonic strategies* (i.e., memory strategies) is an alternative to using written or external aids. A popular method for recalling telephone numbers, license plates, or word lists involves *chunking* (or *clustering*) information (Wilson, 1982). The goal of this technique is to decrease the number of pieces of information to be remembered by grouping items together. For example, the seven separate digits of a phone number can be reduced to three chunks: 734-9561 becomes 734, 95, and 61.

Chunking can also help when a survivor needs to remember a list of words, such as items to purchase at the store. In this situation, a written list is probably the most appropriate strategy, but situations arise that require an alternative strategy. The key to chunking items on a word list is to identify groups or categories. For example, apples, milk, aluminum foil, cheese, broccoli, eggs, and paper towels can be chunked into three categories: produce (apples and broccoli), dairy products (milk, cheese, and eggs), and paper goods (aluminum foil and paper towels).

Quantifying can be used in conjunction with chunking. In quantifying, items to be recalled are visualized or counted. Using the preceding example, the total of seven items formed three groups, two of which included two items and one of which included three items.

Visual imagery is another method to help with recalling specific information. One form of visual imagery is to imagine a familiar building or location and "place" items in various positions within that setting. Using the grocery list example, the person could visualize walking through the store and removing desired items from shelves. Visual imagery is also useful as an organizational strategy. For example, by "placing" the main ideas of a verbal presentation in different rooms of a house, a person can imagine walking from room to room to retrieve the ideas in the correct sequential order. Yet another use for visual imagery involves the learning of names. For example, to assist an individual in learning the name of a coworker, Stephanie, the clinician might draw a picture of steps and a person's knee with the words "step" and "knee" below and the name "Stephanie" across the top (Wilson, 1982).

Storytelling is another useful memory technique for list recall. A person needing to recall several unrelated items can make up a sentence or short story that incorporates all of the words. For example, the vocabulary words *attitude, determination, sarong, unique,* and *cartridge* can form the following story:

> Because of my positive attitude and determination, my mother rewarded me with a new, unique sarong. It had pictures of pen cartridges all over it.

Verbal rehearsal entails repeating aloud the information to be remembered until it is either used or written down. For example, once a person locates a desired phone number in a directory, he or she can repeat it out loud until it is correctly dialed. This technique is even more effective when used in combination with chunking. Rather than verbally rehearsing the seven individual digits in a phone number, the person can chunk the digits into groups, as described previously, and verbally rehearse the three groups.

In *first letter mnemonics*, the first letter of each word is used to form an acronym. Common examples of this include using the word SCUBA to remember "self contained underwater breathing apparatus" and HOMES to remember the names of the Great Lakes (Huron, Ontario, Michigan, Erie, and Superior). However, the acronym does not have to form a real word. For example, first letter mnemonics forming the nonword SCOTE can help a student remember to bring a straw, a compass, an orange, toothpicks, and an eraser to class for a science project.

Finally, the *PQRST* technique (Robinson, 1970) facilitates memory of various types of written information. It uses organized rehearsal to facilitate the comprehension and retention of narratives by outlining an overview process involving the following: **P**review of the passage, formulation of **Q**uestions, **R**eading of the passage, **S**tating answers to wh-questions, and **T**esting oneself on the answers to those questions. The PQRST technique is particularly beneficial to survivors of TBI who return to school following injury.

Executive Functioning

The term *executive functioning* encompasses a number of higher-order cognitive skills: planning, sequencing, coordinating, and initiating and finishing a task or goal. A major precursor to successful treatment of executive functioning relates to insight. When a person lacks insight into his or her own deficits because of restricted reasoning or awareness, verbal explanations are usually fruitless. Sometimes the only way to demonstrate to survivors their current level of functioning is to involve them in controlled situations in which they will fail to some extent. Then the demonstration of alternative strategies to manage the situation appropriately and efficiently may be effective.

Once a survivor reaches Rancho Level VIII (see Appendix 5.B), he or she is likely to acknowledge impairments and their impact on participation in daily activities. At this point, intervention for executive functioning becomes a prominent goal, because survivors typically display increased motivation and desire for reintegration into their former lifestyle. This desire is an outward sign of improved initiation and cognitive recovery. Once an individual has expressed this desire, realistic goal setting—both short term and long term—can begin.

Goal Setting. Goal setting requires a team effort. Although a survivor may generate goals, they may not be realistic ones. Rehabilitation professionals and family members—need to help in the selection of appropriate and achievable goals. Input from family members is particularly helpful because they can provide information about the person's previous lifestyle and recovery process.

Problem Solving. Treatment for problem solving requires two types of intervention. First, survivors of TBI need practice (a) identifying problems and their salient features, (b) generating possible solutions, (c) determining the best solution, (d) organizing the steps to implement the solution, (e) implementing the solution, and (f) evaluating the effectiveness of the solution. These steps are outlined in Figure 6.7 using a hypothetical problem. Second, because TBI survivors often have difficulty transferring practice into real-world situations, they need to participate in simulations of actual problems encountered in day-to-day living. Both with hypothetical situations and real-world simulations, aspects of the problem-solving process can be targeted singly or in combination.

The first step in problem solving is *problem identification*. To address this during individual or group therapy sessions, clinicians often read prefabricated scenarios or generate hypothetical problem situations such as that presented in Figure 6.7. The survivor's task is to identify the problem and salient features of the situation.

Generating solutions is a natural successor to identifying problems. Here, the survivor generates as many solutions as possible regarding a stated problem. The crucial feature of generating solutions is that multiple possibilities exist. Although some solutions may be more appropriate or feasible than others, the exercise of generating solutions should be open-ended, and evaluation of the merit of various solutions comes at a later stage in the problem-solving process (see Figure 6.7).

After the survivor generates multiple potential solutions, the evaluation process begins. The purpose is to *determine the best solution*. At this point, the survivor identifies positive and negative aspects associated with each possible solution. Writing pros and cons on a piece of paper is helpful and provides the individual with a visual reference when determining the best solution. The clinician's job is to provide assistance as needed to ensure that evaluations are thorough and accurate.

Having determined the best solution, the survivor must then *organize the steps* involved in its implementation. Depending on the problem and proposed solution, this step may involve gathering specific items and/or sequencing tasks. For example, if a person owes money and decides that writing a check is the best solution, he or she would need to gather a checkbook, a pen, and proper identification; if a person shatters a jar of jelly on the kitchen floor, materials needed to implement a solution might include shoes (to protect bare feet from broken glass), a dustpan and broom, a trash can, a mop, soap and water, and a bucket. The importance of sequencing the steps is evident for the last scenario; it would not be safe to begin to clean the mess by mopping, followed by using the dustpan and broom, and then putting on shoes. To assist with organization, lists of needed materials and the order for performing activities can be generated.

So the survivor can practice *implementing solutions*, many rehabilitation facilities have kitchens, laundry machines, and rooms set up like apartments. These areas provide opportunities for individuals to engage in problem-solving activities in realistic environments. Hospital gift shops and cafeterias are also potential settings for developing problem-solving skills in real-world situations.

Scenario: You are at a movie with some friends. When you reach into your wallet, you realize you only have a $5.00 bill. The movie costs $7.50 and starts in 10 minutes.

Identify the problem	Generate solutions	Determine best solution	Organize steps	Evaluate solution
You do not have enough money to pay for the movie	Borrow money from a friend	A possible solution, but you feel uncomfortable and embarrassed about borrowing money	You have decided to go to a nearby cash machine Steps:	You spent 5 minutes walking to the cash machine. When you arrived, no one was using the machine so you withdrew $10.00 and walked back to the theater. You purchased a ticket and bought something to drink during the movie. When you walked into the theater, the previews for new movies were showing. Because the theater was dark, you had trouble finding your friends, but by walking up and down the center aisle you found them. You took your seat just as the featured film started.
	Write a check	Not a good solution because the theater does not accept checks	• Check to make sure you have your cash card with you and remember your PIN	
	Use a credit card	Not a good solution because the theater does not accept credit cards	• Ask the cashier at the ticket window where the closest cash machine is	
	Go to a nearby cash machine	A possible solution but, depending on where the cash machine is, you might not make it back in time for the start of the movie	• Tell your friends you need to do something and will be right back	

(continues)

Figure 6.7. Sample problem-solving exercise.

Identify the problem	Generate solutions	Determine best solution	Organize steps	Evaluate solution
	Steal money from someone else waiting in line	Not a good solution because it is not socially acceptable, and you would get into trouble if you got caught	• Ask your friends to go ahead without you but to save you a seat • Walk to the cash machine	
	Ask a stranger to give you money	Not a good solution because it is not socially acceptable	• Wait your turn	
	Sneak into the movie without paying	Not a good solution becaue it is not socially acceptable, and you would get in trouble if you got caught	• Withdraw enough money to pay for the movie and for snacks during or afterward • Walk back to the theater	
	Tell your friends you do not want to go to the movie	Not a good solution becaue it is dishonest, and you really do want to see the movie	• Purchase a ticket • Join your friends in the theater	

Figure 6.7. *Continued.*

If returning to work or school is a therapy goal, simulations of problems that may arise in these settings can usually be enacted as well. Simulations provide the survivor with the opportunity for actual—rather than solely verbal—follow-through and execution of the solution.

After implementing the solution, the survivor needs to *evaluate* how well it worked. Hopefully, the problem is now resolved. If it is not, the reasons need to be determined. Were all of the necessary steps included in the original solution? Were the steps implemented in the appropriate sequence? Did a better solution exist?

Carryover. Ideally, the goal is for a survivor of TBI to generalize rehabilitation strategies to a variety of contexts. Clinicians frequently express concern that generalization of newly learned behaviors across time, settings, and people is difficult; for example, many survivors require assistance with executive functioning on a long-term basis. As a result, ongoing family and caregiver education and training about intervention techniques is an important part of successful carryover. In particular, teaching family members appropriate ways to cue a survivor, instead of doing the task or solving the problem for him or her, is a must.

Moving treatment sessions to functional environments, such as a survivor's home, workplace, or a place of leisure, is another way to promote carryover of learned executive strategies. For example, imagine a survivor who is cognitively and physically ready to return to work but must rely on public transportation because of driving restrictions. Sessions conducted in the therapy room might involve identifying alternate modes of transportation and determining the positive and negative aspects associated with each option. If the clinician and client decide that taking the bus is the best solution, additional sessions might involve learning bus routes, stops, and schedules. An appropriate next step for promoting carryover is providing opportunities for the individual to practice using the designated bus route and stops while accompanied by the clinician or a caregiver. This minimizes anxiety and promotes procedural learning of the task. Gradually, assistance can be faded until the survivor is successfully and independently taking the bus to work. Depending on the person's success, additional routes (e.g., to the supermarket and back) can be added over time.

High-Level Cognitive Processes

Many of the intervention strategies discussed thus far have utilized a functional approach: The treatment occurs within the context of functional and realistic activities. An alternative approach to remediation is a process-specific one in which intervention directly targets cognitive processes that interfere with successful communication (Yorkston & Kennedy, 1999). A process-specific approach lends itself well to intervention targeting high-level impairments affecting critical thinking, drawing inferences, abstract reasoning, and flexibility of thought.

Several published workbooks contain activities to target high-level cognitive skills using a process-specific approach. (Examples of such texts include *Workbook for Reasoning Skills* [Brubaker, 1983], *Workbook for Cognitive Skills* [Brubaker, 1988], *Just for Adults: An Adult Handbook for Language Rehabilitation* [Lazzari, 1990], and *Cognitive-Linguistic Improvement Program* [Ross-Swain, 1992].) *Critical thinking* tasks often involve the identification of relations and associations between two objects or ideas; analyzing analogies such as, "Cramp is to muscle as fracture is to _____," can help to sharpen critical thinking skills. For *drawing inferences,* the clinician might present a short written or verbal scenario (e.g., "John landed hard. The ice felt cold and wet. It looked so easy when other people did it. John hadn't realized that just standing up would be so difficult.") followed by a question requiring inferential thinking in the form of deductive or inductive reasoning (e.g., "What was John doing?"). *Abstract reasoning* exercises can take many forms—some require language skills and some require nonverbal processing. A common type of abstract reasoning using language involves the interpretation of proverbs or idioms (e.g., "Look before you leap" or "Don't cry over spilled milk"). Abstract reasoning using visual perceptual skills might require examination of a sequence of boxes with designs in them and determination of which of four choices comes next in the series. *Flexibility of thought* can be addressed through problems or puzzles that require multiple solutions, such as providing two definitions of "judge" or thinking of multiple uses for a flowerpot.

Pragmatic Behaviors

One way to target deficits associated with verbal and nonverbal pragmatics is by videotaping survivors engaged in conversations. Prior to videotaping, discussion of specific areas in which a survivor has difficulty is helpful. This discussion can include suggestions on how to handle a variety of pragmatic skills: discourse organization, tangential speech, topic shading, selection of appropriate topics, dysprosody, expression of affect, eye contact, proxemics, and interpreting communication partners' behaviors.

Initially, taped conversations should be between a survivor and clinician. When they review the tape, the clinician helps the survivor identify each time an inappropriate behavior occurs. Gradually, the provision of cues can be minimized as the survivor gains skill at recognizing problematic behaviors. With additional practice and progress, clinicians can modify several aspects of the video-feedback technique to increase the degree of difficulty. For example, conversational partners can be varied by involving spouses, friends, or coworkers, and a variety of topics and activities can be introduced as a means of eliciting different types of discourse genres.

Another effective approach for targeting verbal and nonverbal pragmatic behaviors involves participation in group treatment sessions. Group members need not be restricted only to survivors of TBI; survivors of stroke and other acquired neurological disorders may present with similar difficulties and benefit from group treatment.

One approach to structuring group treatment sessions is to assign individuals to watch for other participants' specific communication problems—such as inappropriate topic changes and selections, excessive talking, and interrupting. Another alternative is to have an individual self-monitor for these same types of behaviors. Instances of problematic behaviors can be noted for discussion at a later time or identified and discussed as they occur. As a group, participants then brainstorm appropriate ways to handle various situations.

Summary

Survivors of TBI can display a variety of communication challenges. Although some survivors exhibit behaviors characteristic of traditional aphasia syndromes, the majority have impairments that relate to deficits in the cognitive processes that underlie communication. After several years of searching for an appropriate label, professionals have agreed on the term *cognitive–communication impairment* to identify these challenges.

Effective assessment and treatment of cognitive–communication impairments require clinicians to adopt individualized approaches that incorporate information about a person's preinjury lifestyle and postinjury abilities and goals. Once impairments are identified, the clinician, survivor, and family members work as a team to develop meaningful long-term and short-term goals. Some aspects of cognition and communication may improve rapidly with little intervention; other areas may progress more slowly, with gradual improvements over many years. As a result, ongoing assessment is necessary. This ensures that treatment will target appropriate skills and compensatory strategies to provide survivors with a means of participating in all aspects of life—personal, social, academic, and vocational—throughout the recovery process.

References

Adamovich, B., & Henderson, J. (1992). *Scales of Cognitive Ability for Traumatic Brain Injury*. Itasca, IL: Riverside.

American Speech-Language-Hearing Association. (1991). Guidelines for speech–language pathologists serving persons with language, socio–communicative, and/or cognitive–communicative impairments. *Asha, 33*(Suppl. 5), 21–28.

Baddeley, A., & Wilson, B. A. (1994). When implicit learning fails: Amnesia and the problem of error elimination. *Neuropsychologia, 32*, 53–68.

Ben-Yishay, Y., Piasetsky, E. B., & Rattok, J. (1987). A systematic method for ameliorating disorders in basic attention. In M. J. Meier, A. L. Benton, & L. Diller (Eds.), *Neuropsychological rehabilitation* (pp. 165–181). New York: Churchill Livingstone.

Boller, F., & Vignolo, L. A. (1966). Latent sensory aphasia in hemisphere-damaged patients: An experimental study with the Token Test. *Brain, 89*, 815–830.

Bricolo, A., Turazzi, S., & Feriotti, G. (1980). Prolonged posttraumatic unconsciousness: Therapeutic assets and liabilities. *Journal of Neurosurgery, 52*, 625–634.

Brookshire, R. H., & Nicholas, L. E. (1993). *Discourse Comprehension Test*. San Antonio: Communication Skill Builders.

Brubaker, S. H. (1983). *Workbook for reasoning skills*. Detroit: Wayne State University Press.

Brubaker, S. H. (1988). *Workbook for cognitive skills*. Detroit: Wayne State University Press.

Burns, M. S., Halper, A. S., & Mogil, S. I. (1985). *Rehabilitation Institute of Chicago Evaluation of Communication Problems in Right Hemisphere Dysfunction* (RICE). Rockville, MD: Aspen.

Buschke, H. (1973). Selective reminding for analysis of memory and learning. *Journal of Verbal Learning and Verbal Behavior, 12*, 543–550.

Buschke, H., & Fuld, P. A. (1974). Evaluating storage, retention, and retrieval in disordered memory and learning. *Neurology, 24*, 1019–1025.

Cherney, L. R. (1998). Pragmatics and discourse: An introduction. In L. R. Cherney, B. B. Shadden, & C. A. Coelho (Eds.), *Analyzing discourse in communicatively impaired adults* (pp. 1–7). Gaithersburg, MD: Aspen.

Darley, F. L. (1982). *Aphasia*. Philadelphia: Saunders.

Dirckx, J. H. (Ed.). (1997). *Stedman's concise medical dictionary for the health professions* (3rd ed.). Baltimore: Williams & Wilkins.

Frattali, C. M., Thompson, C. K., Holland, A. L., Wohl, C. B., & Ferketic, M. M. (1995). *Functional assessment of communication skills for adults*. Rockville, MD: American Speech-Language-Hearing Association.

Geschwind, N. (1964). Non-aphasic disorders of speech. *International Journal of Neurology, 4*, 207–214.

Geschwind, N. (1967). The varieties of naming errors. *Cortex, 3*, 97–112.

Glisky, E. L., & Delaney, S. M. (1996). Implicit memory and new semantic learning in posttraumatic amnesia. *Journal of Head Trauma Rehabilitation, 11*(2), 31–42.

Glisky, E. L., Schacter, D. L., & Tulving, E. (1986). Learning and retention of computer-related vocabulary in memory-impaired patients: Method of vanishing cues. *Journal of Clinical and Experimental Neuropsychology, 8*, 292–312.

Goodglass, H., & Kaplan, E. (1983). *Boston Diagnostic Aphasia Examination*. Philadelphia: Lea & Febiger.

Hagen, C. (1999). *Rehabilitation in managed care: Controlling cost, ensuring quality.* Gaithersburg, MD: Aspen.

Hagen, C. (2000, February). *Rancho Los Amigos Levels of Cognitive Functioning–Revised.* Presentation at TBI Rehabilitation in a Managed Care Environment: An Interdisciplinary Approach to Rehabilitation, Continuing Education Programs of America, San Antonio, TX.

Hagen, C., & Malkmus, D. (1979, November). *Intervention strategies for language disorders secondary to head trauma.* Short course presented at the annual meeting of the American Speech-Language-Hearing Association, Atlanta, GA.

Halpern, H., Darley, F. L., & Brown, J. R. (1973). Differential language and neurologic characteristics in cerebral involvement. *Journal of Speech and Hearing Disorders, 38,* 162–173.

Heaton, R. K. (1981). *Wisconsin Card Sorting Test manual.* Odessa, FL: Psychological Assessment Resources.

Helm-Estabrooks, N., & Hotz, G. (1991). *Brief Test of Head Injury.* Itasca, IL: Riverside.

Holloran, S. M., & Bressler, E. J. (1983). *Cognitive reorganization: A stimulus handbook.* Austin, TX: PRO-ED.

Hoogeveen, K. (1993, April). *An educational perspective on TBI.* Presentation at Demystification of TBI: An Educational Perspective of Traumatic Brain Injury, Quality Training Institute, Atlanta, GA.

Hunkin, N. M., Squires, E. J., Aldrich, F. K., & Parkin, A. J. (1998). Errorless learning and the acquisition of word processing skills. *Neuropsychological Rehabilitation, 8,* 433–449.

Hunkin, N. M., Squires, E. J., Parkin, A. J., & Tidy, J. A. (1998). Are the benefits of errorless learning dependent on implicit memory? *Neuropsychologia, 36,* 25–36.

Kaplan, E., Goodglass, H., & Weintraub, S. (1983). *Boston Naming Test.* Philadelphia: Lea & Febiger.

Lawson, M. J., & Rice, D. N. (1989). Effects of training in use of executive strategies and verbal memory problems resulting from closed head injury. *Journal of Clinical and Experimental Neuropsychology, 11,* 842–854.

Lazzari, A. M. (1990). *Just for adults: An adult handbook for language rehabilitation.* East Moline, IL: LinguiSystems.

Malec, J., & Questad, K. (1983). Rehabilitation of memory after craniocerebral trauma: Case report. *Archives of Physical Medicine and Rehabilitation, 64,* 436–438.

Milton, S. B., Prutting, C. A., & Binder, G. M. (1984). Appraisal of communicative competence in head injured adults. *Clinical Aphasiology Conference Proceedings, 14,* 114–123.

Nieman, H., Ruff, R. M., & Baser, C. A. (1990). Computer-assisted retraining in a head-injured individual: A controlled efficacy study of an outpatient program. *Journal of Consulting and Clinical Psychology, 58,* 811–817.

O'Connor, M., & Cermak, L. S. (1987). Rehabilitation of organic memory disorders. In M. J. Meier, A. L. Benton, & L. Diller (Eds.), *Neuropsychological rehabilitation* (pp. 260–279). New York: Churchill Livingstone.

Parente, R., & Anderson-Parente, J. K. (1989). Retraining memory: Theory and application. *Journal of Head Trauma Rehabilitation, 4*(3), 55–65.

Pimental, P. A., & Kingsbury, N. A. (1989). *Mini Inventory of Right Brain Injury.* Austin, TX: PRO-ED.

Robinson, F. P. (1970). *Effective study.* New York: Harper.

Rogers, M. A., Alarcon, N. B., & Olswang, L. B. (1999). Aphasia management considered in the context of the World Health Organization Model of Disablements. *Physical Medicine and Rehabilitation Clinics of North America, 10,* 907–923.

Rosenbek, J. C., LaPointe, L. L., & Wertz, R. T. (1989). *Aphasia: A clinical approach.* Austin, TX: PRO-ED.

Ross, J. D., & Ross, C. M. (1976). *Ross Test of Higher Cognitive Processes.* Novato, CA: Academic Therapy.

Ross-Swain, D. (1992). *Cognitive-linguistic improvement program.* San Diego: Singular.

Ross-Swain, D. (1996). *Ross Information Processing Assessment* (2nd ed.). Austin, TX: PRO-ED.

Ruff, R., Mahaffey, R., Engel, J., Farrow, C., Cox, D., & Karzmark, P. (1994). Efficacy study of THINKable in the attention and memory retraining of traumatically head-injured patients. *Brain Injury, 8,* 3–14.

Russell, E. W. (1975). A multiple scoring method for the assessment of complex memory functions. *Journal of Consulting and Clinical Psychology, 43,* 800–809.

Sarno, M. T. (1980). The nature of verbal impairment after closed head injury. *Journal of Nervous and Mental Disease, 168,* 685–692.

Sarno, M. T., Buonaguro, A., & Levita, E. (1986). Characteristics of verbal impairment in closed head injured patients. *Archives of Physical Medicine and Rehabilitation, 67,* 400–405.

Schmidt, M. (1996). *Rey Auditory Verbal Learning Test: A handbook.* Los Angeles: Western Psychological Services.

Sohlberg, M. M., & Mateer, C. A. (1987). Effectiveness of an attention-training program. *Journal of Clinical and Experimental Neuropsychology, 9,* 117–130.

Sohlberg, M. M., & Mateer, C. A. (1989a). *Introduction to cognitive rehabilitation: Theory and practice.* New York: Guilford Press.

Sohlberg, M., & Mateer, C. A. (1989b). Training use of compensatory memory books: A three stage behavioral approach. *Journal of Clinical and Experimental Neuropsychology, 11,* 871–891.

Spreen, O., & Benton, A. L. (1977). *Neurosensory Center Comprehensive Examination for Aphasia.* Victoria, BC: Neuropsychology Laboratory, Department of Psychology, University of Victoria.

State University of New York at Buffalo. (1997). *Guide for the uniform data set for medical rehabilitation.* Buffalo: Author.

Stone, C. P., Girdner, J., & Albrecht, R. (1946). An alternate form of the Wechsler Memory Scale. *Journal of Psychology, 22,* 199–206.

Thorndike, R. L., Hagen, E., & Sattler, J. (1986). *Stanford-Binet Intelligence Scale–Fourth Edition.* Chicago: Riverside.

Wechsler, D. (1945). A standardized memory scale for clinical use. *Journal of Psychology, 19,* 87–95.

Wechsler, D. (1997a). *Wechsler Adult Intelligence Scale–Third Edition.* San Antonio, TX: Psychological Corporation.

Wechsler, D. (1997b). *Wechsler Memory Scale–Third Edition.* San Antonio, TX: Psychological Corporation.

Wilson, B. (1982). Success and failure in memory training following a cerebral vascular accident. *Cortex, 18,* 581–594.

Woodcock, R. W., & Johnson, M. B. (1989). *Woodcock-Johnson Psycho-Educational Battery– Revised: Tests of Cognitive Ability.* Allen, TX: DLM Teaching Resources.

World Health Organization. (1999). *International classification of functioning, disability and health* (Beta-2 draft, full version). Geneva: Author.

Yorkston, K. M., & Kennedy, M. R. (1999). Treatment approaches for communication disorders. In M. Rosenthal, E. R. Griffith, J. S. Kreutzer, & B. Pentland (Eds.), *Rehabilitation of the adult and child with traumatic brain injury* (3rd ed., pp. 284–296). Philadelphia: Davis.

Dysarthria and Traumatic Brain Injury

David R. Beukelman, Rebecca Burke, and Kathryn M. Yorkston

Receiving a consultation request referring an individual with "dysarthria associated with TBI" tells even the most experienced clinician very little about what to expect when that client arrives for the first appointment. The clinician knows that the *dysarthria* label means that the client is likely to have problems executing the movements required for speech production. Beyond this basic fact, a long list of clinically important elements remains unknown. For example, is the dysarthria accompanied by other communication disorders such as apraxia or cognitive–communication impairments? What type of dysarthria does the client exhibit? Is it characterized by weakness, by incoordination, or by both? How severe is the problem? Is the client unable to produce any speech sound, or is the problem minimal—limited, perhaps, to reductions in speaking rate and naturalness? In what communication situations does the client wish to participate? Is the client's communicative participation limited to basic needs in a sheltered environment, or does participation involve a variety of roles, such as student, employee, or family member responsible for household management? The list of possible factors that need to be considered in the intervention plan is extensive.

As is apparent from the other chapters in this volume, the impact of TBI on communication is highly variable. This chapter attempts to construct a framework for clinical decisions regarding this heterogeneous population. First, because clinicians most frequently make predictions about the extent and course of recovery from dysarthria associated with TBI, the chapter reviews information about the prevalence and natural course of the condition along with common speech characteristics. Next, a framework based on the World Health Organization (WHO) model of disablement (WHO, 1999) is introduced as a means of organizing the many consequences of dysarthria including the impaired physiologic mechanism, changes in speech, and altered patterns of communicative participation. Finally, a staging system is presented that identifies the appropriate course of intervention for speakers with differing levels of dysarthria severity ranging from profound to mild.

Dysarthria Associated with TBI

Prevalence and Natural Course

The prevalence of dysarthria associated with TBI is not completely understood. However, a number of clinical researchers have contributed to our current knowledge base. Rusk, Block, and Lowmann (1969) reported that approximately one third of 96 survivors of TBI demonstrated dysarthria during the early stages of their recovery. Sarno, Buoaguro, and Levita (1986) reported that one third of their subjects with severe TBI demonstrated dysarthria. Olver, Ponsford, and Curran (1996) reported that motor speech disorders were present in 34% of their sample in a 5-year follow-up study. Yorkston, Honsinger, Mitsuda, and Hammen (1989) completed a survey of 151 persons with TBI. They found that the prevalence of dysarthria changed as a function of time postonset. Of those in acute rehabilitation, 45% reported mild to moderate dysarthria, and 20% reported severe dysarthria. Of those in outpatient settings, 12% demonstrated mild and moderate dysarthria, and 10% reported severe dysarthria. For children, Ylvisaker (1986) reported that 10% of children and 8% of adolescents continued to produce unintelligible speech during follow-up studies.

Dysarthria has often been reported as one of the long-term sequelae of severe TBI. The course of recovery for persons with severe communication disorders following TBI is, as yet, poorly understood. Dongilli, Hakel, and Beukelman (1992) studied a group of individuals who were nonspeaking when they entered acute rehabilitation. The communication disorders of over half of these individuals resolved during the middle stages of cognitive recovery—especially during Levels V and VI of the Rancho Los Amigos Levels of Cognitive Functioning (I to X) (see Appendix 5.B in Chapter 5). These authors found that individuals whose severe communication disorder persisted after Level VI demonstrated either a severe dysarthria or a severe specific language disorder.

In the case of severe dysarthria, strong evidence is emerging from the literature that important changes in speech performance can occur with ongoing speech intervention many years after the onset of TBI (Enderby & Crow, 1990; Jordon & Murdoch, 1990; Jordon, Ozanne, & Murdoch, 1988; Keatley & Wirtz, 1994; Light, Beesley, & Collier, 1988; Najensen, Sazbon, Feifelzon, Becker, & Schechter, 1978; Workinger & Netsell, 1992). For example, in a long-term study of 4 individuals with TBI and severe brain stem impairment, few spontaneous gains were made within the first 18 months, and substantial changes in function were noted as long as 48 months postinjury (Enderby & Crow, 1990). Workinger and Netsell (1992) reported the case study of an individual who gradually became a functional speaker after using an augmentative and alternative communication (ACC) system for 13 years following his TBI. Light et al. (1988) reported on the experiences of an adolescent with TBI who initially used an AAC system and became a functional speaker 3 years after her injury. Of course, other survivors recover little functional speech or manage interactions with familiar persons in familiar settings with natural speech but still require AAC with unfamiliar speakers or in difficult communicative situations.

At this point, little is known to guide clinicians in predicting the return of functional speech in persons with severe dysarthria following TBI. Therefore, individuals with TBI, their family members, and the clinicians who serve them must carefully monitor a survivor's progress to determine whether the return to use of natural speech is an option. Although examples exist of recovery of functional speech many years following TBI, only a few studies document the persistent nature of dysarthria following TBI. Thomsen (1984) reported that all of the individuals who demonstrated dysarthria 4 months after injury continued to demonstrate dysarthria 10 to 15 years later. This author did not indicate whether the severity of dysarthria had changed over that time period. Rusk et al. (1969) reported that half of the survivors with dysarthria made significant improvement in speech performance. *This te importance of treatment*

Speech Characteristics

The neurological injuries associated with TBI are diverse and depend on a variety of factors. Because injury can occur to different portions of the brain, the neuropathologies associated with dysarthria vary, and the subsequent speech characteristics vary across survivors. In their investigation of speakers with TBI, Theodoros and Murdoch (1994) identified four specific types of dysarthria (flaccid, ataxic, hypokinetic, and spastic) and four mixed dysarthria types (spastic ataxic, spastic hypokinetic, spastic flaccid, and flaccid ataxic). Most specifically, they identified the features of ataxic dysarthria in 41% of their TBI group; however, the subtype of mixed spastic–ataxic dysarthria appeared in 30% of the sample and was the most frequently occurring type of dysarthria. These authors reported a few speakers with symptoms of hypokinetic and hyperkinetic dysarthria following assumed damage to the basal ganglia and upper brain stem nuclei. Marquardt, Stoll, and Sussman (1990) concluded that spastic dysarthria is the most prevalent form of dysarthria following TBI.

Many different speech symptoms are exhibited by speakers with dysarthria following TBI. The extensive variability among speakers makes generalizations difficult. Because of this variability, speech–language pathologists must perform individualized assessments to plan intervention programs. The following section presents a framework for intervention based on the World Health

Organization's model of disablement (WHO, 1999). For a detailed discussion of the speech symptoms demonstrated by persons with dysarthria following TBI, the interested reader is referred to Theodoros, Murdoch, and Chenery (1994), Murdoch and Theodoros (1999), and McHenry (1996).

A Framework for Intervention

Because dysarthria associated with TBI can take many forms, no single intervention or type of intervention is appropriate for all speakers. The following section describes a framework for initial assessment and treatment planning for individuals with dysarthria associated with TBI. The framework is based both on the model of disablement and principles of staging intervention according to disorder severity.

The Model of Disablement

To deal with the variability observed in the dysarthria of individuals with TBI, use of the World Health Organization's model of disablement is helpful. This framework, also called *International Classification of Impairments, Activities, and Participation* (WHO, 1999), helps the intervention team understand the range of consequences associated with health conditions. It is particularly useful because it not only contains elements related to the biologic or physiologic consequence of the condition but also addresses psychosocial consequences of dysarthria. The following definitions of three critical elements of this model have important implications for dysarthria intervention:

1. *Impairment level* refers to a loss or abnormality of a body structure or of a physiological or psychological function. For dysarthria, the impairment involves weakness, spasticity, or incoordination of the area subsystems of speech (respiratory, laryngeal, velopharyngeal, and oral articulatory function).

2. *Activity level* refers to the nature and extent of functioning and generally reflects the individual's overall ability to perform functional activities such as speaking, walking, eating, and so on. In the dysarthria field, the overall indicators of the activity level typically have been (a) overall intelligibility of speech, (b) speaking rate, and (c) speech naturalness.

3. *Participation level* refers to the nature and extent of a person's involvement in life situations. The key word in this definition is *situations*—social, educational, vocational, or therapeutic events. This level of disorder deals with the social involvement of an individual with dysarthria. The level of social involvement is dependent on the individual's preferences, opportunities, and capabilities.

Impairment, activity, and participation levels need to be assessed to understand the full impact of dysarthria following TBI. As an example, consider the case of a teenager with mild–moderate dysarthria resulting from TBI. The adolescent exhibited an impairment characterized by a slightly breathy voice, reduced voice loudness, slightly hypernasal speech, and somewhat imprecise oral articulation. His limitations at the level of activity (speaking) included a reduction in speech intelligibility in adverse speaking situations, a slight reduction in speaking rate to compensate for his neurological impairments, and a noticeable reduction in speech naturalness. Given the social complexity of his educational situation (i.e., high school), this young man experienced a complicated participation disability. When he interacted with familiar persons in relatively optimal conditions, his communication was quite effective; however, when he was in adverse speaking situations, such as in large classrooms, among groups of students, or in noisy hallways, his communication effectiveness was reduced even with familiar listeners. Consequently, he participated minimally in group and classroom situations. He also reported that a small group of students devalued him because of his speech disorder. Although some of his consequences of TBI—such as slight cognitive and memory limitations—were not immediately apparent to others, his dysarthric speech was obvious the moment a person interacted with him.

Effective interventions for persons with dysarthria due to TBI involve assessment and, when appropriate, interventions at each of the three levels of disorder. A more detailed discussion is provided in the assessment and intervention sections of this chapter.

Assessing the Consequences of Dysarthria

The assessment of survivors of TBI with communication disorders is an ongoing process. Recovery is a long-term, dynamic process with a progression of recovery possibly occurring over several years. The initial assessment has several different goals. The first is the differential diagnosis of the communication disorder. The questions posed during this aspect of the assessment are (a) What types of communication problems are exhibited—cognitive–linguistic, specific language, and/or motor speech disorders? and (b) What is the relative severity of each of these problems?

Chapter 6 provides a more complete description of issues related to the differential diagnosis of various communication disorders. When dysarthria is present, the second goal of assessment is a description of the type of dysarthria, that is, assigning a label, such as *flaccid*, *spastic*, *ataxic*, *mixed*, and so on. See Duffy (1995) for a complete description of this topic.

The final phase of the initial assessment concerns the staging of intervention. *Staging* is the sequencing of management to address current problems and anticipate future ones. Staging strategies are commonly employed in medical practice to guide intervention decisions. For example, persons with cancer have their malignant tumors staged by an assessment team before interventions are prescribed. This system guides oncologists to utilize appropriate interventions for patients. In the dysarthria field, the appropriate selection and sequencing of interventions has been problematic. The following staging strategy is offered as a guideline to assist clinicians with these decisions. Staging is based on a speaker's performance at the activity and participation levels of the World Health Organization's model of disablement.

Assessments typically begin with an evaluation of overall speech performance (activity level) in optimized speaking and listening environments. Information about speech intelligibility, speaking rate, naturalness, listener effort/fatigue, and acceptance allows for staging the functional performance level of the individual. It also fosters understanding of the impact of TBI on overall speech function. An additional aspect of the assessment involves having the speaker and his or her frequent listeners estimate communication effectiveness in a variety of communication situations. Specific assessment strategies are outlined below.

Speech Intelligibility

The authors measure speech intelligibility objectively using the *Sentence Intelligibility Test* (Yorkston, Beukelman, & Tice, 1996), which is a computerized version of the *Assessment of Intelligibility of Dysarthric Speech* (Yorkston & Beukelman, 1981a). These measures provide information about the intelligibility of sentences as well as the speaking rate at which these sentences are produced. Typically, these tests are used with adults and adolescents who can read the stimuli. For young children, the Index of Augmented Speech Comprehensibility in Children (I-ASCC; Dowden, 1997) is useful. This is an intelligibility test for single words with vocabulary at the second-grade level or lower.

Speaking Rate

As mentioned before, speaking rate is an overall measure of speech activity. Because of the extent of interaction between connected speech intelligibility and speaking rate in some dysarthric speakers—especially those with ataxic dysarthria—measuring speaking rate is important. The *Sentence Intelligibility Test* (Yorkston et al., 1996) measures speaking rate for sentence-length stimuli, and the Pacer/Tally Software Application measures speaking rate for paragraph-length stimuli (Beukelman, Yorkston, & Tice, 1997). In the latter application, the speaker reads one of a number of standard passages from a computer screen. The computer measures the time from beginning to end of the passage and automatically computes speaking rate in words per minute or in syllables per second.

Speech Naturalness

Speech naturalness is a measure of the extent to which speech deviates from the expected based on a person's gender and age. In clinical settings, speech naturalness is usually measured perceptually using a rating scale. It is generally rated both for speech that is read aloud and for spontaneous speech.

Listener Effort, Fatigue, and Acceptance

Recently, clinicians have become aware of an additional set of factors that require measurement during assessment of activity—listener effort, fatigue, and acceptance. Following the transcription of the speech intelligibility test, listeners rate on a 7-point scale the effort required to transcribe the sample. In addition, they rate the amount of fatigue they would experience when listening to the individual speak for 15 minutes. Finally, they rate on a 7-point scale their acceptance of the speaker as a potential communication partner. Typically, listener acceptance questions deal with people's willingness to interact with the person with dysarthria or the extent to which they would avoid interacting with him or her.

Communication Effectiveness

Yorkston, Beukelman, and Tice (1999) developed a communication effectiveness questionnaire (see Figure 7.1). This questionnaire contains 8 standard communication effectiveness questions that are asked of the speaker and, when possible, of frequent listeners (e.g., family members, peers, or caregivers). Depending upon the participation pattern of an individual (e.g., employment or volunteer work), 10 additional questions probe communication effectiveness in educational, recreational, or employment situations.

Stages of Dysarthria Intervention

With the information obtained during the initial assessment, speakers with dysarthria due to TBI are assigned to one of five stages, which range from no useful speech (Stage 1) to no detectable speech disorder (Stage 5). More complete descriptions of Stages 1 through 4 follow.

(*text continues on page 144*)

Name: _____ Date: _____

Person completing the survey: _____ **Speaker** _____ **Family/Friend:** _____

Section One
This is an evaluation of how effectively the speaker communicates in various social situations. Please read the statement describing each of the following situations and indicate how successfully you feel that the speaker is able to communicate. If you feel that communication is very effective, circle the "7." If communication cannot occur at all in a situation, circle a "1." Feel free to use any number on the scale.

1. Having a conversation with a few friends (at home or bedside).
   Not at   1 2 3 4 5 6 7   Very
   All Able   ═══════════════════   Effective

2. Participating in a conversation with strangers in a quiet place.
   Not at   1 2 3 4 5 6 7   Very
   All Able   ═══════════════════   Effective

3. Conversing with a familiar person over the telephone.
   Not at   1 2 3 4 5 6 7   Very
   All Able   ═══════════════════   Effective

4. Conversing with a stranger over the telephone.
   Not at   1 2 3 4 5 6 7   Very
   All Able   ═══════════════════   Effective

5. Being part of a conversation in a noisy environment (social gathering).
   Not at   1 2 3 4 5 6 7   Very
   All Able   ═══════════════════   Effective

6. Speaking to a friend when you are emotionally upset or when you are angry.
   Not at   1 2 3 4 5 6 7   Very
   All Able   ═══════════════════   Effective

7. Having a conversation while traveling in a car.
   Not at   1 2 3 4 5 6 7   Very
   All Able   ═══════════════════   Effective

8. Having a conversation with someone at a distance (across the room).
   Not at   1 2 3 4 5 6 7   Very
   All Able   ═══════════════════   Effective

(continues)

Figure 7.1. Communicative Effectiveness Survey. *Note.* From Phoneme Identification Task: A Computer Program (computer software), by K. M. Yorkston, D. R. Beukelman, and R. Tice, 1999, Lincoln, NE: Tice Technology Services. Copyright 1999 by Tice Technology Services. Reprinted with permission.

Section Two

Please read the statements describing the following situations. If you feel that the statement describes a frequently occurring or important communication situation for the speaker, make an "X" to the left of the item number. Next, for each statement that you have chosen, indicate how successfully you feel that communication is in each situation. Add contexts that are unique to your situation in Items 16 through 18.

___ 9. Speaking in front of a small group without a microphone.

Not at   1   2   3   4   5   6   7   Very
all Able   Effective

___ 10. Conversing with someone who is somewhat hard of hearing.

Not at   1   2   3   4   5   6   7   Very
all Able   Effective

___ 11. Conversing through the outdoor speaker system with an employee at a fast-food restaurant or at a gas station.

Not at   1   2   3   4   5   6   7   Very
all Able   Effective

___ 12. Having a long conversation over an hour in length.

Not at   1   2   3   4   5   6   7   Very
all Able   Effective

___ 13. Speaking outdoors.

Not at   1   2   3   4   5   6   7   Very
all Able   Effective

___ 14. Communicating at work (   ).

Not at   1   2   3   4   5   6   7   Very
all Able   Effective

___ 15. Speaking to young children.

Not at   1   2   3   4   5   6   7   Very
all Able   Effective

___ 16. Other: _____

Not at   1   2   3   4   5   6   7   Very
all Able   Effective

___ 17. Other: _____

Not at   1   2   3   4   5   6   7   Very
all Able   Effective

___ 18. Other: _____

Not at   1   2   3   4   5   6   7   Very
all Able   Effective

Figure 7.1. *Continued.*

Stage 1: No Useful Speech

Some individuals with TBI produce no useful speech. Stage 1 is defined as the absence of useful speech that may result from a number of factors including poor cognition or arousal, severe motor deficits, or severe language deficits.

Speech and Communicative Participation

Typically, individuals at this stage require augmentative and alternative communication (AAC) intervention to meet their basic communication needs (see Chapter 8). Because natural speech is not functional, communicative participation in rehabilitation activities is dependent on AAC devices and techniques and the structure provided by active communication partners.

Building the Physiologic Foundations for Speech

In addition to using AAC devices, many individuals at Stage 1 receive intensive therapy to assist them in regaining neuromotor control as the basis of future speech performance. Usually, this intervention focuses on the physiological building blocks for speech (e.g., Case Example: Building Physiologic Support for Speech, later in this chapter). Typically, this approach follows a strategy of initially focusing on each of the speech subsystems and gradually combining subsystem function to support the production of speech. Assessment and intervention techniques for the respiratory, phonatory, and velopharyngeal systems are described in the following sections along with techniques to enhance early speech sound production.

Managing the Respiratory System. Many individuals with severe dysarthria cannot produce functional speech because of severe respiratory impairment. Clinical observation of an individual's breathing patterns during speech attempts provides an initial indication of respiratory status. The primary components being studied include loudness and breathing patterns. *Loudness* has a direct relationship with subglottal air pressure; as subglottal air pressure increases or decreases, loudness also increases and decreases. Further information on the normal physiology of respiration is available in Yorkston, Beukelman, Strand, and Bell (1999), Folkins and Kuehn (1982), and Hixon (1973). *Breathing pattern* refers to the pattern and timing of inhaling and exhaling during speech. Aspects of normal breathing movement include speech respiratory patterns (i.e., quick preparatory inhalation with long exhalation), point of lung volume for inhalation, and the location in the respiratory cycle where inhalations occur. Abnormal breathing patterns include exaggerated respiratory movements (i.e., excessive shoulder movement) and running out of air. Informal assessment of movement can be accomplished by placing one hand over the diaphragm and the other over the rib cage. This gives a gross estimation of respiratory movements.

Although some aspects of respiratory function can be inferred from listening to and watching speech production, perceptual assessment alone may be insufficient for treatment planning. Supplementing perceptual assessment with physiologic measurements allows the clinician to understand the respiratory system in isolation from other speech subsystems. For example, respiratory impairments may be exaggerated by weakness in the laryngeal and velopharyngeal subsystems. One measure of respiratory support is subglottal air pressure, the energy source for speech. It can be measured directly through a tracheotomy tube or based on intraoral pressure during production of a voiceless stop consonant such as /t/ or /p/. Because the glottis is open during /p/ and the nasal and oral cavity are closed, intraoral pressure is an estimate of subglottal air pressure (Yorkston, Beukelman, Strand, & Bell, 1999). An aerodynamic measurement system[1] provides a measure of air pressure level via a tube positioned intraorally, through the corner of the mouth. Normal adult subglottal air pressure is between 4 and 8 cm H_2O (Hixon, 1993). Any concern about nasal air leakage due to poor velopharyngeal closure can be addressed with a nose clip, whereas oral leakage due to a poor lip seal can be overcome through a face mask with a cork in the opening and a small hole drilled for the tubing.

Movement patterns during respiration for speech can be measured through the use of the magnetometer system (Hixon, Mead, & Goldman, 1976) and the respitrace unit (Hunker, Bless, & Weismer, 1981). The respitrace system is a transduction system that relays changing circumference of the chest and abdomen. It consists of two coils of insulated wire glued to cotton mesh bands placed on the person's torso (Yorkston, Beukelman, Strand, & Bell, 1999). The respitrace system totals the rib cage and abdominal movements to estimate total lung volume changes. It displays results as either movement-by-time or movement-by-movement (Abbs, Hunker, & Barlow, 1983; Putnam & Hixon, 1984). Individuals with dysarthria may exhibit reduced vital capacity and inappropriate or excessive lung volumes. After determining that respiratory impairment limits speech function, a number of intervention techniques are available. These are reviewed in the following section.

Establishing consistent subglottal air pressure. The *adapted blow bottle* (Hixon, Hawley, & Wilson, 1982) is an effective biofeedback system that can be used in a respiratory intervention program. A water bottle can be modified by adding an extended length of tubing to the straw and applying a measurement strip to the outside of the bottle from 0 to 12 cm (top to bottom). The

---

[1]Aerowin, Neuro Logic, Inc., 2888 Douglas Way, Caxenovia, NY 13035 (Phone: 315/655-2295). See also Aerophone II, Kay Elemetrics Corp. 2 Bridgewater Lane, Lincoln Park, NJ 07035-1488 (Phone: 973/628-6200).

speaker blows into a straw that has been placed at the desired depth (e.g., 5 cm H_2O) so that bubbles rise to the surface. This can be done in the clinical setting and at home as part of a daily speech therapy regimen. Netsell and Daniel (1979) reported success using a similar device (a U-tube manometer) to train individuals with severe head injuries to generate and sustain functional air pressures for speech. Their client could actually generate 10cm H_2O for 10 seconds within eight 20-minute sessions (an increase from 1 or 2 cm H_2O for less than 3 seconds). However, a "5 for 5 rule" is frequently applied; this rule suggests that a speaker who can generate 5 cm of water pressure for 5 seconds should have sufficient respiratory support for phonation (Netsell & Hixon, 1978).

Eliminating abnormal respiratory behaviors. Individuals with cognitive deficits due to TBI may maintain abnormal breathing patterns such as taking a breath after every word despite having the physiologic ability to produce longer utterances. Others may adopt very unusual patterns of speech breathing such as speaking on inhalation. Maladaptive behaviors need to be identified and eliminated.

Inspiratory checking. Inspiratory checking is a technique of controlling airflow through the larynx by using inspiratory muscles to counter the elastic recoil of the expiratory system (Netsell, 1995; Netsell & Hixon, 1992). This technique requires speakers to inhale deeply and then let the air out slowly as they speak. By capitalizing on the passive recoil pressures of the lungs, speakers use their inspiratory muscle forces to maintain a relatively steady subglottal air pressure level. This is a technique recommended for individuals who overdrive their respiratory system causing release of excessive airflow from the lungs.

Respiratory prosthesis. Before recommending respiratory prosthetic devices, medical approval is required, because these devices are contraindicated and can even be dangerous for individuals with head injuries who present inspiratory weakness. *Abdominal binders* provide support for individuals with intact diaphragmatic innervation but limited innervation of the expiratory muscles (Yorkston, Beukelman, Strand, & Bell, 1999). Rosenbek and LaPointe (1985) describe an *expiratory board* or paddle that the individual can lean into when exhaling.

Establishing Voluntary Phonation. Severe TBI may result in an individual's being unable to produce phonation voluntarily during the early phases of Stage 1. Phonation may initially occur during nonspeech activities such as coughing or laughing, or in response to a painful stimulus. When this happens, the posture should be noted and further phonation encouraged. Once initial phonation occurs, the treatment focus shifts to developing voluntary phonation by cueing the individual to sustain the sound once it is started (e.g., "Keep coughing"). *Pushing and pulling activities* (Prator & Swift, 1984) like pushing down on the armrests of a chair, pushing downward against mounted overhead slings (Rosenbek, 1984), or pulling against mounted bicycle handlebars (Yorkston, Beukelman, Strand, & Bell, 1999) are options. Vowel differentiation and intelligibility drills, as described later, are then implemented.

Postural adjustments. The most effective posture to achieve phonation varies depending on the individual and the type of dysarthria present. Input from occupational and physical therapists is a valuable source of possible strategies. The individual who has weak respiratory support (i.e., flaccid dysarthria) may benefit from a supine position set up by using a wheelchair or lawn chair with an adjustable back (Collins, Rosenbek, & Donahue, 1982). The individual with excessive muscle tone (i.e., spastic dysarthria) may benefit from a position that reduces the abnormal muscle tone. The individual with weak respiratory support and a slumped position (i.e., hypokinetic dysarthria) may benefit from sitting upright.

Laryngeal efficiency. Laryngeal efficiency is reflected in how adequately the airstream is valved by the vocal folds. If the vocal folds do not close adequately, the result is *hypoadduction;* on the other hand, if they close too tightly, the result is *hyperadduction.* Hypoadduction often causes a breathy, weak, and thin vocal quality. McHenry (1995) reported that 55% of males and 75% of females with severe head injuries evidenced reduced laryngeal airway resistance manifested as breathiness. Hyperadduction causes a strained strangled voice quality (Theodoros & Murdoch, 1996).

Increasing loudness. For survivors of TBI in Stage 1, the reestablishment of voluntary phonation is an important initial intervention goal. After this is accomplished, a second goal is to develop phonation of sufficient loudness and duration to support conversational speech. The techniques employed to increase loudness are dependent upon the type of vocal fold function and underlying dysarthria. Behavioral training focusing on coordination of respiration and phonation can help increase loudness. For example, behavioral training can include having the individual start phonation at the appropriate point in the respiratory cycle and increase generation of subglottal air pressure. The pushing and pulling activities described above also promote increased loudness. Additional techniques include having the individual push or pull his or her hands together while phonating. Once the individual has achieved optimal medial compression of the vocal folds, he or she needs to adjust subglottal air pressure to avoid overdriving the system, which will increase vocal roughness.

Velopharyngeal Intervention To Support Speech Sound Production. Many survivors of TBI with Stage 1 dysarthria experience impairment of velopharyngeal function. After establishing respiratory support for speech and voluntary phonation and before intervention can focus on articulatory improvement, the status of the velopharyngeal mechanism must be assessed. As will be discussed in the following section, early articulation intervention for survivors of TBI with Stage 1 dysarthria usually focuses on the production of vowels and simple consonant–vowel combinations. If the palate rests on or near the tongue so that production of vowel sounds is severely nasalized, the speaker will not differentiate sounds. Under these conditions, a *palatal lift* is often used to lift the soft palate so that vowels can be produced. A detailed discussion of velopharyngeal assessment and palatal lift fitting is provided in the section describing Stage 2 intervention.

Early Speech Sound Production. During Stage 1, articulation treatment usually focuses on the survivor's production of a number of different vowel and consonant sounds, single words, and short phrases. Once respiratory support for speech and consistent voluntary phonation have been reestablished, the focus of intervention turns to producing specific vowel and consonant sounds that can be distinguished from one another. This usually begins with *contrastive production drills* or production of sound groups such as /a/, /o/, /u/, and so on. The speaker is encouraged to produce the vowels so that a listener can distinguish each from the others. As is reviewed in much greater detail by Yorkston, Beukelman, Strand, and Bell (1999), contrast drills are gradually expanded to include consonant–vowel combinations and eventually single words.

Some survivors of TBI experience such excessive muscle tone during speech efforts that their production of sounds and words is limited. In this case, strategies to reduce excessive tone may be appropriate. *Tone reduction* can be attempted through biofeedback training by using surface electrodes either targeting a specific muscle (Netsell & Cleeland, 1973; Rubow, Rosenbek, Collins, & Celesia, 1984) or overall muscle tone (Finley, Niman, Standley, & Ender, 1976). Reduction of tone in a specific muscle group has also been accomplished through botulinum toxin injections (Schulz & Ludlow, 1991). Medications can reduce muscle spasticity but have an uncertain effect on articulation (Duffy, 1995; Rosenfield, Viswanath, Herbrick, & Nudelman, 1991). Tone reduction through pharmacological intervention should be attempted only with the support of the medical team, because the side effects of antispasticity medications can interfere with other functions such as swallowing.

Some survivors cannot produce specific consonant sounds because their neuromuscular control is so weak that articulatory movements are insufficient to achieve the appropriate targets in a timely manner. *Strengthening exercises* are usually not necessary for persons with TBI, because the strength demands for speech are so low. However, if extensive weakness is present, strengthening exercises—such as bilabial closure with electromyographic biofeedback (Linebaugh, 1983)—may be appropriate; however, research indicates that speech only requires 10% to 20% of maximum force of lip movement (A. Barlow & Abbs, 1983). Strengthening exercises involving a number of daily repetitive drills to increase strength are only indicated for individuals presenting with a flaccid dysarthria (Yorkston, Beukelman, Strand, & Bell, 1999). Rosenbek and LaPointe (1985) caution against delaying other intervention approaches, such as working on speech tasks, while performing strengthening exercises.

Stage 2: Natural Speech Supplemented by AAC

Some individuals with TBI produce some understandable speech but experience frequent communication breakdowns. In these situations, natural speech must be supplemented by AAC techniques. During Stage 2, natural speech can carry part of the communication load; however, communication is often easier if speech is supplemented with alphabet cues or techniques to establish the topic (see, e.g., the case example on building physiologic support for speech). The primary intervention goals during Stage 2 are (a) to establish the situations in which natural speech is effective, (b) to integrate the use of AAC strategies with emerging natural speech, and (c) to continue to improve natural speech performance by reducing physiologic impairment.

Participation

Once again, clarifying the participation expectations is important. In Stage 2, clinicians need to identify situations in which survivors of TBI will use AAC only, because their natural speech is inadequate—for example, when talking with strangers during community activities. Identifying those situations in which natural speech can play a major communicative role—such as when communicating with familiar listeners in routine situations like therapy activities or self-care—is also important. Depending on a speaker's cognitive skills, partners may take more or less responsibility for structuring communicative interactions.

Speech Intervention

When focusing on improving functional activity during Stage 2, the goal is to improve speech by making it easier for listeners to understand. Initially, this is accomplished by teaching the individual with TBI to supplement speech with cues to assist the listener. Later, speech intervention involves techniques that encourage the speaker to produce clearer speech with increased articulatory precision.

Case Example: Building Physiologic Support for Speech

Mike could not speak when he arrived at the rehabilitation center. His natural speech was limited to vocalizations when he laughed and cried, and he could not voluntarily produce phonation. He exhibited a very severe dysarthria.

Mike communicated by looking at objects of choice and, in response to questions from his communication partner, by gazing up to signal "yes" and down to signal "no." As his cognitive status improved, Mike demonstrated that he could use eye pointing to choose words and phrases that were printed on a clear plastic communication board (i.e., an e-trans system). In time, he regained sufficient control of one of his arms to point to letter, word, and phrase choices on a communication board. Because he still could not speak as he neared the end of Rancho Level VI, the decision was made to purchase an electronic AAC device for him. He spelled his messages completely accurately; however, he made it quite clear that he was not interested in learning the abbreviation codes necessary to retrieve partial or complete messages. Clearly, Mike's spelling and message formulation abilities were sufficient to meet his daily communication needs through AAC.

Once Mike's immediate communication needs were met with an AAC system, he and his parents communicated their strong desire that Mike be given the opportunity to reestablish functional speech. Eight years later, Mike had become such an effective speaker that he no longer used his AAC system except in very adverse communication situations. His speech intervention program first involved reestablishing voluntary control of his respiratory system by using an adapted blow bottle. Next, he focused on the development of voluntary control of phonation. Then, his family assisted him in several years of intelligibility drills to improve the understandability (intelligibility) of his speech.

Mike and his family deserve a great deal of credit for their tenacity. Under the guidance of a speech–language pathologist who supervised their efforts, they provided the daily motor practice that Mike required to reestablish motor control of his speech mechanism. They also deserve credit because they remained open to the possibility that Mike might not regain functional speech. Periodically, the supervising speech–language pathologist reviewed the family's diary to evaluate whether Mike was continuing to improve. In time, Mike, his family, and his clinician had to make the difficult decision to discontinue intervention. Although Mike successfully regained natural speech that functioned to meet many of his communication needs, not all persons with severe dysarthria are able to do this.

Supplemented Speech. Several forms of speech supplementation exist. One is alphabet supplementation. In alphabet supplementation, the speaker identifies on an alphabet board or an AAC system the first letter of each word as it is spoken. Because many individuals with TBI retain spelling ability, identification of the first letter of words while speaking is a manageable task. Several clinical outcome reports demonstrate the considerable positive impact of alphabet supplementation on the intelligibility of spoken messages by survivors of TBI. Hustad, Yorkston, and Beukelman (1999) provide a review of this research. In another report, Beukelman and Yorkston (1977) describe a survivor of TBI whose speech intelligibility was 31% without alphabet supplementation but improved to 72% when using the technique. One of the benefits of alphabet supplementation early in recovery is that it gives survivors opportunities to speak more frequently than if they talked only during their therapy or their practice sessions. The following case example describes use of speech supplementation. An example of an alphabet (and topic) supplementation board is provided in Figure 7.2.

A second type of speech supplementation involves *topic identification.* Typically, a topic board (see Figure 7.2) contains a listing of frequently discussed subjects. If the speaker can make the listener aware of the topic under discussion, the intelligibility of severely dysarthric speech is typically enhanced considerably. Research in this area suggests that for persons with natural speech intelligibility between 10% and 50%, the increase in speech intelligibility experienced during topic supplementation ranges from 30% to 40% (Dongilli, 1994). Many individuals with TBI struggle with topic identification because of the high cognitive demands associated with analyzing a conversation and determining the topic. Topic supplementation appears to be more difficult for survivors of TBI than alphabet supplementation; however, when it is successful, it has a substantial impact on the communication effectiveness of people with severe dysarthria.

The third type of speech supplementation involves *repair of communication breakdowns.* During Stage 2, speech is highly distorted, and communication breakdowns may occur even with alphabet or topic supplementation. One of the goals during this phase of intervention is to teach survivors and their frequent communication partners strategies to resolve communication breakdowns utilizing AAC strategies or supplemented speech strategies. Typically, most communication breakdowns can be resolved with AAC strategies.

Intervention to Enhance Speech Precision. An important goal of Stage 2 is to increase the precision, and thus the intelligibility, of natural speech. This may be accomplished through the use of *contrastive production* and *intelligibility drills.* During these exercises, speakers are encouraged to take advantage of their

---

 Case Example: Speech Supplementation

After Mike had reestablished voluntary control of respiration and phonation, he could produce approximations of a limited number of words. Early on, he was largely unintelligible, unless he provided his listener with additional information. Perhaps because his AAC system was spelling based, he indicated a strong interest in using the alphabet supplementation strategy. In the beginning, his communication breakdown rate overwhelmed his listeners, and they insisted that he use his AAC system as a communication breakdown resolution strategy. After attempting to vocalize a word or phrase a few times, he would frequently produce the utterance with his AAC system. In time, his supplemented speech became more understandable and his need for breakdown resolution subsided. During this time, Mike made little effort to assist his listeners by establishing the topic of his message or indicating when he intended to transition from one topic to another. Despite efforts to encourage him to use topic clarification strategies, he found this task very difficult. He still launched into a narrative with little preparation offered to his listeners. Throughout Stage 2, Mike continued to work with his family on intelligibility drills in an effort to improve the intelligibility of his speech. Toward the end of Stage 2, he was fitted with a palatal lift to reduce the air escaping through his nasal cavity when he attempted to produce pressure consonants. Given his respiratory limitations, the palatal lift improved his efficiency in using his limited air supply.

---

ability to modify production depending on the adequacy of the final speech end-product. Rather than have speakers change specific movement patterns, clinicians provide speakers with information about the adequacy of production and ask them to make the necessary changes in motor performance to improve the perceived speech output. This approach allows speakers to make whatever changes they can in the execution of speech movements to compensate for their neuromotor impairments.

Some speakers in Stage 2 can improve their articulation considerably by adjusting their *speaking rate*. This is particularly true for survivors of TBI with an ataxic component to their dysarthria. By reducing their habitual speaking rate, these individuals can often improve the level of coordination required for intelligible speech. Some speakers find the Pacer/Tally software (Yorkston,

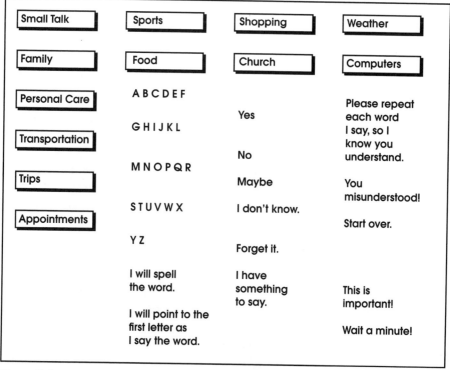

Figure 7.2. Alphabet–topic board used in speech supplementation.

Beukelman, & Tice, 1997) helpful to achieve initial changes in speaking rate. Of course, in time, the optimal speaking rate needs to be habitualized.

Physiologic Intervention

During Stage 2, emphasis on minimizing the physiologic impairment continues. The overall goals are (a) to establish consistent respiration function during speech, (b) to optimize phonation stability, and (c) to compensate for velopharyngeal impairment.

Establishing Consistent Respiratory Function for Speech. The primary respiratory goal for Stage 2 is to assist speakers to reestablish appropriate lung volume for speech and involves reaching targeted levels both for the upper and lower ends of the lung volume range. During Stage 1, speakers with TBI regain sufficient respiratory support for consistent phonation and the initial production of a limited number of words. However, many still demonstrate important respiratory limitations for speech. Some retain a pattern of inhaling to excessively high lung volume prior to speech. Others speak with very low lung volume. Intervention in Stage 2 attempts to return the speaker consistently to a target respiratory range, typically from 65% to 35% of lung volume. Some speakers return to this range with behavior instruction, while others require more specific biofeedback such as a display of lung volume. Use of a respitrace system with an attached oscilloscope can be effective for this purpose (Yorkston, Beukelman, Strand, & Bell, 1999).

Optimizing Phonation Function. Improved *vocal flexibility* is an important goal of physiologic intervention for some speakers with dysarthria. Normal speakers can fine tune their vocal productions by varying pitch, loudness, and breath group lengths. Individuals with TBI and dysarthria frequently cannot make these fine adjustments and may exhibit reduced vocal flexibility, frequently called *monotonous speech.* Measurements of vocal flexibility include both perceptual judgments and acoustic features such as fundamental frequency range, peak, and slope of fundamental frequency changes (Yorkston, Beukelman, Strand, & Bell, 1999).

Vocal quality, another important goal of intervention, is dependent on the type of dysarthria an individual exhibits. Some dysarthrias—such as the flaccid or spastic types—display a consistent alteration in vocal quality. Speakers with flaccid dysarthria consistently display a breathy voice quality, while speakers with spastic dysarthria have strained–strangled or harsh voice qualities. Others, such as ataxic dysarthric speakers, experience irregular quality that may be associated with irregular respiratory effort. A speaker with ataxic dysarthria may be overdriving the laryngeal mechanism and, if so, should be instructed to speak with less effort. This can be facilitated either through direct instruction and feedback from a sound level meter or through monitoring intraoral air pressure during speech. Effortful closure techniques such as pushing and pulling may be appropriate for those with laryngeal flaccidity.

Managing Velopharyngeal Weakness. Disorders of the velopharyngeal mechanism are common among survivors of TBI. Intervention is crucial because of the influence of *velopharyngeal incompetence* on other speech subsystems. For example, velopharyngeal incompetence can exaggerate poor respiratory support and inefficient laryngeal valving. Velopharyngeal impairment frequently takes the form of weakness due to flaccidity or a combination of spasticity and flaccidity. The timing of velopharyngeal movement may also be a problem for some speakers with ataxic dysarthria. However, the focus of the following section is on velopharyngeal impairment characterized by weakness. Additional resources include Croft, Shprintzen, and Rakoff's (1981) discussion of valving mechanisms in normal speakers; Kuehn and Kahane's (1990) review of velopharyngeal anatomy, histology, and physiology; Dworkin and Johns's (1980) review of the management of velopharyngeal incompetence in dysarthria; Liss,

Kuehn, and Hinkle's (1994) discussion of direct training of velopharyngeal musculature; and Bedwinek and O'Brian's (1985) provision of patient selection profiles for the use of speech prostheses in adult disorders.

Assessment. As a first step in assessment, the clinician listens for a variety of features associated with velopharyngeal dysfunction, including hypernasality or hyponasality, nasal emissions, and articulation error patterns. Although hypernasality and hyponasality are changes in resonance properties, nasal emission is the abnormal airflow through the nasal cavity when producing pressure consonants such as /b/, /p/, /f/, and /v/. This is not subject to dialectal differences. Therefore, it is a more accurate indication of velopharyngeal incompetence than hypernasal resonance, although the two may co-occur.

Velopharyngeal impairment may result in a pattern of articulation errors in which voiced consonants—such as /b/, /g/, and /d/—are perceived as nasals. A gross estimation of velopharyngeal function can be obtained by occluding the nose to prevent air escape and listening to the individual's loudness and articulation precision (Yorkston & Beukelman, 1991). Because judging the relative contribution of velopharyngeal functioning is difficult (as compared, e.g., to reduced respiratory support), instrumental analysis should supplement perceptual assessment.

The most common instrumental techniques are *aerodynamic measurements* and *direct visualization* via an endoscope. The specific technique employed depends on a number of factors including the speaker's level of cognitive function. For example, a confused individual who is emerging from coma may not tolerate direct visualization of the velopharyngeal mechanism. Aerodynamic measures estimate the overall contribution of velopharyngeal resistance rather than providing a direct measure of velopharyngeal movement. An *airflow meter* (such as the pneumotachometer) captures the amount of nasal emission through a nose mask, which it displays across a wire screen. An *air pressure transducer* measures intraoral air pressure through a flexible polyethylene tube placed in the oral cavity next to the tongue and converts oral airflow into an electrical voltage. Velopharyngeal resistance is then calculated based on simultaneous measurements of nasal airflow and intraoral airflow (S. M. Barlow, Suing, Grossman, Bodmer, & Colbert, 1989; Warren & DuBois, 1964; Warren & Ryon, 1967). The analysis is interpreted as being within normal limits if no nasal emission of air occurs during voiceless plosives—such as /p/—and the intraoral air pressure is about 7 cm H_2O.

Endoscopic equipment is used for direct visualization of the velopharyngeal mechanism. The endoscope is made of flexible tubing attached to a light source and a viewing lens. It is inserted through the nose after application of a topical anesthetic. It allows for viewing soft palate and pharyngeal wall movement during rest breathing, speaking, and swallowing (Miyazaki, Matsuya, & Yamaoka,

1975; Shprintzen, 1995). The structures can be viewed directly or from a video camera attached to the viewing end. A number of research articles have supported the usefulness of the endoscopic procedure (D'Antonio, Chait, Lotz, & Netsell, 1987; Ibuki, Karnell, & Morris, 1983; Karnell, Ibuki, Morris, & Van Demark, 1983; Shprintzen, 1995). The endoscopic procedure can also be helpful in fitting a palatal lift.

Palatal lifts. A palatal lift is an acrylic appliance fitted by a prosthodontist to cover the hard and soft palate. It lifts the soft palate and provides a surface for the lateral walls to contact. The retentive portion is fastened to the maxillary teeth (Yorkston & Beukelman, 1991; Yorkston, Beukelman, Strand, & Bell, 1999). Palatal lifts are fitted over several days or weeks because they usually require several adjustments to maximize speech production and ensure oral comfort.

For speakers with velopharyngeal incompetence due to weakness, a palatal lift prosthesis may be helpful. This intervention may occur during Stage 1 or Stage 2. For survivors of TBI who have limited ability to produce and practice differentiated vowel and consonant sounds because the flaccid palate rests on the posterior tongue, the palatal lift may be fit early in treatment, after the establishment of consistent voluntary phonation. For speakers who can differentiate vowel sounds in Stage 1, palatal lift intervention may be delayed until Stage 2, when increased speech intelligibility requires improved production of pressure consonants and reduced excessive hypernasality.

Determining candidacy for palatal lifts involves a number of decisions (Bedwinek & O'Brian, 1985; Yorkston, Beukelman, Strand, & Bell, 1999). Palatal lifts are appropriate for individuals with severe velopharyngeal dysfunction not modified by behavioral treatment approaches. Fitting of a palatal lift early in recovery from TBI can prevent the individual from overdriving the respiratory systems and encourage use of residual speech capabilities (Beukelman & Yorkston, 1991). It is most successful if velopharyngeal dysfunction is an isolated problem relative to other speech subsystems, but this occurs in only a small subgroup of individuals with dysarthria (Yorkston, Beukelman, Strand, & Bell, 1999).

Palatal lifts are not recommended for individuals who are not motivated or cooperative (Dworkin & Johns, 1980; Gonzalez & Aronson, 1970), individuals with a severely spastic soft palate, individuals who cannot manage oral secretions due to swallowing difficulties, or children under the age of 4 years. The fitting process is complicated for individuals who are edentulous or whose neurological status is changing. Because individuals who have sustained a TBI have a changing neurological status, the palatal lift has to be adjusted accordingly to ensure a proper fit.

Initially, palatal lifts may be uncomfortable. As a result, a *desensitization program* is sometimes beneficial for those with increased oral sensitivity, a hyperactive gag response, or spasticity of the soft palate. A number of desensitization programs have been proposed involving tactile desensitization over a 2- to 3- week period (Daniel, 1982) and application of topical anesthetic gels (Brand, Matsko, & Avart, 1988). Brand and colleagues (1988) reported their attempts to fit a palatal lift for an individual with TBI. Initially, the individual continually dislodged the device, and a desensitization program was unsuccessful; however, once a topical gel anesthetic was applied, the individual tolerated wearing the lift for 3 to 4 hours at a time.

The goals of palatal lift fitting for individuals with severe dysarthria include a series of speech outcomes such as improving the production of pressure consonants while maintaining production of nasal consonants and decreasing hypernasality. Other goals include swallowing without pain, breathing through the nose, and rotating the head without pain.

Stage 3: Speech Intelligibility Is Reduced in Some Situations

During Stage 3, natural speech is usually the primary means of communication, although dysarthria is still obvious. Most individuals in Stage 3 no longer use AAC strategies except for resolving communication breakdowns in challenging communication situations. The primary intervention goals during Stage 3 are (a) to learn to structure communication situations so that both listeners and speakers can function optimally; (b) to improve intelligibility and naturalness of speech; and (c) to optimize speech breathing patterns, voice quality, and velopharyngeal and articulatory function.

Participation

Stage 3 intervention involves the participation of speakers and their listeners in learning to optimize communication situations (see the following case example on optimizing communication situations). Although speech is adequate to meet most daily communication needs, comprehension still demands considerable effort on the part of listeners. Therefore, strategies are needed to optimize the communication situation. For example, speakers should reduce ambient noise by muting television sets or radios. Whenever possible, conversations should take place in quiet settings—such as conferences rooms—rather than in areas frequented by many people. When meeting with friends, a quiet restaurant is preferable to noisier situations such as the food court of a shopping mall. Students should arrange conversations with teachers or professors in their offices rather than in hallways or classrooms. Also, Stage 3 often involves specific education of frequent listeners or teaches the speaker with TBI to instruct listeners how to maximize communication effectiveness.

Case Example: Optimizing Communication Situations

Although Mike made remarkable progress, he remains a Stage 3 speaker in that he still experiences difficulty being understood in adverse speaking situations. He now resides in an assisted living center. When the living room of the facility is noisy with other residents and their guests, Mike has difficulty being understood. Usually, his listeners suggest that they move to a quieter area on the patio, in the hall, or in an adjoining conference area. For some time after Mike became a functional speaker, he continued practicing to improve his speech. However, progress was difficult for him and his family to detect. Together, they agreed that he had done an excellent job and that he no longer needed to work on his speech.

Enhancing Speech

The Stage 3 activity level focuses primarily on improving speech intelligibility and speech naturalness by highlighting aspects of speech that interfere with these overall speech characteristics. The goal is to increase the precision of oral articulation and the prosodic aspects of speech. Typically, this involves controlling speaking rate, using respiratory patterns that correspond to the grammatical form of utterances, and learning techniques to signal word prominence in a natural way. In addition, speakers with TBI are taught to monitor their listeners to determine when communication breakdowns occur and to attempt to speak more clearly in those situations so that further breakdowns do not occur.

Impairment

Respiration Intervention to Normalize Breath Patterning. As discussed earlier, speakers with severe dysarthria due to TBI usually experience respiratory limitation during Stages 1 and 2. By Stage 3, most have reestablished minimal respiratory support for connected speech; however, several goals for respiratory intervention remain. First, intervention may be necessary to retrain speakers regarding the appropriate point in utterances to take breaths. Due to earlier respiratory limitations, some survivors will have learned to speak using very short breath group units. Now that their respiratory control has improved, they need instruction and practice breathing at phrase, clause, and sentence boundaries. This instruction usually begins by having the speaker read passages aloud in which breath groups have been marked. Next, the speaker may read texts that contain extensive conversation such as plays. Role-playing conversational exchanges are also effective in training breath patterns. Finally, feedback can be provided by reviewing audiotapes or videotapes of these training activities.

Laryngeal Intervention. Improving laryngeal coordination involves both timing the respiratory and laryngeal systems and making articulation distinctions. Timing of the respiratory and laryngeal systems involves starting phonation at the beginning of the exhalation phase of respiration for speech. A respitrace unit or other respiratory monitoring system can provide feedback by displaying the respiratory signal on one channel and an acoustic waveform on the other. The timing can then be displayed for biofeedback. Traditional voice therapy techniques to reduce laryngeal hyperadduction and increase airflow may also be appropriate.

Velopharyngeal Intervention to Maintain Optimal Function. Palatal lift intervention is still required for some Stage 3 TBI survivors. Usually, the lift will initially have been fitted in Stage 1 or 2; during Stage 3 the lift will likely need to be maintained and refitted for optimal performance.

Behavioral intervention for mild velopharyngeal impairment may be considered, although some controversy exists about its effectiveness. Pushing exercises have been proposed (Froeschels, 1943; Froeschels, Kastein, & Weiss, 1955; Ruscello, 1982), but no current research indicates that strengthening the soft palate improves speech (Shelton, Hahn, & Morris, 1968). Recently, some innovative work has been reported using *continuous positive airway pressure* (CPAP), an air pressure flow device (traditionally used for individuals experiencing sleep apnea) that delivers air to the nose from a hose and mask. The air pressure creates resistance that the soft palate muscles must work against to obtain velopharyngeal closure (Kuehn, 1991). The goal is to increase the strength of the velopharyngeal muscles that provide closure, while the individual practices speech drills of sounds including vowels, nasals, and pressure consonants. Advantages over a palatal lift are comfort, convenience, and active participation by the individual with dysarthria and his or her caregivers (Kuehn & Wachtel, 1994). Kuehn and Wachtel (1994) report the effectiveness of this procedure for a speaker with dysarthria years after TBI. He wore a palatal lift but continued to demonstrate substantial hypernasality (4 on a 5-point scale). This score decreased to 2 within 4 weeks of CPAP therapy, and this rating was maintained 1 year after CPAP therapy.

Rate control is an additional therapy method that may be effective for individuals with mild impairment in velopharyngeal functioning. Slowing the rate allows more time to achieve velopharyngeal closure and reach articulatory points that can result in increased speech intelligibility. Yorkston and

Beukelman (1981b) reported that this approach was effective for subjects with ataxic dysarthria contributing to hypernasality.

Oral Articulation Intervention for "Clear Speech." During Stage 3, articulatory intervention focuses on assisting the speaker to utilize clear speech strategies (Pinchey, Dublach, & Braida, 1985, 1986, 1989). Nondisabled speakers usually use these strategies when they talk in adverse conditions or to a person with a hearing impairment. The strategies include (a) speaking more clearly, (b) speaking at a slightly reduced rate, and (c) speaking with appropriate loudness. Obviously, if one of these strategies results in reduced intelligibility or naturalness, that strategy should be discontinued. In addition, assessment should identify any specific residual articulatory error patterns. The specific residual patterns vary from person to person; however, as an example, Rosenbek and LaPointe (1985) point out that articulation distinctions are most often difficult for voiced–voiceless pairs (e.g., /t/ and /d/) and initial /h/ production. Exaggeration of other aspects of minimal pairs (e.g., vowel duration) can help to make sounds distinct. Finally, during Stage 3, speakers are often taught to take increased responsibility for monitoring the precision of their speech so that they can speak more clearly in adverse speaking situations, with persons who have difficulty understanding them, or with strangers. In effect, these individuals are learning to shift back and forth between conversational and clear speech depending on the demands of the situation.

Stage 4: Obvious Speech Disorder with Intelligible Speech

During Stage 4, dysarthria persists, but it does not impact speech intelligibility; typically, only speaking rate and naturalness are affected. Many individuals with Stage 4 dysarthria following TBI do not progress beyond this level to regain normal speech; however, a few do.

Participation

Typically, Stage 4 participation requires that individuals be taught to implement good speaking strategies in natural contexts. This means that they must carefully introduce their topic, speak in grammatically predictable sentences, and avoid situations involving particularly adverse speaking environments. Because their dysarthria is still apparent, some Stage 4 speakers find it useful to introduce themselves to new listeners by acknowledging their speech disability and encouraging the listener to indicate if he or she has difficulty understanding a message so that it can be clarified.

The extent to which speech naturalness contributes to a speaker's disability level varies depending on a number of factors. For example, some individuals may speak with reduced naturalness; however, because their listeners can understand them easily and are familiar with them, their residual speech patterns affect overall communication only minimally. On the other hand, unnaturalness can be an issue if a speaker interacts with the public or in social contexts that are judgmental of speech performance. Recall the teenager mentioned earlier in this chapter; his speech was perceived as unnatural by his peers in high school, and he was socially stigmatized by a small group of fellow students. Listener and speaker interviews or questionnaires can serve to rate a dysarthric speaker's overall speech naturalness.

Enhancing Speech

Stage 4 speakers with TBI typically focus on improving speech naturalness. This involves managing *intonation patterning, breath–pause patterning,* and *stress patterning* to enhance the overall naturalness of speech.

Assessment begins with a perceptual analysis of how natural the speech is perceived on a 7-point scale (Darley, Aronson, & Brown, 1975). Robin, Klouda, and Hug (1991) suggested stimuli appropriate for assessing prosody including the speaker's ability to produce emotion (e.g., happy, sad, question, neutral), emphatic stress (e.g., "*Don* shot the *puck* to *Kent*"), and syntactic juncture in complex sentences (e.g., "If Harry went to the bank, Ann will be very angry"). Assessment of naturalness also includes determination of breath patterns and where they are in the context of the sentence's syntax; for example, does the speaker produce only one or two words per breath despite the respiratory capability to do otherwise, or does the sentence structure need to be altered to compensate for a severely restricted respiratory system?

Intervention strategies to improve naturalness differ considerably depending on the type of dysarthric pattern that an individual exhibits. For example, if a person has primarily ataxic dysarthria and tends to stress equally each syllable of words, the focus of intervention will be to reduce the stress on unstressed syllables and maintain stress at the appropriate level for stressed syllables. For someone with primarily flaccid dysarthria, intervention will be almost the opposite. The clinician may encourage the person to stress the important syllables of a word and allow the unimportant syllables to remain unstressed.

An awareness of the importance of *prosodic elements* of speech is critical for individuals regardless of their dysarthria severity level, but it is particularly important for speakers in Stage 4. Based on assessment information, materials match the speaker's current cognitive level and respiratory–phonatory abilities.

For example, written stimulus materials may be short if the person's respiratory status is severely compromised or long if the person has adopted a maladaptive system of too few words per breath group. Treatment continues by having the person say a sentence reflecting a certain prosodic pattern with input from the clinician concerning the appropriateness of stress and naturalness. The goal is to obtain the best possible speech based on the individual's current speech capacity (Yorkston, Beukelman, Strand, & Bell, 1999, p. 475). Possible compensatory strategies include emphasizing the target word (e.g., a person may be encouraged to use long pauses to signal stressed words) and reducing the number of suprasegmental features that signal stress.

Some individuals realize during Stage 4 that their speech characteristics will remain unchanged for a long period of time. If this is the case, intervention may need to focus on counseling to lead the speaker with TBI and his or her family members to some acceptance of this persistent and probably chronic level of disability.

Physiologic Intervention

The nature of physiologic intervention for dysarthria changes from stage to stage. Readers will recall that in Stage 1 the emphasis is on establishing the physiologic foundations for speech using, for the most part, nonspeech activities. In Stage 2, focus turns to the enhancement of physiologic subsystems during speech. In Stage 3, less emphasis is on the individual subsystems; rather, intervention seeks to refine overall aspects of speech production such as rate and naturalness. During Stage 4, relatively limited focus is placed on individual speech subsystems. Typically, at this point in recovery, the intervention focuses on overall speech performance and on naturalness.

Summary

Several points warrant reemphasis; first, because recovery from dysarthria associated with TBI progresses over an extended period of time (usually years), a communication intervention needs to meet both short-term and long-term communication needs. Even though clinicians cannot predict a long-term recovery of speech, waiting months or even years to determine whether natural speech will return and allowing the individual to remain with minimal or no communication ability in the interim is inappropriate. Standard practice for persons with TBI is to meet their current needs through AAC strategies or supplemented speech strategies while working to develop the basis for useful natural speech in the future. Second, no evidence suggests that implementing AAC or supplemented speech strategies negatively impacts the recovery of functional speech, unless the goal for functional speech is abandoned by the AAC user, his or her family, and the intervention team. Again, the recovery of natural speech occurs over an extended period of time and numerous clinical reports support the effectiveness of systematic motor speech intervention for these individuals. Third, a variety of factors outside of speech production—particularly the cognitive limitations of the individual—influence intervention for dysarthria associated with TBI. Throughout intervention, adjustments to instructional techniques must accommodate cognitive limitations. Fourth, at this time, clinicians find it difficult to make accurate predictions regarding who with severe dysarthria associated with TBI will recover substantially and who will not. Typically, decisions about whether to terminate intervention are based upon indices of progress and survivor acceptance of involvement in an intervention program rather than on predictive characteristics. Perhaps this will change in the future. Finally, both AAC-based and natural-speech–based communication intervention programs for persons with TBI have been demonstrated to be effective in improving communication and performance participation.

References

Abbs, J., Hunker, C., & Barlow, S. (1983). Differential speech motor subsystem impairments with suprabulbar lesions: Neurophysiological framework and supporting data. In W. Berry (Ed.), *Clinical dysarthria* (pp. 21–56). San Diego, CA: College-Hill.

Barlow, A., & Abbs, J. (1983). Force transducers for the evaluation of labial, lingual, and mandibular motor impairments. *Journal of Speech and Hearing Disorders, 26,* 616–621.

Barlow, S. M., Suing, G., Grossman, A., Bodmer, P., & Colbert, R. (1989). A high-speed data acquisition and protocol control system for vocal tract physiology. *Journal of Voice, 3,* 283–293.

Bedwinek, A. P., & O'Brian, R. L. (1985). A patient selection profile for the use of speech prosthesis in adult disorders. *Journal of Communication Disorders, 18*(3), 169–182.

Beukelman, D. R., & Yorkston, K. M. (1977). A communication system for the severely dysarthric speaker with an intact language system. *Journal of Speech and Hearing Disorders, 42,* 265–270.

Beukelman, D. R., & Yorkston, K. M. (1991). *Communication disorders following traumatic brain injury: Management of cognitive, language, and motor impairments.* Austin, TX: PRO-ED.

Beukelman, D. R., Yorkston, K. M., & Tice, R. (1997). *Pacer/Tally rate measurement software.* Lincoln, NE: Tice Technology Services.

Brand, H. A., Matsko, T. A., & Avart, H. N. (1988). Speech prosthesis retention problems in dysarthria: Case report. *Archives of Physical Medicine and Rehabilitation, 69,* 213–214.

Collins, M., Rosenbek, J., & Donahue, E. (1982). The effects of posture on speech in ataxic dysarthria. *Asha, 24,* 767.

Croft, C. B., Shprintzen, R. J., & Rakoff, S. J. (1981). Patterns of velopharyngeal valving in normal and cleft palate subjects: A multi-view videofluoroscopic and nasendoscopic study. *Laryngoscope, 91,* 265–271.

D'Antonio, L., Chait, D., Lotz, W., & Netsell, R. (1987). Perceptual–physiologic approach to evaluation and treatment of dysphonia. *Annals of Otology, Rhinology and Laryngology, 2,* 182–190.

Daniel, B. (1982). A soft palate desensitization procedure for patients requiring palatal lift prostheses. *Journal of Prosthetic Dentistry, 48,* 565–566.

Darley, F. L., Aronson, A. E., & Brown, J. R. (1975). *Motor speech disorders.* Philadelphia: Saunders.

Dongilli, P. (1994). Semantic context and speech intelligibility. In J. Till, K. Yorkston, & D. Beukelman (Eds.), *Motor speech disorders: Advances in assessment and treatment* (pp. 175–192). Baltimore: Brookes.

Dongilli, P., Hakel, M., & Beukelman, D. (1992). Recovery of functional speech following traumatic brain injury. *Journal of Head Trauma Rehabilitation, 7,* 91–101.

Dowden, P. (1997). Augmentative and alternative communication decision making for children with severely unintelligible speech. *Augmentative and Alternative Communication, 13,* 48–58.

Duffy, J. R. (1995). *Motor speech disorders: Substrates, differential diagnosis, and management.* St. Louis, MO: Mosby.

Dworkin, J. R., & Johns, D. F. (1980). Management of velopharyngeal incompetence in dysarthria: A historical review. *Clinical Otolaryngology, 5,* 61–74.

Enderby, P., & Crow, E. (1990). Long-term recovery patterns of severe dysarthria following head injury. *British Journal of Disorders of Communication, 25,* 341–354.

Finley, W. W., Niman, C., Standley, J., & Ender, P. (1976). Frontal EMG biofeedback training of athetoid cerebral patients: Report of six cases. *Biofeedback of Self Regulation, 1,* 169–182.

Folkins, J., & Kuehn, D. P. (1982). Speech production. In N. Lass, L. McReynolds, J. Northern, & D. Yoder (Eds.), *Speech, language, and hearing: Volume 1* (pp. 246–285). Philadelphia: Saunders.

Froeschels, E. (1943). A contribution to the pathology and therapy of dysarthria due to certain cerebral lesions. *Journal of Speech Disorders, 8,* 301–321.

Froeschels, E., Kastein, S., & Weiss, D. A. (1955). A method of therapy for paralytic conditions of the mechanisms of phonation, respiration, and glutination. *Journal of Speech and Hearing Disorders, 20,* 365–370.

Gonzalez, J., & Aronson, A. (1970). Palatal lift prosthesis for treatment of anatomic and neurologic palatopharyngeal insufficiency. *Cleft Palate Journal, 7,* 91–104.

Hixon, T. (1973). Respiratory function in speech. In F. Minifie, T. Hixon, & F. Williams (Eds.), *Normal aspects of speech, hearing, and language* (pp. 73–126). Englewood Cliffs, NJ: Prentice Hall.

Hixon, T. (1993). *Clinical evaluation of speech breathing disorders: Principles and methods—Telerounds.* Tucson, AZ: National Center for Neurogenic Communication Disorders.

Hixon, T., Hawley, J., & Wilson, J. (1982). An around-the-house device for the clinical determination of respiratory driving pressure. *Journal of Speech and Hearing Disorders, 47,* 413–415.

Hixon, T., Mead, J., & Goldman, M. (1976). Dynamics of the chest wall during speech production: Function of the thorax, rib cage, diaphragm, and abdomen. *Journal of Speech and Hearing Research, 19,* 297–356.

Hunker, C., Bless, D., & Weismer, G. (1981, November). *Respiratory inductive plethysmography: A clinical technique for assessing respiratory function for speech.* Paper presented at the annual convention of the American Speech-Language-Hearing Association, Los Angeles.

Hustad, K., Yorkston, K., & Beukelman, D. (1999). Optimizing communication effectiveness. In K. Yorkston, D. Beukelman, E. Strand, & K. Bell (Eds.), *Management of motor speech disorders in children and adults* (pp. 483–537). Austin, TX: PRO-ED.

Ibuki, K., Karnell, M. P., & Morris, H. L. (1983). Reliability of the nasophayrngeal fiberscope (NPF) for assessing velopharyngeal function. *Cleft Palate Journal, 20,* 97–104.

Jordon, F. M., & Murdoch, B. E. (1990). Unexpected recovery of functional communication following a prolonged period of mutism post-head injury. *Brain Injury, 4,* 101–108.

Jordon, F. M., Ozanne, A. E., & Murdoch, B. E. (1988). Long-term speech and language disorders subsequent to closed head injury in children. *Brain Injury, 2,* 179–185.

Karnell, M. P., Ibuki, K., Morris, H. L., & Van Demark, D. R. (1983). Reliability of the nasopharyngeal fiberscope (NPF) for assessing velopharyngeal function: Analysis of judgement. *Cleft Palate Journal, 20,* 199–208.

Keatley, A., & Wirtz, S. (1994). Is 20 years too long? Improving intelligibility in longstanding dysarthria—A single case treatment study. *European Journal of Disorders of Communication, 29,* 183–201.

Kuehn, D. P. (1991). New therapy for treating hypernasal speech using continuous positive airway pressure (CPAP). *Plastic and Reconstructive Surgery, 88,* 959–966.

Kuehn, D., & Kahane, J. (1990). Histologic study of the normal human soft palate. *Cleft Palate Journal, 27,* 26–35.

Kuehn, D. P., & Wachtel, J. M. (1994). CPAP therapy for treating hypernasality following closed head injury. In J. A. Till, K. M. Yorkston, & D. R. Beukelman (Eds.), *Motor speech disorders: Advances in assessment and treatment* (pp. 207–212). Baltimore: Brookes.

Light, J., Beesley, M., & Collier, B. (1988). Transition through multiple augmentative and alternative communication systems: A three-year case study of a head injured adolescent. *Augmentative and Alternative Communication, 4,* 2–14.

Linebaugh, C. (1983). Treatment of flaccid dysarthria. In W. H. Perkins (Ed.), *Dysarthria and apraxia* (pp. 59–67). New York: Thieme-Stratton.

Liss, J. M., Kuehn, D. P., & Hinkle, K. P. (1994). Direct training of velopharyngeal musculature. *Journal of Medical Speech–Language Pathology, 2,* 243–251.

Marquardt, T., Stoll, J., & Sussman, H. (1990). Disorders of communication in traumatic brain injury. In E. D. Bigler (Ed.), *Traumatic brain injury: Mechanisms of damage, assessment, intervention, and outcome* (pp. 181–205). Austin, TX: PRO-ED.

McHenry, M. A. (1995). Laryngeal airway resistance following traumatic brain injury. In D. Robin, K. M. Yorkston, & D. R. Beukelman (Eds.), *Disorders of motor speech: Recent advances in assessment, treatment, and clinical characterization* (pp. 229–240). Baltimore: Brookes.

McHenry, M. (1996). Motor speech disorders. In R. Gillis (Ed.), *Traumatic brain injury rehabilitation for speech–language pathologists* (pp. 223–250). Boston: Butterworth-Heinemann.

Miyazaki, T., Matsuya, P., & Yamaoka, M. (1975). Fiberscopic methods for assessment of velopharyngeal closure during various activities. *Cleft Palate Journal, 12,* 107–114.

Murdoch, B. E., & Theodoros, D. G. (1999). Dysarthria following traumatic brain injury. In S. McDonald, L. Togher, & C. Code (Eds.), *Communication disorders following traumatic brain injury* (pp. 211–234). Hove, East Sussex, UK: Psychology Press.

Najensen, T., Sazbon, L., Feifelzon, J., Becker, E., & Schechter, I. (1978). Recovery of communication functions after prolonged traumatic coma. *Scandinavian Journal of Rehabilitation Medicine, 10,* 15–21.

Netsell, R. (1995). Speech rehabilitation for individuals with unintelligible speech and dysarthria: The respiratory and velopharyngeal systems. *Special Interest Divisions: Neurophysiology and Neurogenic Speech Language Disorders, 5*(4), 6–9.

Netsell, R., & Cleeland, C. (1973). Modification of lip hypotonia in dysarthria using EMG feedback. *Journal of Speech and Hearing Disorders, 38,* 131–140.

Netsell, R., & Daniel, B. (1979). Dysarthria in adults: Physiologic approach in rehabilitation. *Archives of Physical Medicine and Rehabilitation, 60,* 502–508.

Netsell, R., & Hixon, T. (1978). A noninvasive method for clinically estimating subglottal air pressure. *Journal of Speech and Hearing Disorders, 43,* 326–330.

Netsell, R., & Hixon, T. (1992). Inspiratory checking in therapy for individuals with speech breathing dysfunction. *Asha, 34,* 152.

Olver, J., Ponsford, J., & Curran, C. (1996). Outcome following traumatic brain injury: A comparison between 2 and 5 years after injury. *Brain Injury, 10,* 841–848.

Pinchey, M., Dublach, N., & Braida, L. (1985). Speaking clearly for the hard of hearing I: Intelligibility differences between clear and conversational speech. *Journal of Speech and Hearing Research, 28,* 96–103.

Pinchey, M., Dublach, N., & Braida, L. (1986). Speaking clearly for the hard of hearing II: Acoustic characteristics of clear and conversational speech. *Journal of Speech and Hearing Research, 29,* 434–446.

Pinchey, M., Dublach, N., & Braida, L. (1989). Speaking clearly for the hard of hearing III: An attempt to determine the contribution of speaking rate to differences in intelligibility between clear and conversational speech. *Journal of Speech and Hearing Research, 32,* 600–603.

Prator, R. & Swift, R. (1984). *Manual of voice therapy.* Boston: Little, Brown.

Putnam, A. H. B., & Hixon, T. (1984). Respiratory kinematics in speakers with motor neuron disease. In M. R. McNeil, J. C. Rosenbek, & A. E. Aronson (Eds.), *The dysarthrias: Physiology, acoustics, perception, management* (pp. 36–68). San Diego, CA: College-Hill.

Robin, D. A., Klouda, G. V., & Hug, L. N. (1991). Neurogenic disorders of prosody. In M. P. Cannito & D. Vogel (Eds.), *Treating disordered speech motor control: For clinicians by clinicians* (pp. 241–271). Austin: PRO-ED.

Rosenbek, J. (1984). Treating the dysarthric talker. *Seminars in Speech and Language, 5,* 359–384.

Rosenbek, J. C., & LaPointe, L. L. (1985). The dysarthrias: Description, diagnosis, and treatment. In D. Johns (Ed.), *Clinical management of neurogenic communication disorders* (pp. 97–152). Boston: Little, Brown.

Rosenfield, D., Viswanath, N., Herbrick, K., & Nudelman, H. (1991). Evaluation of the speech motor control system in amyotrophic lateral sclerosis. *Journal of Voice, 5,* 224–230.

Rubow, R. T., Rosenbek, J. C., Collins, M. J., & Celesia, G. G. (1984). Reduction of hemifacial spasm and dysarthria following EMG biofeedback. *Journal of Speech and Hearing Disorders, 49,* 26–33.

Ruscello, D. (1982). A selected review of palatal training procedures. *Cleft Palate Journal, 19,* 181–194.

Rusk, H., Block, J., & Lowmann, E. (1969). Rehabilitation of the brain-injured patient: A report of 157 cases with long-term follow-up of 118. In E. Walker, W. Caseness, & M. Critchley (Eds.), *The later effects of head injury* (pp. 327–332). Springfield, IL: Thomas.

Sarno, M., Buoaguro, A., & Levita, E. (1986). Characteristics of verbal impairment in closed head injured patients. *Archives of Physical Medicine and Rehabilitation, 79,* 3–9.

Schulz, G. M., & Ludlow, C. L. (1991). Botulinum treatment for orolingual–mandibular dystonia: Speech effects. In C. A. Moore, K. M. Yorkston, & D. R. Beukelman (Eds.), *Dysarthria and apraxia of speech: Perspectives on management* (pp. 227–242). Baltimore: Brookes.

Shelton, R. L., Hahn, E., & Morris, H. L. (1968). Diagnosis and therapy. In D. C. Spriestersbach & D. Sherman (Eds.), *Cleft palate and communication* (pp. 225–227). New York: Academic Press.

Shprintzen, R. (1995). Instrumental assessment of velopharyngeal valving. In R. Shprintzen & J. Bardach (Eds.), *Cleft palate speech management: A multidisciplinary approach* (pp. 221–246). St. Louis, MO: Mosby-Year Book.

Theodoros, D., & Murdoch, B. (1994). Laryngeal dysfunction in dysarthric speakers following severe closed head injury. *Brain Injury, 8,* 667–684.

Theodoros, D. G., & Murdoch, B. E. (1996). Differential patterns of hyperfunctional laryngeal impairment in dysarthric speakers following severe closed head injury. In D. A. Robin, K. M. Yorkston, & D. R. Beukelman (Eds.), *Disorders of motor speech: Assessment, treatment, and clinical characterization* (pp. 205–227). Baltimore: Brookes.

Theodoros, D., Murdoch, B., & Chenery, H. (1994). Perceptual speech characteristics of dysarthric speakers following severe closed head injury. *Brain Injury, 8,* 101–124.

Thomsen, I. V. (1984). Late outcome of severe blunt head injury: A 10 to 15 second follow-up. *Journal of Neurology, Neurosurgery, & Psychiatry, 47,* 260–268.

Warren, D. W., & DuBois, A. (1964). A pressure-flow technique for measuring velopharyngeal orifice area during continuous speech. *Cleft Palate Journal, 4,* 38–49.

Warren, D. W., & Ryon, W. E. (1967). Oral port constriction, nasal resistance, and respiratory aspects of cleft palate speech: An analog study. *Cleft Palate Journal, 4,* 38–49.

Workinger, M., & Netsell, R. (1992). Restoration of intelligible speech 13 years post-head injury. *Brain Injury, 6,* 183–187.

World Health Organization. (1999, June 24). *International classification of impairments, activities, and participation: Beta-1 draft for field trials, Beginner's guide* [Online]. Available: http://www.who.int/msa/mnh/ems/icidh/

Ylvisaker, M. (1986). Language and communication disorders following pediatric head injury. *Journal of Head Trauma Rehabilitation, 1,* 48–56.

Yorkston, K., & Beukelman, D. (1981a). *Assessment of intelligibility of dysarthric speech.* Austin, TX: PRO-ED.

Yorkston, K. M., & Beukelman, D. R. (1981b). Ataxic dysarthria: Treatment sequences based on intelligibility and prosodic considerations. *Journal of Speech and Hearing Disorders, 46,* 398–404.

Yorkston, K. M., & Beukelman, D. R. (1991). Motor speech disorders. In D. R. Beukelman & K. M. Yorkston (Eds.), *Communication disorders following traumatic brain injury: Management of cognitive, language, and motor impairments* (pp. 251–315) Austin, TX: PRO-ED.

Yorkston, K. M., Beukelman, D. R., Strand, E. A., & Bell, K. R. (1999). *Management of motor speech disorders in children and adults.* Austin, TX: PRO-ED.

Yorkston, K., Beukelman, D., & Tice, R. (1996). Sentence Intelligibility Test: A Computer Program [Computer software]. Lincoln, NE: Tice Technology Services.

Yorkston, K. M., Beukelman, D., & Tice, R. (1997). Pacer/Tally: A computer program [Computer software]. Lincoln, NE: Tice Technology Services.

Yorkston, K. M., Beukelman, D. R., & Tice, R. (1999). Phoneme Identification Task: A Computer Program [Computer software]. Lincoln, NE: Tice Technology Services.

Yorkston, K., Honsinger, M., Mitsuda, P., & Hammen, V. (1989). The relationship between speech and swallowing disorders in head-injured patients. *Journal of Head Trauma Rehabilitation, 4,* 1–16.

Augmentative and Alternative Communication and Assistive Technology
Bridging Cognitive and Communication Gaps for Survivors of TBI

Karen Hux and Michelle Gutmann

The recovery process for survivors of TBI involves regaining independence in a wide range of cognitive and physical domains. With respect to augmentative and alternative communication (AAC) and assistive technology (AT) for cognitive and communication purposes, the domains of greatest importance include speech, memory, and reading and writing skills. As such, AAC and AT techniques and strategies are commonly implemented at various stages of recovery from TBI. Because the TBI recovery process is often unpredictable—for example, sometimes a long period of time without noticeable improvement is followed by a period of rapid improvement—AAC and AT techniques should be evaluated and possibly altered frequently to reflect a person's evolving abilities and needs.

This chapter provides general information about assessing and implementing AAC and AT strategies and techniques for both pediatric and adult populations with TBI. Before addressing specific AAC and AT strategies appropriate for use during various stages of recovery, two other issues need consideration: (a) the necessity for expertise from individuals with a variety of professional backgrounds and (b) general guidelines for assessment. Following discussion of these two issues, the AAC and AT options within the domains of speech production, memory, and literacy skills will be discussed.

Team Composition

Because of the varied patterns of deficits displayed by survivors of TBI, the selection and implementation of AAC and AT interventions often require the expertise of individuals from a wide variety of professions. Table 8.1 lists some professionals who may comprise the intervention team and the roles they are likely to assume. In some cases, additional professionals such as social workers, medical specialists, and neuropsychologists may be added to the team.

Given the constraints of time and rehabilitation funding, orchestrating the collaboration among a group of professionals can be a difficult and time-consuming process. Because of the direct association between communication

Augmentative and alternative communication (AAC) has been defined as "any approach designed to support, enhance, or augment the communication of individuals who are not independent communicators in all situations" (Beukelman, Yorkston, & Dowden, 1985, p. 3).

Traditionally, AAC has included both low technology and high technology options. The distinction between the two often depends on the level of sophistication of the system and whether electronics are involved. In general, low technology options include those systems that can be made from materials readily available, such as paper and pencil, and that *do not* support either voice or print output; high technology options typically include systems with voice and/or print output or systems that are programmable.

Assistive technology (AT) has been defined as "aided tools to improve the skills, abilities, lifestyle, and independence of individuals with disabilities" (Glennen, 1997, p. 6).

AT includes devices or systems such as adapted computers, eyeglasses, closed-caption televisions, wheelchairs, and environmental control systems. AAC tools and techniques are a part of AT. Because of the focus and scope of this chapter, AT techniques and strategies discussed will be limited to those related to cognitive and communicative functioning.

concerns and AAC and AT interventions, speech–language pathologists often coordinate a team's efforts. In all instances, successful AAC and AT interventions for people with TBI begin with skilled, function-based assessments by all professionals involved. The team can then use these assessments to make sound clinical decisions about the implementation of AAC and AT technology.

General Assessment Principles

How and When To Assess

Because of the changing nature of survivors' profiles, AAC and AT assessment is an ongoing endeavor. Although all assessments aim to yield as much information as possible, initial assessments need not be as comprehensive as assessments aimed at selecting a system for long-term or permanent use. This is not to suggest that initial assessments should be shallow; rather, in the initial stages of recovery, basic communication needs can often be met by relatively simple systems for which assessment is minimal. However, because of the constraints introduced by cognitive and communication impairments, assessment for any kind of AAC or AT system must include attention to details such as the types of cueing that are helpful and the compatibility of system features with a survivor's current strengths and challenges.

Table 8.1
Contributing Professionals and Their Roles in Implementing AAC
and AT Interventions

Profession	Role description
Speech–language pathologist	Assesses face-to-face and written communication
	Often coordinates efforts for AAC or AT system implementation
	Conducts intervention for motor speech and cognitive–communication impairments
Occupational therapist	Deals with issues regarding seating and positioning
	Conducts switch assessment
	Conducts intervention for upper limb and visual perceptual deficits that affect AAC or AT selection
	With the physical therapist, assesses the need for and implements powered mobility devices
	May assume responsibility for some technology-related issues
Physical therapist	Deals with issues regarding seating and positioning
	Conducts intervention for switch access
	With the occupational therapist, assesses the need for and implements powered mobility devices
Rehabilitation engineer	Devises complex technical solutions to various individual problems
	Provides technical consultation to other team members as needed
Technologist	Sets up and implements technological systems
	Provides technical support

As a survivor emerges from posttraumatic amnesia and progresses through the early stages of recovery, the use of multiple AAC and AT systems is likely. Rapid changes in AAC and AT systems and strategies may be necessary as motor function and cognitive and communication abilities improve. To avoid the expense of technical systems that may be appropriate only for short periods of time, systems used during early recovery phases should come from AAC and AT loan libraries whenever possible. Borrowing devices from loan libraries also provides a period during which professionals can evaluate a survivor's potential to master and implement a particular system. Loan libraries may be available through state departments of education or rehabilitation facilities.

With continued recovery, persistent cognitive and communication challenges become apparent, and a survivor's AAC and AT needs become more stable. Table 8.2 delineates several issues that professionals need to consider when selecting devices for long-term use by people with TBI. Additional general information about performing assessments is available in textbooks such as *Augmentative and Alternative Communication: Management of Severe Communication Disorders in Children and Adults* (Beukelman & Mirenda, 1998), *Handbook of Augmentative and Alternative Communication* (Glennen & DeCoste, 1997), and *The Handbook of Assistive Technology* (Church & Glennen, 1992).

Alternate Access

Often survivors of TBI have cognitive or physical impairments that limit or prevent them from using traditional methods of accessing computers or communication systems. When direct selection (e.g., via a keyboard, a mouse, or simple pointing) is not possible, alternate access is required. *Alternate access* includes any method of indirect selection that permits operation of an AAC or AT device or system; the most frequently used methods in-

Table 8.2
Issues and Variables Affecting the Selection of AAC and AT Systems

Issue	Variables
Physical features of device	Portability (size and weight)
	Aesthetic appeal
	Size of display
	Number of keys
Organizational format	Representational set
	Selection set
Interaction of system features with cognitive and communication impairments	Methods of encoding
	Methods of retrieval
	Rate enhancement strategies
	Organizational format
Physical and Cognitive Access	High or low tech
	Direct or indirect selection

volve (a) communication facilitators, (b) voice recognition technology, and (c) single-switch and multiple-switch devices. In all instances, something other than direct touch or pointing allows the client to access items on a display or device. Table 8.3 summarizes and defines various alternate access techniques and devices. Notice that when switches are used for alternate accessing, multiple scanning options are available; an occupational therapist's determination of the site for switch placement is pivotal to success.

The Continuum of Speech Recovery

Regaining functional speech is a major marker in the recovery process for people with TBI and their families. Most survivors relied on natural speech as their primary mode of communication prior to injury. A sudden decrease or abolition of natural speech ability may be extremely distressing and is an example of one of the many lifestyle changes to which people with TBI must adapt. Furthermore, losing the use of natural speech after having relied on it previously is emotionally very different from never having had natural speech ability. Consequently, in addition to noting physical, motor, and cognitive limitations, professionals developing and implementing AAC and AT techniques and devices with survivors of TBI must be highly aware of a person's emotional status and attitude toward the use of alternative methods of communication.

Clinician Beware

The introduction of AAC interventions to a person with TBI is often met with disapproval and rejection; after all, speech is of primordial importance, and most survivors of TBI desire to work toward its return. Although this may be a justifiable goal, professionals must bear in mind and try to impress upon survivors and their families that functional communication is equally important. Often people with TBI and their families are wary of the introduction of AAC options for fear of suppressing natural speech recovery. This reaction is understandable and predictable; communication by any means other than natural speech may seem foreign or unnatural. However, the reaction is not justified; the use of AAC options tends to speed rather than slow the return of natural speech.

Family members and injured persons face a myriad of changes and decisions resulting from TBI. Many feel overwhelmed by the need to make yet another decision—this time to choose a method of communication. Because

(*text continues on page 176*)

Table 8.3
Definitions and Features of Alternate Access Systems

Alternate access	Definition	Features
Communication facilitators	Designated person(s) trained to facilitate communication	Requires training on type and operation of AAC system(s) and/or strategies Facilitator needs to be familiar with TBI survivor
Voice recognition	Method of input in which a person's voice serves as the interface between person and machine. Voice recognition is implemented by way of specific hardware and software.	Supports word processing and environmental control Length of training and calibration for each user differs from system to system Voice characteristics need to be stable Successful for some people with mild to moderately severe dysarthria Heavy cognitive demands on users
Switches	Mechanical interface between an individual and an electronic device	A means for people with limited motor control and/or emerging cognitive abilities to control communication systems Uses a single, consistent, repetitive motor movement for activation
Linear scanning	Scanning method in which communication choices (e.g., symbols, letters, or words) are presented one at a time in a line-by-line pattern	Item-by-item choice presentation Slow scanning process Limited cognitive demands required of users

Method	Description	Considerations
Circular scanning	Scanning method in which communication choices (e.g., symbols, letters, or words) are presented one at a time in a circular pattern	Typically appear on specially designed circular devices Slow scanning process because users must wait while the scanning arm sweeps around to the desired point Limited cognitive demands required of users Works best with a limited set of communication choices
Row–column scanning	Scanning method in which communication choices (e.g., symbols, letters, or words) are scanned from top to bottom, beginning from the leftmost margin. Scanning proceeds row by row down the face of the device. Users select a target row via switch activation. Within a selected row, items are scanned singly from left to right. A final selection is made by a second switch activation when the desired target is reached.	Requires visual and attentional vigilance by users Requires sufficient motor coordination to make at least two switch activations Requires careful organization of targets to ensure those used frequently are easiest and quickest to access
Group–item scanning	Scanning methods in which groups of communication choices (e.g., symbols, letters, or words) are presented. When a group is selected, individual communication choices within the group are presented either row by row or column by column.	Requires multiple switch activations for selection of a single communication target High cognitive demands on users because of embedding of targets within quadrants of AAC system Requires careful organization of targets to ensure those used frequently are easiest and quickest to access

What is functional speech?

Functional speech refers to the use of oral language to support daily communication needs. In many ways, functional speech is a threshold concept; it does not imply that natural speech is sufficient to support all communication needs, but it is adequate for at least some communicative interactions. For example, a person with functional speech may successfully engage in conversations about familiar topics and with familiar partners given a relatively noise-free environment but not have adequate speech to relate highly specific or technical information to novel communication partners. Many factors—such as fatigue, speech intelligibility, speaking environment, stress level, cognitive status, premorbid linguistic proficiency, and the degree to desire to communicate—may affect the adequacy of communication skills at any given time and, hence, the status of functional speech.

communication by speech is the expected outcome for most survivors, recognition of the need for another means of communication can bring to the surface feelings of "violation of expectation." This violation of expectation phenomenon and the powerful emotions it evokes almost invariably make acceptance of AAC interventions a gradual process with intermittent, if not frequent, relapses. The loss, or potential loss, of speech as the primary means of communication is emotionally very significant. Sensitivity on the part of professionals and many adjustments on the part of the person with TBI and those in his or her environment are necessary to move toward acceptance of AAC.

Sometimes people react to the introduction of AAC with anger and resentment. These feelings can be manifested in a "slay the messenger" attitude directed at the clinician for introducing AAC options and the underlying implication that speech is not a viable option. Persistence, patience, and an understanding of the emotional pathology can be powerful tools in a clinician's arsenal when faced with such a situation. Indeed, clinicians may find themselves counseling families and survivors. Ultimately, the proper time to implement and withdraw AAC interventions is a clinical judgment call.

Awareness of the grieving and adjustment process and the challenges associated with proposing AAC interventions can help to minimize frustration for clinicians. Providing general information as people request it is often helpful; in this way, survivors and family members can digest and assimilate information at a palatable rate. Similarly, clinicians may find it helpful to enlist survivors and family members as co-diagnosticians and as active members in the process when exploring communication options. The perspective provided by significant others can be invaluable in the therapy process, and, by involving survivors and family members in the decision-making process, they often feel more invested in assessment and treatment programs.

Speech Recovery

The return of natural speech may be possible for some survivors of TBI, but its restitution may not occur for a protracted period of time. For some survivors, a period of posttraumatic mutism (the inability to produce any vocalization) occurs after they emerge from coma (see Chapter 7). This period may last for a few days or may last indefinitely. Fortunately, a relatively small number of survivors experience extended periods of mutism; for the remainder, mutism is a temporary stage during the speech recovery process (Dongilli, Hakel, & Beukelman, 1992; Ladtkow & Culp, 1992; Levin et al., 1983). During the period of mutism, functional personal communication and the relearning of specific communication skills are pivotal components of the rehabilitation process. Clinicians must advocate for AAC interventions to reestablish, as soon as possible, functional communication (DeRuyter & Becker, 1988).

Once mutism resolves, survivors may experience other types of motor speech challenges such as dysarthria, apraxia, or neurogenic stuttering (see Chapter 7). Yorkston, Honsinger, Mitsuda, and Hammen (1989) reported that 10% of adult TBI outpatients receiving treatment following a period of inpatient therapy continued to have nonfunctional communication secondary to motor speech disorders. Although these challenges can occur as additions to cognitive or linguistic deficits impairing communicative functioning, the present focus will be solely on disruptions to speech production; the use of AAC and AT strategies and devices to address cognitive limitations will be addressed in a later section of this chapter. The following sections describe a variety of AAC and AT strategies and

How does the grieving process associated with loss of natural speech ability relate to the grieving process associated with death?

People with TBI and their families may go through a grieving process with respect to the loss of the ability to communicate by natural speech. This grieving process is similar to that encountered when dealing with other types of loss and can entail one or more of the five stages of grief outlined by Kubler-Ross (1969): denial, anger, bargaining, depression, and acceptance. The major difference between grieving speech loss and grieving death concerns the certainty of the outcome and the period of time over which the process occurs. With death, an endpoint exists; with the loss of natural speech, survivors of TBI and their families must struggle with not knowing whether recovery will occur—either in part or in full—and what the time frame is for the recovery process. In addition, survivors and their families must deal with multiple losses (e.g., physical disabilities, sensory losses, changes in interpersonal relationships, changes in vocational aspirations), so several grieving processes may exist simultaneously.

devices to assist individuals in maximizing their communication potential during various stages of recovery. To assist in this, Hagen's five stages of dependence and independence concerning the recovery of communicative functions provide a framework (C. Hagen, personal communication, 1999). These stages include the following:

- Unable Communicators—persons with severe communication disorders who cannot communicate through verbal or nonverbal modalities.

- Assisted Communicators—persons who can communicate only when a listener is present who is familiar enough with them to understand the meaning of idiosyncratic forms of communication (e.g., speech sounds, gestures, communication boards, facial expressions).

- Limited Communicators—persons who can communicate verbally or through the use of technology using single words, phrases, or simple sentences. In some cases, individuals have challenges in organization or problem solving that make supervision necessary.

- Limited Community Communicators—persons who are functional communicators in familiar and nonstressful environments that provide allowances for slowed information processing and/or verbal language deficits.

- Community Communicators—persons who communicate with ease as speakers or listeners and in all settings.

The concept of listener co-construction of messages (Stuart, Lasker, & Beukelman, 2000) serves to broaden Hagen's framework by incorpo-

What is the difference between being mute and being nonspeaking?

Mutism implies that a person cannot produce any vocalizations. In contrast, nonspeaking implies that a person cannot produce words with sufficient intelligibility for others to understand consistently. Because a person who is mute is, by definition, also nonspeaking, some professionals use the terms interchangeably. However, for the purpose of this chapter, the terms retain their distinct meanings.

rating the notion that listeners or conversation partners can play an active role in the communication process by helping to construct a speaker's message. Survivors displaying communication behaviors consistent with the first four stages of recovery rely on listener co-construction of messages to varying degrees. For *unable communicators*, listeners are likely to co-construct the majority of messages because of the survivors' inability to communicate through conventional means. Listeners or communication partners must interpret any gesture, vocalization, or movement that may have communicative intent. The more familiar a communication partner is with the survivor, the greater the accuracy of his or her interpretation. *Assisted communicators* also rely heavily on listener co-construction of messages. A survivor in this stage has more communication options than unable communicators, but the partner still interprets and completes the majority of communicative attempts. In addition, the partner attempts to repair frequent communication breakdowns.

As survivors progress to the level of *limited communicators*, they demonstrate more skill in conveying messages, but organizational problems that can hinder communication persist. Listeners must be careful to allow the survivor as much independence as possible without compromising the communication process; however, communication breakdowns continue to be frequent. Co-construction techniques that are particularly useful at this stage involve reviewing and fine-tuning survivors' message intents to minimize breakdowns and confusion. Finally, *limited community communicators* benefit from listener co-construction of messages during stressful or unfamiliar situations. Because people at this stage are independent communicators in some situations, the level of listener co-construction is considerably lower than in previous stages; however, conversational repair is still a necessity on some occasions, and listeners must still assume an active role in the communication process.

AAC and AT Strategies During Recovery Stages

Unable Communicators

Usually, the reason for a survivor of TBI being mute or nonspeaking is either (a) low levels of arousal, alertness, or responsiveness secondary to cognitive dysfunction or (b) persistent motor deficits across functions necessary to support speech (i.e., respiration, phonation, articulation, and resonance). Individuals who are unable communicators because of low levels of arousal are typically in Levels I to III of the Rancho Los Amigos Levels of Cognitive Functioning (Hagen, 2000; see Appendix 5.B in Chapter 5). Because of the extent of cognitive deficits during this early period of recovery, temporary AAC and AT interventions are common. In contrast, individuals who are unable communicators because of persistent *motor deficits* can be at any stage of cognitive functioning on the Rancho Levels and are in need of long-term or permanent AAC and AT interventions. For both groups, the most frequently used AAC and AT techniques and strategies include systems for indicating yes or no responses, single-switch devices for controlling electronic equipment, and eye gaze communication systems (see the later case example on intervention for a person with locked-in syndrome).

Yes or No Systems. Yes or no systems are typically one of the first means by which a survivor can convey basic needs and respond to questions. The systems are among the most basic of AAC strategies because they do not involve any technology, instead relying on a movement that the person can execute reliably and consistently. The most common yes or no systems use eye blinks (e.g., one blink for "yes" and two blinks for "no"), head nods and shakes, or hand squeezes (e.g., one squeeze for "yes" and two squeezes for "no"). People with severe motor control deficits that prevent use of these systems may use less common and more idiosyncratic systems such as opening the mouth to indicate "yes" and keeping it closed to indicate "no."

Two critical elements must be in place to ensure the success of a yes or no system. First, the survivor must be able to produce the specified motor response consistently and reliably. Second, the communication partner must pose only yes or no questions; a mute or nonspeaking person relying solely on a yes or no system for communication cannot answer questions that require description, reasoning, or elaboration.

Single-Switch Devices. Low technology systems—such as single-switch loop tapes—are another early AAC intervention with survivors of TBI. These systems are often helpful in stimulating arousal (see Chapter 5). For example, the survivor can gain access to auditory material—such as music, a favorite comedian, or a simple message—by repeatedly activating a switch connected to an auditory playback system. Selection and placement of an appropriate type of switch is dependent on identification of a body site over which a survivor has reliable and consistent motor control.

Although single-switch devices are deceptively simple, they can fulfill an important role in the rehabilitation process. First, they support reestablishment of basic cause–effect relations. Second, they provide an introduction to low-level technological interventions, including the use of switches to facilitate interaction. Third, they promote the use of familiar and favored auditory stimuli that can have a soothing, yet gently stimulating, effect on a survivor.

Eye Gaze Systems. Another type of intervention for persons who are unable communicators is the use of eye gaze communication systems that rely heavily on communication partners' interpretations based on the eye gaze behaviors of people with TBI. In many situations, the system is formalized only to the extent that people in the environment know that the survivor communicates by looking in the direction of desired items or persons. The mute or nonspeaking person conveys the topic of conversation, and the communication partner co-constructs the message by assigning words to accompany and verify the visual signal.

More sophisticated eye gaze communication systems involve transfer of linguistically coded information through the visual channel. These systems—often referred to as *eye transfer communication systems* or *e-tran*—provide a means of communication that, although bulky, is relatively precise. Typically, an e-tran system includes a Plexiglas frame situated in front of a user, in the middle of which is a circular or rectangular hole through which the user and conversational partner can establish eye contact (see Figure 8.1). On the Plexiglas are symbols for communication—either alphabetic, pictorial, or a combination of the two.

In e-tran's simplest form, the user gazes at the target symbol or letter, and the communication partner "reads" the message. To facilitate use of the system, the arrangement displayed for the user is commonly duplicated on the communication partner's side of the Plexiglas. Although communication transfer is slow, it can nonetheless be quite accurate, and the system provides the user with relative control over his or her communication.

More complicated e-tran systems require partner-assisted scanning in which the communication partner must scan through exemplars within an area of the display frame or within a given category of semantically related exemplars. For example, an e-tran system may have a number of pictures or symbols grouped together in one region of the display frame. The role of the communication partner is to verbalize the options, while the survivor uses a yes or no response to indicate when the communication partner has reached the desired target. In this way, the e-tran user establishes the general topic of conversation, and the communication partner determines the specific communication target. For example, a user may visually scan pictures of leisure activities and the communication partner verbally labels each option in sequence (e.g., music, television, outside activities) as the user's gaze passes over them. For users who need extensive selection sets, the system can incorporate multiple coding systems. For instance, color or numeric coding can support categorization by topic or by part of speech, depending on the abilities and preferences of the user.

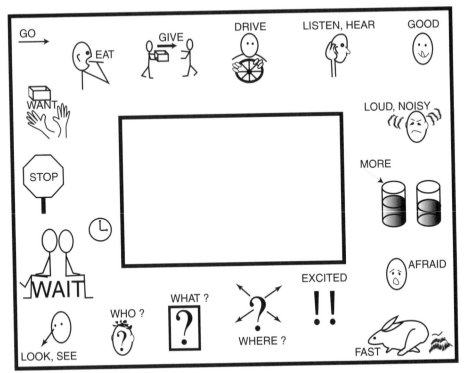

Figure 8.1. Example of an e-tran system.

Assisted Communicators

AAC strategies and devices typically used with assisted communicators include basic *communication boards* and simple *voice output communication aids* (VOCAs). Persons at this level need considerable support with virtually all communication tasks. Due to heavy reliance on listener co-construction of messages at this stage, the chosen communication system must be easy to implement. Similarly, the constant need for interpretation by familiar listeners mandates that any AAC system lend itself to ready adaptation to a variety of conversational needs.

Basic Communication Boards. Basic communication boards are displays that provide graphic representations (i.e., pictures, symbols, or letters) of frequently needed words, phrases, or concepts. Boards are arranged to be convenient for individual users. For example, display items can be arranged horizontally, vertically, in an arc, or in some combination thereof to facilitate physical and visual access. Because inclusion of personally relevant items can provide motivation

Case Example: AAC Intervention for a Person with Locked-in Syndrome

Tom was 22 years old when he sustained a severe TBI as a result of a fall at work. He was comatose for 3 weeks and minimally responsive for another 8 months. Despite regaining consistent arousal and awareness after that point, Tom remained mute and unable to perform volitional body movements. As the extent of his physical disability became apparent, Tom was diagnosed with locked-in syndrome. The only volitional control he had over body movements was opening and closing his eyes and jaw. However, despite this devastating motor impairment, Tom's cognitive functioning was relatively intact. He responded to humor and sarcasm and enjoyed listening to conversations about current events.

Tom's first communication system was to use eye blinks to provide yes or no responses. Although this provided a way to respond to questions posed by others, it did not give Tom any means of initiating communication or picking his own topics of conversation. Likewise, e-tran systems did not provide Tom with sufficient freedom to express the extent of his thoughts and communicative intents. To address this dilemma, Tom's speech–language pathologist provided him with an alphabet display and a dry erase board. The alphabet display included four rows of letters organized according to their frequency of use in English—that is, the most commonly used letters (i.e., S, R, T, E, A, O) appeared in the top row and the least commonly used letters (i.e., Z, X, V, Q) appeared in the bottom row. After considerable training with Tom, his family, and caregivers, Tom learned to use the alphabet display to spell words letter by letter. Jaw opening to indicate "yes" and no movement to indicate "no" was Tom's most reliable means of selecting letters as a communication partner first listed letter rows and then individual letters within a row to spell each word. As Tom confirmed letter choices, his communication partner wrote them on the dry erase board. Although the process was slow, Tom finally had a means of expressing his thoughts and engaging in communicative interactions with others.

for using a communication board, family members and survivors often play pivotal roles in determining the display content.

Simple Voice Output Communication Aids (VOCAs). VOCAs are dedicated AAC devices that support face-to-face communication. They typically range from very simple devices with limited messaging capability to highly sophisticated devices with nearly limitless messaging capacity. VOCAs support communication by providing a synthetic voice (i.e., synthesized speech) or by speaking messages that have been recorded onto them (i.e., digitized speech). Each VOCA is different in terms of the number of messages it can support, the type of voice output it uses, the type of selection set and representation set it supports, the type of display it has, and its portability and cosmesis. Table 8.4 defines some of the common terminology associated with VOCAs.

Table 8.5 provides a summary of some of the AAC systems commonly used by TBI survivors. Features of systems frequently used with persons who are assisted communicators are notable for their simplicity. Systems are typically limited with respect to number of communication targets and the accessing methods.

Limited Communicator

For limited communicators, those persons at the next stage of Hagen's (C. Hagen, personal communication, 1999) hierarchy, the AAC choices may include some of the options outlined in Table 8.5 as well as some of those listed in Table 8.6. When options from Table 8.5 are selected, they are used with a higher number of targets and a more sophisticated type of representation.

Limited Community Communicator

For survivors of TBI who are limited community communicators, AAC systems may include some of those used by assisted communicators and limited communicators as well as more sophisticated systems such as those listed in Table 8.7. Systems used at this stage tend to be conventional and to rely minimally on listener interpretation. Communication often consists of phrase-length and sentence-length utterances.

Communicators at this level and beyond can utilize strategies such as alphabet supplementation and topic cues in addition to other AAC techniques and devices. To perform *alphabet supplementation*, the speaker points to the first letter of a word as he or she verbalizes it (Beukelman & Yorkston, 1977). This assists the listener in understanding intended words as well as providing the speaker with a mechanism to facilitate slowing the rate of speech. Alphabet supplementation requires a survivor to have relatively intact spelling skills and sufficient metacognitive ability to recognize appropriate times to invoke the strategy. While alphabet supplementation is used *during* communicative exchanges, topic cues are provided *prior* to a communication exchange. With *topic cues*, the speaker typically points to one of several topic words or pictures on a communication board to provide context for the conversation for lis-

Table 8.4

Terminology Associated with VOCAs

Feature	Definition
Portability	Extent and ease with which a user can transport a device from place to place
Cosmesis	Aesthetic appeal
Adaptability	Extent to which a device supports alternate means of access
LED	Light-emitting diode: The light on a device that often accompanies selection of a target; potential targets light up on devices that support item prediction
Display type	
LCD	Liquid crystal display: Type of display on which letters or symbols appear to the user and sometimes to the conversation partner
Dynamic	Display that supports changes of the selection set when activated or whose indicator changes after each selection
Fixed	Display that has symbols affixed to a specific surface and are invariant with respect to location
Representation set	The way in which words, ideas, and concepts are depicted on an AAC system, and the symbols, pictures, and so on, that comprise the "language" of the AAC user
Selection set	The actual array of choices available on a system; typically more limited on systems with fixed/static displays than on systems with dynamic displays
Overlay	A template used to arrange the symbols, letters, or words; usually comprised of a grid (e.g., 4 × 8, 4 × 12), although locations can be sized according to need

teners (Hustad & Beukelman, 2000). Common topics include recreation, family, friends, medical issues, home life, vacations, and hospital/rehabilitation activities.

Community Communicator

Some community communicators rely solely on natural speech, but others are totally or partially dependent on AAC to meet their communication needs. When AAC systems serve as the primary means of communication, community communicators maximally exploit system capabilities (as illustrated in the case

Table 8.5

Examples of AAC Systems for Assisted Communicators

AAC System	Features
BigMac[a]	Single message output system
	Supports digitized speech
	Easily programmable
Message Mate[b]	Direct access or scanning[c]
	Digitized speech
	Stores up to 40 messages
Communication boards	Limited number of targets
	Representational sets may include photos, line drawings, and traditional orthography
	May contain multiple pages
Gestural communication	Often idiosyncratic gestures
	Comprehension is highly dependent on listener familiarity

[a]Available from AbleNet, Inc., 1081 10th Avenue, SE, Minneapolis, MN 55414.
[b]Available from Words+, Inc., 40015 Sierra Highway, Building B-145, Palmdale, CA 93550.
[c]One- and two-switch scanning available.

example on AAC intervention for a community communicator). For example, the survivor may employ all available levels of a device, use many of the memory features, and generate novel messages using orthography. Similarly, a survivor at this level who uses a multipurpose or integrated system will likely use it in a skilled and competent way for both spoken and written communication. Because survivors of TBI who are community communicators are skilled in each of the four tenets of communicative competence outlined by Light (1989)—linguistic competence, operational competence, social competence, and strategic competence—they function independently with respect to communication in virtually all situations. The survivor requires minimal or no listener co-construction of messages or cueing to repair communication breakdowns.

Recovery of Memory

The construct of memory is integral to a discussion of recovery from TBI. The status of memory functioning following TBI affects AAC and AT in two ways. First, survivors with substantial memory deficits need compensatory systems

Table 8.6
Examples of AAC Systems for
Limited Communicators

AAC System	Features
Lightwriter SL-35[a]	Portable
	Supports spelling (unlimited novel message generation)
	Stores up to 26 messages in memory (240 characters in length each)
	10 DecTalk voices
	Dual-sided screen
Alphatalker[a]	Icon-based communication system
	Digitized and synthesized voices
	Supports alternate accessing system
	Cells large enough to support picture-based communication
	48 target cells
	Rate enhancement features
DeltaTalker[a]	Icon-based communication system
	Rate enhancement features
	Digitized and synthesized speech
	128 target cells
Canon Communicator[b]	Primarily a print output device
	Supports limited number of digitized messages
	Memory for at least 26 phrases for print output
	Highly portable, cosmetically appealing device
Simple writing systems	Canon Communicator
	Magic slates, white boards
	Computers with basic word-processing software
Voice amplification	Systems to amplify voice
	Most systems do not attenuate dysarthric speech, but newer ones may

[a]Available from Prentke-Romich Company, 1022 Heyl Road, Wooster, OH 44691.
[b]Available from Canon Information Technology Services, P.O. Box 2338, Chesapeake, VA 23327.

Table 8.7
Examples of AAC Systems for
Limited Community Communicators

AAC System	Features
Dynavox, Dynamyte[a]	Dynamic display device
	Symbol-based communication system
	10 DecTalk voices
	Highly customizable and programmable
Multipurpose/Integrated systems	Computer-based systems used for written and face-to-face communication
	Careful software selection is critical for successful implementation
	Considerations such as weight, access, screen matrix type, voice, and battery life are important
Multimodal systems	Combine aspects of speech and AAC/AT as needed
	Invocation of different modes of communication is often contextually bound and situation specific
	AAC strategies include but are not limited to use of gestures, body language, communication displays, and alphabet supplementation
Low technology backup	All AAC users must have a reliable low technology backup system (e.g., communication display or notebook) for use when their AAC system is not available

[a]Available from Dynavox Systems, LLC, 2100 Wharton Street, Suite 400, Pittsburgh, PA 15203.

to facilitate learning and participation in daily activities. AT directed at compensating for memory deficits makes a crucial contribution to academic, vocational, and community reintegration processes. Second, the memory challenges of survivors with communication deficits requiring the support of AAC strategies affect the extent to which such systems can be implemented successfully. The following sections provide information about (a) the use of AT to compensate for memory deficits and (b) the effect of memory impairments on the implementation of AAC systems.

Case Example: AAC Intervention for a Community Communicator

Marilyn was a vivacious and attractive 28-year-old woman when both she and her husband were involved in a serious car accident: A truck broadsided their car as they were on their way home from visiting family. An ambulance rushed Marilyn to the hospital from the scene where she had lost consciousness and had sustained facial and bodily injuries. Marilyn remained in a coma for 3 weeks. Once she regained consciousness and was medically stable, she began rehabilitation. Marilyn remained hospitalized for almost 1 year after the accident.

By nature quite outspoken, Marilyn could not speak at all after the accident. After first regaining consciousness, she used eye blinks to communicate "yes" and "no." As she progressed cognitively and physically, Marilyn and her speech–language pathologists discovered that her spelling skills were intact, and she began communicating by typing on a laptop computer. Using her dominant right hand, Marilyn typed messages using all five fingers; use of her left hand was limited to performance of two key operations such as shifting. She used commercially available word-processing software and exploited the speaking capabilities of the computer as a rudimentary voice output device.

As Marilyn's status improved and she became increasingly mobile, she found that her laptop computer was cumbersome and detracted from her independence. She wanted a device that allowed her to type messages but was more portable and had a better quality voice than her laptop computer. She saw an occupational therapist and a speech–language pathologist for a complete AAC assessment to explore options for face-to-face communication.

After exploring several devices that were portable and supported direct selection as a means of accessing orthography, Marilyn chose the LightWRITER® SL-35 because of the dual-sided screen, the quality of the female voice, and the unit's cosmesis. The device was obtained, and training in its use was provided both to Marilyn and her husband. At her last visit, Marilyn enthusiastically typed, "I love it!" She had independently stored messages in the memory and had discovered some of the features that had not been shown to her.

This device fit Marilyn's needs at the time at which she obtained it. However, as her abilities continued to improve with ongoing rehabilitation, additional issues arose. Specifically, Marilyn needed counseling to deal with balancing her reliance on a VOCA with her ongoing, but slow, improvement in regaining natural speech. As her independence increased, her AAC needs shifted—sometimes increasing and sometimes decreasing. Also, Marilyn needed ongoing technical maintenance of her AAC device.

Compensating for Memory Deficits

Memory aids for survivors of TBI include many commonly used and commercially available items such as calendars, journals, logs, daily planners, and maps. Many of these are tools that noninjured people use to organize and streamline their daily tasks and routines. The distinction between how noninjured people and people with TBI use such memory aids is in their level of dependence on the tools and their need for direct training to use them effectively.

A common type of memory aid is a *memory book* (sometimes referred to as a memory prosthesis). A memory book can supplement extant memory. Several groups of researchers have documented the effectiveness of memory books to facilitate performance of everyday activities by survivors of TBI with memory deficits ranging from mild to severe (Burke, Danick, Bemis, & Durgin, 1994; Carney et al., 1999; Cicerone et al., 2000; Schmitter-Edgecombe, Fahy, Whelan, & Long, 1995; Sohlberg & Mateer, 1989; Zencius, Wesolowski, & Burke, 1990). Professionals have found that they can enhance survivors' acceptance of memory books by addressing psychosocial issues (e.g., family support, team "buy-in" to system use) and by using commercially available items that do not stigmatize and that are aesthetically appealing (Fluharty & Priddy, 1993). This is consistent with Wolfensberger's "normalization principle," which encourages "the utilization of means which are as culturally normative as possible, in order to establish and/or maintain external behaviors and characteristics which are as culturally normative as possible" (as cited in Fluharty & Priddy, 1993, p. 85).

A recently developed alternative to memory books is the use of electronic organizers. Given the popularity of electronic organizers among the general population, the fact that their cost will likely come down over time, and their normal appearance, this is a memory aid option worthy of consideration. However, as with any technical system, professionals must carefully balance the needs and capabilities of survivors with system features and requirements. Electronic organizers do not provide the same versatility that memory books do in terms of level of complexity and accommodation of limitations relating to cognitive and physical access.

Both professionals and family members tend to exert considerable pressure on survivors to use memory aids. Despite this pressure, the literature supports selective implementation. Studies have shown that specific features of the training protocols used to encourage device use influence the effectiveness of memory aids. Specifically, Fluharty and Priddy (1993) reported a case study in which a survivor more readily accepted a commercially available memory aid when the training stressed the unobtrusiveness of the memory aid and the frequency with which other people use similar systems. Burke and his colleagues (1994) reported that the customization of a memory book—with survivors as active participants in the customization process—helped the survivor view the book as an aid to independence rather than as a prosthetic device. Burke and colleagues also highlighted the advantage of involving persons from the discharge environment when implementing memory aids to serve two functions: (a) to enhance their familiarity with the aid and with the survivor's use of it and (b) to facilitate transfer from the therapeutic to the discharge environment.

The type of memory required to perform various training protocols varies. Donaghy and Williams (1998) reported on a training protocol that capitalizes on three residual cognitive strengths of survivors of TBI: immediate attention, procedural memory, and reliance on old learning. By combining these skills in a five-level training protocol emphasizing procedural memory, Donaghy and Williams demonstrated that individuals with severe memory impairments can successfully use individualized memory books. Similarly, Sohlberg and Mateer (1989) reported on a training process emphasizing procedural memory and automaticity. The training procedure includes three phases critical for mastering new skills—acquisition, application, and adaptation—and an efficiency building component to ensure that skills are learned sufficiently for survivors to use them automatically.

Effects of Memory Impairment on Learning and Implementing AAC and AT Systems

Survivors of TBI often have difficulty using any but the most rudimentary, low-technology AAC and AT systems until the resolution of posttraumatic amnesia (see Chapter 5). After emerging from posttraumatic amnesia, persistent anterograde amnesia is the memory impairment that has the most deleterious effect on the learning and use of AAC and AT systems. However, despite this amnesia, survivors can successfully implement strategies and devices if professionals provide compensatory strategies involving strong visual cueing and if they select very simple systems for initial mastery. Implementation of even rudimentary systems can facilitate survivors' level of attention, use of language, and participation in therapy.

Memory impairments other than anterograde amnesia also negatively affect learning and mastery of AAC and AT systems. Strengths and challenges in procedural memory, short-term memory, long-term memory, metamemory, and prospective memory interact in different permutations to influence survivors' success with various systems. For example, short-term memory impairment may negate the possibility of using abbreviation expansion with VOCAs—a strategy that relies on the user inputting short codes or abbreviations to retrieve longer messages. Similarly, prospective memory impairment may preclude a user from planning for a communication event for which preprogrammed messages may be appropriate; impairment of metamemory may detract from a user's ability to plan appropriately for using an AAC system by remembering to charge the system, add words to a display, or select appropriate messages given a conversational context.

Despite the deleterious effects of memory impairments on the use of AAC and AT tools, people with TBI can benefit substantially from the incorporation of such systems into an integrated treatment program. The use of low technology AAC and AT interventions with survivors of TBI has a long history (Ladtkow & Culp, 1992). Of particular importance is the use of devices that can function in the hybrid role of memory aid and communication device. For example, memory books can facilitate communication by providing users with an array of conversational topics. Similarly, simple communication notebooks or boards arranged by topic can serve as memory prompts for participation in daily events. The mere act of carrying a memory book or AAC system can be a potent reminder to engage with the tool and, as such, can serve both as a memory and communication prosthesis.

Recovery of Literacy

The recovery of reading and writing skills follows much the same trajectory as recovery of face-to-face communication. TBI sustained in adolescence and beyond may impinge on literacy skills already developed and automatized to some degree. In contrast, TBI in very young children may predate the acquisition of literacy skills, and this necessitates special considerations; depending on a child's educational program, introduction to traditional orthography may follow a typical trajectory that involves paper-and-pencil tasks and multisensory approaches, or, for a child with physical and cognitive impairments, the acquisition of literacy skills may be totally dependent on AT—the child may use a computer and specialized software for all of his or her writing needs (see the case example on ACC-supported literacy intervention).

Programs Supporting Reading and Writing

Differences exist between the reading skills of individuals who sustain injuries prior to the acquisition of literacy and those who sustain injuries later in development. In addition to group differences related to injury severity, Ewing-Cobbs, Fletcher, Levin, Iovino, and Miner (1998) found that children injured in early stages of literacy development achieved significantly lower reading recog-

Case Example: AAC-Supported Literacy Intervention

Kaitlin sustained brain damage from Shaken Baby Syndrome. Prior to age 2 years 3 months, her development had been entirely normal. Following violent shaking at the hands of her birth mother, Kaitlin was hospitalized with a moderate to severe TBI. Reports indicated that she did not lose consciousness at the time of injury but became listless, agitated, and cried inconsolably. The extent of her injury was initially unclear; only later did it become obvious that she had a dense right hemiplegia, left hemiparesis, severely delayed expressive language development, visual impairment, and motor speech deficits.

Kaitlin entered daycare when she was 4 years old. A petite girl with long hair and short bangs, she sat in a wheelchair with an attached tray table. She scanned the busy preschool environment and reached out to both children and adults with her left hand.

Kaitlin's vocalizations consisted of undifferentiated vowel sounds, a high-pitched squeal to indicate pleasure and delight, and attempts to approximate familiar monosyllabic words (e.g., *eat, drink, sing*). She had been exposed to black-and-white line drawings as well as color-enhanced Picture Communication Symbols (Mayer-Johnson™) for communication. She had a limited display on her tray and requested activities when prompted to do so. Kaitlin loved music and hummed along with familiar tunes. Her teacher encouraged her to sing the alphabet song, and, as her familiarity increased, Kaitlin first mouthed and then whispered individual letters when cued. In addition, Kaitlin enjoyed listening to stories and looking at the accompanying pictures. She played with large plastic letters when they were presented to her, but this play had little to do with literacy.

As she neared school age, the delay in Kaitlin's oral language development impinged on the development of her written language and literacy. What was needed was intervention to augment both Kaitlin's face-to-face and written communication. Because of her severe communication limitations, hemiplegia, and compromised visual status, Kaitlin needed alternative access and specialized software to interact with a computer. Her teachers determined that software supporting large print, auditory read-back of text, and graphics to accompany written words was most appealing to Kaitlin. An added benefit of the software was that it supported customizable features. Over time, Kaitlin's teachers and family realized that the combination of print and auditory read-back was facilitating Kaitlin's face-to-face communication as evidenced by her tendency to imitate words and phrases as they were read to her by the computer.

nition, spelling, and arithmetic scores following injury than children injured during later stages of development. The researchers concluded that skills in a rapid stage of development were more vulnerable to disruption or dissolution by neurological insult than more well-established skills. This conclusion confirmed the finding of Shaffer, Bijur, Chadwick, and Rutter (1980) who reported that children less than 8 years of age with histories of coma and cortical injury experienced a higher prevalence of reading disorders than did their older counterparts. Hence, literacy skills are more vulnerable to injuries sustained during elementary school years than ones sustained during adolescence or adulthood.

Reading comprehension develops more slowly than word decoding skills and, therefore, is particularly susceptible to disruption from injuries sustained during childhood. Barnes, Dennis, and Wilkinson (1999) reported two findings regarding reading comprehension following TBI: (a) Children injured prior to age 6.5 years experienced more difficulty with word decoding and reading comprehension than children who sustained injuries in the early primary grades, and (b) children who sustained injuries during early primary grades were at greater risk for reading comprehension difficulties than children injured in late primary grades.

All of these findings about literacy development and recovery following TBI support the general notion that survivors struggle more with new learning than with relearning of previously mastered skills. However, individuals who sustain injuries after having acquired normal literacy skills still may experience multiple challenges associated with reading and writing tasks. For these individuals, decoding words, comprehending short and relatively simple reading passages, and writing individual words or short sentences may be minimally impaired; however, performance of literacy tasks requiring a high level of organization and integration of information—such as those typically required in high school and college—may be lacking.

Commercially available programs to support written communication may be of interest both for young children who sustain injuries prior to the acquisition of literacy skills and for adolescents and adults who sustain injuries after becoming literate. However, careful evaluation of programs to determine whether they meet educational and vocational needs—as opposed to merely recreational needs—is a necessity. As a guide, Hunt-Berg, Rankin, and Beukelman (1994) recommended evaluation of several aspects of literacy software when considering its use by children with special needs. Their recommendations of particular relevance to survivors of TBI include those related to speech output for auditory read-back of text, spell checking and spelling assistance, word cueing and prediction, organizational assistance, and grammatical assistance. Predictably, attention to a survivor's physical, cognitive, and visual status is necessary when previewing software.

Features such as grammar and spell checking are commonly available in word processing software packages and can be useful tools in supporting the writing needs of survivors of TBI. More specialized features—such as word prediction, linguistic prediction, and abbreviation expansion—can increase a survivor's speed of communication. Other specialized features—such as auditory read-back of text—can facilitate attention to the details of message construction and content. Ancillary programs may assist people with TBI in their organization of written information and in their use of calendar functions. In a similar vein, magnification programs provide assistance for users with acuity and/or perceptual deficits that make typical screen layouts difficult to handle visually. Finally, some literacy and word processing software, as well as much dedicated software, supports cognitive retraining. Lynch (1998) provides a thorough review of this subject.

Alternate Accessing Systems

When a survivor has physical limitations, alternate computer access may need to be explored. Options include many of those identified in the section on natural speech recovery, such as indirect accessing via scanning or voice input. In addition, specialized software can support alternate accessing via (a) customization of the rate of text and graphics presentation, (b) inclusion of auditory feedback (e.g., for letters, words, or phrases), (c) customization of on-screen keyboards, and (d) the ability to interface with different types of switches. Again, careful assessment by a team of specialists is necessary to ensure that evaluation of physical, cognitive, visual, and communicative aspects of a survivor's profile is complete. Designated team members then need to determine accessing options that meet the survivor's needs. The decision-making process regarding AAC and AT systems in general, and accessing options in particular, needs to be driven by software demands; otherwise, the hardware and method of access may be incompatible with the software required. Whenever necessary, professionals should seek help from technological experts during the exploration of options for a written communication system.

For individuals who have difficulty using direct or traditional indirect methods of access, *speech recognition technology* may provide another option (see the following case example on speech recognition technology). Speech recognition is a technology whose use is fairly widespread in terms of the general public and has been gaining popularity in the disabled community (e.g., for people with carpal tunnel syndrome). However, the application of speech recognition technology to persons with communication disorders is a relatively recent development. Preliminary research shows that at least some individuals who can

Case Example: Speech Recognition Technology

Laura was a talented and popular high school student until a car accident in the middle of her junior year resulted in severe TBI. Although she returned to school 8 months after the accident, she still had weakness on her right side, balance problems, tremors in both arms, ataxic dysarthria, and cognitive deficits. An additional year of therapy, medication, and individualized academic instruction failed to alleviate her physical and cognitive impairments. Laura's hopes of attending college were dwindling, primarily because her motor impairments impeded timely completion of written assignments.

In an attempt to compensate for her right hemiparesis, Laura had begun using her nondominant left hand to learn one-handed typing while still in high school. The tremors in her left hand, however, prevented her from excelling with this method, and, after several months of training, her typing speed was no better than 10 to 12 words per minute. Frustrated with her lack of progress, Laura entered a research program 18 months after injury to explore the use of speech recognition technology as an alternative means of access. The major concern of the researchers was whether a speech recognition system could be trained to understand Laura's breathy and inconsistent voice and imprecise articulation.

During the next several months, Laura worked with three speech recognition systems, two of which used discrete speech production and one of which used continuous speech production. Her preference was for the continuous speech system, Dragon NaturallySpeaking. After multiple training sessions, the system achieved a recognition accuracy rate of approximately 80% when Laura read prepared sentences or when she generated novel sentences. Although this accuracy level was not equal to that achieved by nondysarthric speakers and required many corrections of misinterpreted words and phrases, Laura reported satisfaction with the system. The decreased need to concentrate on controlling her hands reduced her fatigue when performing writing tasks sufficiently that she felt she could once again make plans to attend college.

speak but are dysarthric can use speech recognition as a method of input for written communication (Hux, Rankin-Erickson, Manasse, & Lauritzen, 2000; Manasse, Hux, & Rankin-Erickson, 2000; Rosen & Yampolsky, 2000; Thomas-Stonell, Kotler, Leeper, & Doyle, 1998). For speakers with dysarthria who also have motor impairments affecting use of their arms or hands, speech recognition technology can provide a primary or secondary point of interface for written communication. That is, speech recognition can be used as the only means of access or as an additional means of access implemented when fatigue becomes an issue.

Recent research suggests that certain system features require careful calibration to optimize the use of speech recognition technology by people with dysarthria (Rosen & Yampolsky, 2000), and the training time required for calibration is extended in most documented cases of implementation. One important component of implementation is the need to attend to vocal hygiene—an issue that is particularly important for persons with dysarthria (Manasse et al., 2000). As a result, a speech–language pathologist should always participate in the calibration and implementation of speech recognition with survivors of TBI who have dysarthria.

Although speech recognition technology undoubtedly confers unique advantages as a method of access because of its approximation of normalcy and because of its increasing use by nondisabled individuals, disregarding the cognitive complexity of this technology is a dangerous pitfall for those working with survivors of TBI. The high levels of metacognitive and metalinguistic awareness required by speech recognition technology effectively make cautious assessment indispensable when considering this type of system for people with TBI.

Summary

The AAC and AT needs of people with TBI are many and complex. The need for a professional team to address the AAC and AT needs of survivors is paramount, in terms of both assessment and treatment implementation. System selection, means of alternate access, the broad applicability of AAC and AT systems in the rehabilitation process, and the need for ongoing assessment as physical, cognitive, and linguistic recovery proceeds are all points that require attention. Restitution of communicative function across multiple levels of cognitive and communicative ability is a vital part of rehabilitation. Given this, AAC and AT interventions for survivors of TBI are critical and require attention through all stages of the recovery process.

References

Barnes, M. A., Dennis, M., & Wilkinson, M. (1999). Reading after closed head injury in child-hood: Effects on accuracy, fluency, and comprehension. *Developmental Neuropsychology*, 15(1), 1–24.

Beukelman, D. R., & Mirenda, P. (1998). *Augmentative and alternative communication: Management of severe communication disorders in children and adults*. Baltimore: Brookes.

Beukelman, D. R., & Yorkston, K. M. (1977). A communication system for the severely dysarthric speaker with an intact language system. *Journal of Speech and Hearing Disorders*, 42, 265–270.

Beukelman, D. R., Yorkston, K., & Dowden, P. A. (1985). *Communication augmentation: A casebook of clinical management*. San Diego, CA: College-Hill Press.

Burke, J. M., Danick, J. A., Bemis, B., & Durgin, C. J. (1994). A process approach to memory book training for neurological patients. *Brain Injury*, 8, 71–81.

Carney, N., Chestnut, R. M., Maynard, H., Mann, N. C., Patterson, P., & Hefland, M. (1999). Effect of cognitive rehabilitation on outcomes for persons with traumatic brain injury: A systematic review. *Journal of Head Trauma Rehabilitation*, 14, 277–307.

Church, G., & Glennen, S. (1992). *The handbook of assistive technology*. San Diego, CA: Singular.

Cicerone, K. D., Dahlberg, C., Kalmar, K., Langenbahn, D. M., Malec, J. F., Bergquist, T. F., Felicetti, T., Giancino, J. T., Harley, J. P., Harrington, D. E., Herzog, J., Kneipp, S., Laatsch, L., & Morse, P. A. (2000). Evidence-based cognitive rehabilitation: Recommendations for clinical practice. *Archives of Physical Medicine and Rehabilitation*, 81, 1596–1615.

DeRuyter, F., & Becker, M. R. (1988). Augmentative communication: Assessment, system selection, and usage. *Journal of Head Trauma Rehabilitation*, 3(2), 35–44.

Donaghy, S., & Williams, W. (1998). A new protocol for training severely impaired patients in the usage of memory journals. *Brain Injury*, 12, 1061–1076.

Dongilli, P. A., Hakel, M. E., & Beukelman, D. R. (1992). Recovery of functional speech following traumatic brain injury. *Journal of Head Trauma Rehabilitation*, 7(2), 91–101.

Ewing-Cobbs, L., Fletcher, J. M., Levin, H. S., Iovino, I., & Miner, M. E. (1998). Academic achievement and academic placement following traumatic brain injury in children and adolescents: A two-year longitudinal study. *Journal of Clinical and Experimental Neuropsychology*, 20, 769–781.

Fluharty, G., & Priddy, D. (1993). Methods of increasing client acceptance of a memory book. *Brain Injury*, 7(1), 85–88.

Glennen, S. L. (1997). Introduction to augmentative and alternative communication. In S. L. Glennen & D. C. DeCoste (Eds.), *Handbook of augmentative and alternative communication* (pp. 3–19). San Diego, CA: Singular.

Glennen, S. L., & DeCoste, D. C. (1997). *Handbook of augmentative and alternative communication*. San Diego, CA: Singular.

Hagen, C. (2000, February). *Rancho Los Amigos Levels of Cognitive Functioning–Revised*. Presentation at TBI Rehabilitation in a Managed Care Environment: An Interdisciplinary Approach to Rehabilitation, Continuing Education Programs of America, San Antonio, TX.

Hunt-Berg, M., Rankin, J. L., & Beukelman, D. R. (1994). Ponder the possibilities: Computer-supported writing for struggling writers. *Learning Disabilities Research and Practice*, 9, 169–178.

Hustad, K. C., & Beukelman, D. R. (2000). Integrating AAC strategies with natural speech in adults with chronic speech intelligibility challenges. In D. Beukelman, K. Yorkston, &

J. Reichle (Eds.), *Augmentative communication for adults with acquired neurologic disorders* (pp. 86–106). Baltimore: Brookes.

Hux, K., Rankin-Erickson, J. L., Manasse, N. J., & Lauritzen, E. (2000). Accuracy of three speech recognition systems: Case study of dysarthric speech. *Augmentative and Alternative Communication, 16*, 186–196.

Kubler-Ross, E. (1969). *On death and dying.* New York: Macmillan.

Ladtkow, M. C., & Culp, D. M. (1992). Augmentative communication with traumatic brain injury. In K. M. Yorkston (Ed.), *Augmentative communication in the medical setting* (pp. 139–243). Tucson, AZ: Communication Skill Builders.

Levin, H. S., Madison, C. F., Bailey, C. B., Meyers, C. A., Eisenberg, H. M., & Faustino, C. G. (1983). Mutism after closed head injury. *Archives of Neurology, 40*, 601–606.

Light, J. (1989). Toward a definition of communicative competence for individuals using augmentative and alternative communication systems. *Augmentative and Alternative Communication, 5*, 137–144.

Lynch, W. J. (1998). Software update 1998: Commercial programs useful in cognitive retraining. *Journal of Head Trauma Rehabilitation, 13*(5), 91–94.

Manasse, N. J., Hux, K., & Rankin-Erickson, J. L. (2000). Speech recognition training for enhancing written language generation by a traumatic brain injury survivor. *Brain Injury, 14*, 1015–1034.

Rosen, K., & Yampolsky, S. (2000). Automatic speech recognition and a review of its functioning with dysarthric speech. *Augmentative and Alternative Communication, 16*, 48–60.

Schmitter-Edgecombe, M., Fahy, J. F., Whelan, J. P., & Long, C. J. (1995). Memory remediation after severe closed head injury: Notebook training versus supportive therapy. *Journal of Consulting and Clinical Psychology, 63*, 484–489.

Shaffer, D., Bijur, P., Chadwick, O. F. D., & Rutter, M. L. (1980). Head injury and later reading disability. *Journal of the American Academy of Child Psychiatry, 19*, 562–610.

Sohlberg, M., & Mateer, C. (1989). Training use of compensatory memory books: A three-stage behavioral approach. *Journal of Clinical and Experimental Neuropsychology, 11*, 871–891.

Stuart, S., Lasker, J. P., & Beukelman, D. R. (2000). AAC message management. In D. R. Beukelman, K. M. Yorkston, & J. Reichle (Eds.), *Augmentative and alternative communication for adults with acquired neurologic disorders* (pp. 25–54). Baltimore: Brookes.

Thomas-Stonell, N., Kotler, A., Leeper, H. A., & Doyle, P. C. (1998). Computerized speech recognition: Influence of intelligibility and perceptual consistency on recognition accuracy. *Augmentative and Alternative Communication, 14*, 51–56.

Yorkston, K. M., Honsinger, M. J., Mitsuda, P. M., & Hammen, V. (1989). The relationship between speech and swallowing disorders in head-injured patients. *Journal of Head Trauma Rehabilitation, 4*(4), 1–16.

Zencius, A., Wesolowski, M. D., & Burke, W. H. (1990). A comparison of four memory strategies with traumatically brain-injured clients. *Brain Injury, 4*, 33–38.

Swallowing Disorders Associated with Traumatic Brain Injury

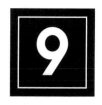

Nancy Manasse and Rebecca Burke

 Case Example: Acute Status

Chad and some other Navy Seals were training on parachute jumps. Once the plane reached the appropriate elevation, the men exited in an orderly and precise manner, parachutes packed tightly on their backs. After Chad jumped, another less-experienced Seal followed him; unfortunately, the other Seal did not allow enough time to pass between Chad and himself. As the second man began free-falling, his body ripped through Chad's parachute. Chad lost consciousness when the man's knee hit him in the head; he free-fell 3,000 feet to the ground.

The landing impact left Chad with multiple fractures, internal injuries, and a severe TBI. He remained in a vegetative state for several weeks, during which time a feeding tube was inserted to meet his nutritional needs. Even after Chad regained normal consciousness, he could not take any food or liquid by mouth for months. A speech–language pathologist helped Chad learn to implement exercises and compensatory strategies to increase the strength and range of motion of the muscles involved in swallowing.

Speech–language pathologists are the primary professionals responsible for addressing swallowing disorders. This chapter focuses on the speech–language pathologist's role in identifying and treating dysphagia (i.e., swallowing problems) secondary to TBI. The first section of the chapter provides an overview of normal and disordered swallowing processes, including information about alternative feeding methods. The second part details the assessment and treatment of swallowing problems associated with various stages of recovery from TBI and explores some ethical considerations.

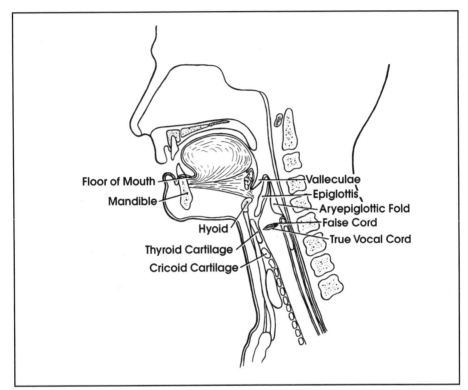

Figure 9.1. Side view of the oral and pharyngeal and associated anatomical structures of the adult. *Note.* From *Evaluation and Treatment of Swallowing Disorders* (p. 16), by J. A. Logemann, 1998, Austin, TX: PRO-ED. Copyright 1998 by PRO-ED. Reprinted with permission.

Overview of Normal and Disordered Swallowing

Speech–language pathologists must understand the processes involved in normal swallowing to understand abnormal swallow responses. Toward this end, Figure 9.1 provides a sagittal view of the oral and pharyngeal structures of the adult, and Figure 9.2 provides a sagittal view of the oral and pharyngeal structures of the infant. The anatomical structures associated with swallowing are identified and labeled in each. Size and structure are the predominant characteristics differentiating the anatomy of infants from adults (Arvedson, 1996; Siktberg & Bantz, 1999). During years 3 through 6, structural growth of the face and skull, enlargement of the oral and pharyngeal cavities, and descent of the larynx and hyoid bone occur. This, combined with improved mastication,

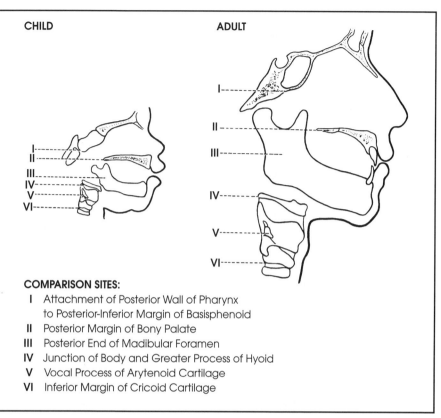

CHILD   ADULT

COMPARISON SITES:
  I   Attachment of Posterior Wall of Pharynx
      to Posterior-Inferior Margin of Basisphenoid
 II   Posterior Margin of Bony Palate
III   Posterior End of Madibular Foramen
 IV   Junction of Body and Greater Process of Hyoid
  V   Vocal Process of Arytenoid Cartilage
 VI   Inferior Margin of Cricoid Cartilage

Figure 9.2. Side view of the oral and pharyngeal and associated anatomical structures of the infant. *Note.* From *Evaluation and Treatment of Swallowing Disorders* (p. 38), by J. A. Logemann, 1998, Austin, TX: PRO-ED. Copyright 1998 by PRO-ED. Reprinted with permission.

results in a more mature swallowing process similar to that of the adult (Kramer & Eicher, 1993).

The adult swallow includes four phases: the oral preparatory phase, the oral phase, the pharyngeal phase, and the esophageal phase. However, the infant's swallow is typically described as having only three phases: the oral phase, the pharyngeal phase, and the esophageal phase. The division of a swallow into these phases is relatively arbitrary, because a normal swallow response requires a smooth, coordinated flow from one phase to the next. Excluding the esophageal phase, the swallowing process takes approximately 2 to 3 seconds to complete. Figures 9.3 and 9.4 are schematics of the swallowing process beginning with propulsion of the bolus posteriorly by the tongue and ending with the bolus passing through the esophagus for the adult and child, respectively.

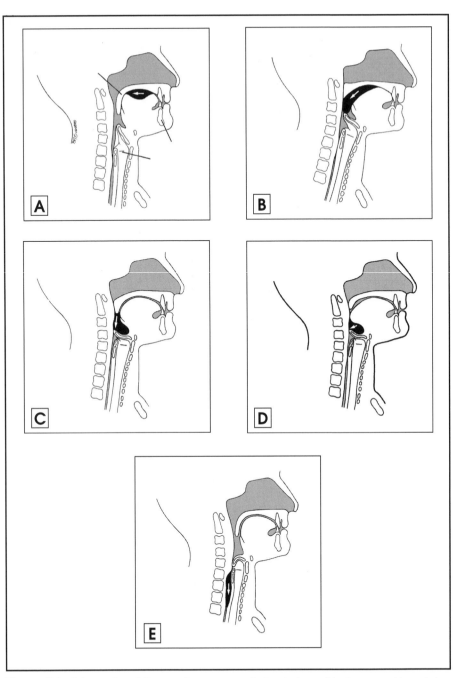

Figure 9.3. Schematic of the swallow process. Lateral view of bolus propulsion during the swallow, beginning with the voluntary initiation of the swallow by the oral tongue (A); the triggering of the pharyngeal swallow (B); the arrival of the bolus in the vallecula (C); the tongue base retraction to the anteriorly moving pharyngeal wall (D); and the bolus in the cervical esophagus and cricopharyngeal region (E). *Note.* From *Evaluation and Treatment of Swallowing Disorders* (p. 28), by J. A. Logemann, 1998, Austin, TX: PRO-ED. Copyright 1998 by PRO-ED. Reprinted with permission.

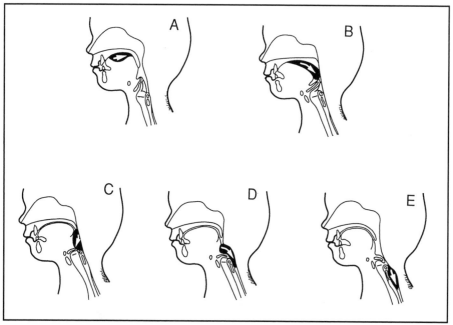

Figure 9.4. Schematic drawing of a child to show phases of normal swallow. Oral phase (A); beginning of pharyngeal phase (B); bolus moving through pharynx (C); bolus entering esophagus (D); bolus in esophagus (E). *Note.* From *Evaluation and Treatment of Swallowing Disorders* (p. 30), by J. A. Logemann, 1998, Austin, TX: PRO-ED. Copyright 1998 by PRO-ED. Reprinted with permission.

A swallowing disorder can occur at one or multiple phases of the swallow process. Several indicators may alert professionals and family members that a problem exists. Some symptoms are easily observable, such as coughing and watery eyes, and occur immediately with eating or drinking. Other physiological symptoms, such as weight loss or a spiked temperature, develop over time. Table 9.1 describes commonly observed signs of impairments related to each phase of swallowing.

Adults

Oral Preparatory Phase

The oral preparatory phase begins with placing food in the mouth. The tongue, cheeks, and teeth contribute to mastication, and an adequate labial seal prevents anterior spillage. Specifically, the tongue and cheeks manipulate the food or liquid bolus while simultaneously preventing the material from dropping into the sulcus—the space between the teeth and lips or cheeks. When the bolus is food as opposed to liquid, breakdown occurs during chewing as the food

Table 9.1

Common Signs and Related Impairments Associated
with Each Swallowing Phase

Swallowing phase	Signs of disorder	Related problems
Oral preparatory phase	Anterior loss from lips	Reduced lip closure
	Poor mastication or munching chewing pattern	Decreased rotary movement of jaws
	Poor retrieval of food from spoon or cup	Reduced lip closure/strength
	Drooling	Reduced lip closure/strength
	Cannot hold a bolus	Reduced tongue shaping
Oral phase	Stasis in sulcus, pocketing	Reduced labial tension/tone
	Slow posterior propulsion of bolus	Reduced lingual coordination
	Premature posterior spillage into pharynx	Reduced tongue control
	Weak suck–swallow pattern[a]	Reduced tongue, lip, and jaw control and coordination
	Tongue thrusting	Decreased coordination
Pharyngeal phase	Coughing before, during, or after swallow reflex	Residue in vallecula
	Choking, gurgly voice quality, red face, watery eyes	Aspiration, reduced laryngeal closure, delayed pharyngeal swallow, reduced closure of airway entrance
	Discomfort in throat during swallowing, solids easier than liquids	Reduced pharyngeal contraction
	Residue in pyriform sinus and/or vallecula	Reduced tongue base posterior movement and peristalsis
	Disruption of breathing pattern[a]	Poor coordination of suck–swallow pattern
Esophageal phase	Reflux, heartburn, liquids handled more easily than solids, burning in mouth and throat	Reduced closure of lower esophageal sphincter

[a] Primarily observed in infants.

mixes with saliva. Finally, the tongue collects and holds the now cohesive bolus (Logemann, 1983; NovaCare Rehabilitation, 1991).

Disorders of the oral preparatory phase are easy to identify because of their visibility. A weak labial seal may result in decreased retrieval of food or liquid from a utensil or cup. Anterior spillage of liquid is also common with reduced lip seal. Decreased lingual strength, range of motion, and coordination may affect the formation or maintenance of a cohesive bolus resulting in residual material spreading throughout the oral cavity or pocketing within the buccal cavity. Some individuals unable to initiate a swallow hold the bolus against their front teeth prohibiting anterior–posterior transit. An additional oral preparatory phase problem is reduced oral sensitivity. This may result in premature loss of material—that is, the bolus falls into the pharyngeal cavity before triggering a swallow response—and possible aspiration (Logemann, 1983).

Oral Phase

The oral phase starts with lingual propulsion of the bolus posteriorly using a rolling, squeezing action. The lateral edges of the tongue elevate to form a chute and the entire tongue compresses the bolus posteriorly as it makes contact with the hard palate. The lips and cheeks ensure the food does not fall into the anterior and lateral sulci. The oral phase ends when the bolus passes the tongue base and the pharyngeal swallow response is triggered (Logemann, 1983; NovaCare Rehabilitation, 1991). Once food or liquid reaches this point, swallowing becomes a reflexive response. The combined oral preparatory and oral phases take 1.5 to 2.0 seconds (Logemann, 1998).

Swallowing problems involving the oral phase center around decreased anterior–posterior propulsion of the bolus. Several factors may contribute to this phenomenon. One such factor is tongue thrust occurring when the tongue presses against or between the teeth in an attempt to initiate a swallow. Another factor is lingual pumping action. This occurs when the tongue base remains in an elevated position as the anterior portion of the tongue repeatedly pushes against the alveolar ridge and teeth. This in turn prevents normal posterior propulsion of the bolus necessary to initiate a swallow response. Other factors include reduced buccal tension and uncoordinated lingual movement resulting in premature loss of food. That is, if a swallow response is not initiated, the bolus may fall into the lateral sulcus or beyond the tongue base into the vallecula or pyriform sinuses creating increased risk for aspiration.

Another related problem that can occur during the oral phase is impaired mastication. Normal chewing behavior occurs as a rotary movement of the jaws. A vertical or munching pattern may occur with decreased strength and coordination of the oral structures and is not an effective means of breaking down food. Furthermore, this weakness creates a need for additional time to complete the mastication process.

Pharyngeal Phase

The pharyngeal phase involves movement of several anatomical structures to protect the airway. Specifically, the velum elevates and retracts to close off the velopharyngeal port and prevent food and liquid from flowing into the nasal cavity; the hyoid bone and thyroid cartilage elevate and rotate anteriorly; and the larynx moves upward and forward closing off access to the airway at three levels—the true vocal folds, the false vocal folds, and aryepiglottic folds—to ensure material does not enter the trachea. The pharyngeal phase takes approximately 1 second and ends when the cricopharyngeal sphincter opens, allowing the bolus to enter the esophagus (Logemann, 1998).

Swallowing problems associated with the pharyngeal phase are harder to detect than those associated with the oral preparatory and oral phases. Common symptoms include residue in the pharyngeal cavity following the swallow, reduced laryngeal elevation, and penetration and aspiration.

Residue in the pharynx occurs when small amounts of food or liquid are trapped in the pyriform sinuses or vallecular space. At a later time, this material may fall into the airway and trigger a choking episode secondary to penetration or aspiration. Reduced laryngeal elevation occurs when the larynx does not completely elevate to meet the tongue base. The result is incomplete airway protection, and the individual may aspirate any residual material left on top of the larynx when breathing is resumed (Logemann, 1998).

Penetration and aspiration can occur before, during, or after initiation of a swallow. Penetration occurs when food or liquid enters the laryngeal vestibule but does not go below the level of the vocal folds. In contrast, aspiration occurs when food or liquid enters the pharynx and continues beyond the level of the vocal folds, entering the trachea. Although many individuals respond with spontaneous coughing when penetration or aspiration occurs, some may not be strong enough to expel the aspirated material. Other people may have reduced sensation precluding their awareness of penetration or aspiration of food or liquid. For these individuals, a spontaneous cough response is absent, and no other immediate signs of aspiration occur. This phenomenon is called silent aspiration. In either case, recurring episodes can lead to aspiration pneumonia if precautions are not implemented.

Several warning signs indicate the presence of aspiration: (a) coughing or choking before, during, or after a swallow; (b) frequent throat clearing; (c) a gurgly vocal quality; and (d) a runny nose and/or watery eyes. In addition, individuals with penetration or aspiration problems may eat slowly, regurgitate food, require extra effort to swallow, or complain of discomfort when swallowing. Silent aspiration is suspected when physiological signs such as abnormal lung sounds, a spiked temperature, or significant weight loss gradually appear.

Disorders of the pharyngeal stage of swallowing may result from delays in the initiation or triggering of the swallow response or from overall weakness or incoordination of the swallowing musculature. A delayed swallow response increases the risk of aspiration because the pharynx remains unprotected with a potential for food or liquid to enter the trachea. Overall weakness affects the coordination and timing of the swallow process and is often associated with incomplete epiglottic inversion, once again resulting in insufficient airway protection.

Esophageal Phase

The esophageal phase begins when the bolus enters the esophagus and ends when it passes into the stomach. The bolus moves through the esophagus in a wavelike fashion referred to as peristalsis. Normal esophageal transit time varies from 8 to 20 seconds (Logemann, 1993).

Although speech–language pathologists are trained to identify and treat disorders of the oral preparatory, oral, and pharyngeal swallowing phases, disorders of the esophageal phase are usually monitored and treated by physicians. Still, speech–language pathologists should be aware of potential esophageal phase problems. These include symptoms associated with gastroesophageal reflux disease—such as complaints of heartburn, reflux, or sore throat—and symptoms indicative of esophageal motility problems, such as complaints of food getting stuck when swallowing. Simple positioning, such as remaining upright after meals for a period of time, may be helpful in eliminating some symptoms; however, many esophageal disorders are treated with medicine. Suspicion of an esophageal problem should be reported to the primary care physician.

Infants

Professionals have long referred to an infant's swallow response as a sequential and rhythmic pattern of sucking, swallowing, and breathing (Logan & Bosma, 1967; Siktberg & Bantz, 1999; Weiss, 1988). The process includes three distinct phases—the oral phase, the pharyngeal phase, and the esophageal phase.

Oral Phase

This phase of an infant's swallow is frequently described as oral suckling or sucking (Arvedson, 1996; Kramer & Eicher, 1993; Logan & Bosma, 1967; Weiss, 1988). Strong buccal, lingual, labial, and jaw movements are used to suck the liquid bolus from a nipple. Successive suckles occur in a rhythmic pattern until the oral cavity is filled with liquid. The tongue then manipulates the bolus posteriorly in a wavelike fashion. Once the bolus reaches the tongue base, the swallow reflex is triggered, marking the beginning of the pharyngeal phase of the swallow.

Siktberg and Bantz (1999) list several signs indicative of oral phase problems in infants. These may include (a) the presence of anterior spillage or drooling associated with a poor labial seal; (b) tongue thrusting resulting from limited lingual control and coordination; or (c) an inefficient suck–swallow–breath pattern resulting from a combination of weak sucking, arrhythmic movements, and lack of jaw stability. Hypersensitivity or hyposensitivity of the lips, cheeks, or tongue may also contribute to swallowing problems in this phase.

Pharyngeal Phase

When the bolus reaches the tongue base, the soft palate elevates, the vocal folds abduct, and the epiglottis rises, providing protection from both reflux and penetration or aspiration. Breathing stops momentarily as the swallow is initiated (Logan & Bosma, 1967). Laryngeal elevation is limited in infants because the larynx is located more superiorly and anteriorly than in adults and is, therefore, already positioned closer to the tongue base (Arvedson, 1996; Logemann, 1998; Siktberg & Bantz, 1999). Pharyngeal peristalsis maneuvers the bolus to the esophagus for the final phase of swallowing.

Symptoms indicative of pharyngeal phase problems in infants may include decreased coordination of the suck–swallow–breath pattern, coughing or choking during feeding, nasal reflux, prolonged meal times, refusal of food, weight loss, and recurrent pneumonia (Arvedson, 1996; Siktberg & Bantz, 1999).

Esophageal Phase

During this final phase of swallowing, the same wavelike movements that occur during the pharyngeal phase propel the bolus through the esophagus to the stomach. Holding the infant at an incline allows gravity to assist in this process (Weiss, 1988).

Potential problems associated with swallowing in infants during this phase may involve gastroesophageal reflux and decreased esophageal motility (Arvedson & Christensen, 1993).

Alternative Feeding Methods

For some, problems may be so severe that swallowing any food or liquid is unsafe. In these cases, a physician designates that the individual shall remain

"NPO" (nothing per os)—that is, he or she is to receive no food or liquid by mouth. Nutritional needs are met using an alternative method of feeding. Whether this alternate feeding method is temporary or permanent depends on the individual recovery pattern.

Adults

Several options exist for alternative methods of feeding. Table 9.2 defines and describes the advantages and disadvantages of four commonly used enteral feeding options: nasogastric tubes (NG-tubes), percutaneous endoscopic gastrostomy tubes (PEGs), gastrostomy tubes (G-tubes), and jejunostomy tubes (J-tubes). In general, PEGs or G-tubes are preferred when the anticipated need for alternative feeding is for an extended period of time; NG-tubes are reserved for use as a short-term alternative. Methods that allow bolus feedings—that is, tube feedings given at specified times rather than continuously throughout the day—have the advantage of making participation in a variety of activities more feasible, because the individual can be disconnected from the feeding unit for periods of time (Annoni, Vuagnat, Frischknecht, & Uebelhart, 1998). Any form of tube feeding places the individual at risk for reflux. Preventative measures—such as elevating the individual's head to a 45° angle for at least 30 minutes after each feeding—minimize the risk of aspiration.

Infants

Alternative options for infants include enteral or parenteral feeding (Young, 1993). Enteral alternatives involve the gastrointestinal tract and use NG-tubes, orogastric tubes (OG-tubes), pyloric tubes, G-tubes, or J-tubes. When selecting an enteral alternative, the guidelines are similar for those used with adults. Because infants are obligate nose breathers, some clinicians favor OG-tubes that are inserted through the oral cavity (Young, 1993). For short-term needs, parenteral feedings that provide nutrition through direct or indirect venous innervation may be preferred.

Swallowing Disorders Associated with TBI

The majority of research related to dysphagia among survivors of TBI involves adults. Swallowing disorders follow TBI in 30% to 61% of cases (Cherney & Halper, 1996; Field & Weiss, 1989; Mackay, Morgan, & Bernstein, 1999). The most common type of disorder associated with TBI—occurring in 81% of survivors with swallowing problems (Lazarus & Logemann, 1987)—is a delayed or

Table 9.2

Advantages and Disadvantages of Alternative Feeding Methods

Feeding method	Definition	Advantages	Disadvantages
Nasogastric tube (NG-tube)	A tube passed through the nose and nasal cavity and inserted into the stomach	Does not require surgery Can be inserted at bedside by a nurse Allows for bolus feedings	Can interfere with speech production and treatment and with swallow physiology Potential irritation of pharyngeal cavity Visible to others Person can easily pull out tube
Percutaneous endoscopic gastrostomy	A tube inserted directly into the stomach using a surgical and endoscopic procedure that does not require major opening of the abdomen	Does not interfere with speech and swallowing Not visible to others Allows for bolus feedings Procedure done in ICU or endoscopy suite versus operating room Procedure is not as invasive as that associated with G-tube or J-tube placement	Procedure is more invasive than that associated with NG-tube placement
Gastrostomy tube (G-tube)	A tube that is surgically inserted through an external opening in the abdomen and extends to the stomach	Does not interfere with speech and swallowing Not visible to others Allows for bolus feedings Procedure is less costly than J-tube	Requires a surgical procedure 7% rate of postoperative complications (Shellito & Malt, 1985)
Jejunostomy tube (J-tube)	A tube that is surgically inserted through an external opening in the abdomen and extends to the small intestine	Does not interfere with speech and swallowing Not visible to others	Does not allow for bolus feedings Requires a surgical procedure 7% rate of postoperative complications (Shellito & Malt, 1985)

absent swallow response. Aspiration occurring before swallow initiation is the most common form of aspiration among survivors of TBI (Lazarus & Logemann, 1987).

Research documenting the presence of dysphagia among neurologically impaired infants and children primarily includes subjects with diagnoses other than TBI. These include disorders such as cerebral palsy, mental retardation, or other less common syndromes (Arvedson, Rogers, Buck, Smart, & Msall, 1994; Tanaguchi & Moyer, 1994). However, Tanaguchi and Moyer (1994) reported that children with a primary diagnosis of TBI were 5 times less likely to develop pneumonia than children with other diagnoses. They attributed this to the acute nature of the injury, the likelihood for improvement over time, and closer monitoring by medical professionals. Additional research pertaining to swallowing disorders among infants and children following TBI is needed. Professionals must be careful when interpreting research that is primarily associated with adults, as these findings may not directly apply to younger populations (Arvedson, 1996).

Hypermetabolism

Individuals with severe TBI often experience hypermetabolic and hypercatabolic states placing them at risk for malnutrition and infection due to immunosuppression. The effect of head injury on metabolic response goes above and beyond that experienced by individuals with severe injuries without head trauma (Petersen, Jeevanandam, & Harrington, 1993). From 1 week to 1 year postinjury, survivors of TBI experience caloric and protein needs twice normal levels. Without appropriate dietary changes, significant weight loss, loss of muscle mass, and muscle atrophy can occur. Early nutritional intervention and physical therapy can help minimize these problems.

Similar metabolic disruptions may also occur in individuals with mild TBIs. Gross, Kling, Henry, Herndon, and Lavretsky (1996) found abnormal cerebral metabolic rates in 20 of 20 patients with mild TBIs. Abnormal metabolic rates were significantly correlated with overall clinical complaints (e.g., attention disorders) and overall neuropsychological test results. Medical professionals must consider the risk of hypermetabolism and appropriate nonoral feeding alternatives for managing its presence. Although responsibility for this issue lies primarily with the physician, the speech–language pathologist should be familiar with the condition and its potential implications.

Return to Oral Intake

Limited research exists on the timing for resumption of oral intake following a period of nonoral feeding. However, level of cognitive functioning and the ability to handle oral secretions are two measures that may provide some information for appropriately timing the return to oral intake. Research indicates that an association exists between level of cognitive functioning and resumption of oral intake. Yorkston, Honsinger, Mitsuda, and Hammen (1989) found that as cognition improves, the occurrence of swallowing disorders decreases. More specifically, other researchers have documented that feeding trials and resumption of oral intake often do not occur until the survivor reaches Rancho Level IV or higher (Mackay et al., 1999; see Appendix 5.B in Chapter 5 for information about Rancho Levels). In fact, Mackay et al. (1999) found that complete feeding via oral intake did not occur until Rancho Level VI. Additionally, the inability to manage one's oral secretions safely is a clear indication that food or liquid will not be safely swallowed either. Hence, once management of secretions improves, the individual is another step closer to resuming oral intake.

The continuation of nonoral feedings may be short term for some and long term for others. When the situation is long term, swallowing should be reassessed annually or if a noticeable change in functioning occurs. Logemann and Ylvisaker (1998) reported that some children with TBI may safely resume oral intake even years after injury. Adamovich (1990) reported that patients with persistent swallowing disorders often improve more quickly after removal of the NG tube. Reasons may include alleviation of irritation caused by the tube and allowance of normal pharyngeal closure.

The resumption of oral intake is a major rehabilitation goal that allows the survivor to once again enjoy both the nutritional and social benefits of eating. Although some indicators suggest when oral intake may resume, research in this area is limited; professionals must consider each survivor's current level of functioning and weigh the associated benefits and risks of oral intake.

Assessment

Figure 9.5 provides a flowchart to guide speech–language pathologists through the basics of swallowing assessment and treatment for survivors of TBI. The chart provides details regarding (a) the information speech–language pathologists need to obtain about an individual's level of function, (b) resources for accessing information, and (c) questions to lead the professional through each step of the assessment and treatment process. This chart serves as only a general frame of reference; the following sections provide more detailed information.

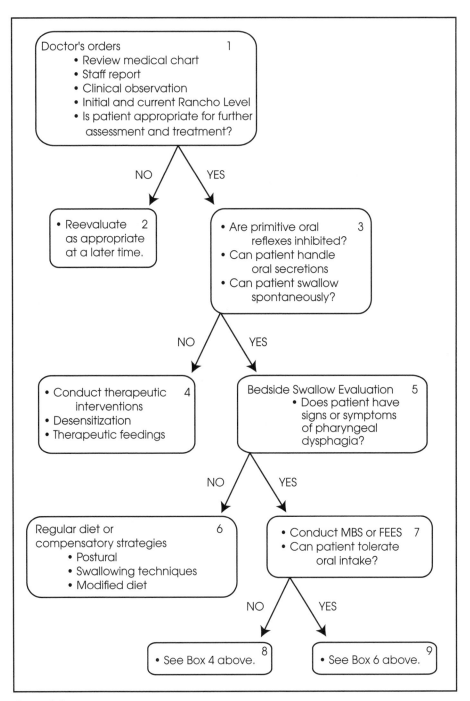

Figure 9.5. Decision-making tree for swallowing assessment and treatment.

Gathering Information

Figure 9.5, Panel 1 lists the steps involved in the information gathering phase of swallowing assessment. Prior to direct interaction with a survivor, the speech–language pathologist should review the medical chart to become familiar with the person's medical history and current level of functioning. For infants, a detailed history pertaining to premorbid feeding skills should be obtained from the parent (Rowe, 1999). Documentation of coma, a history of tracheostomy or mechanical ventilation, and impaired cognitive functioning are red flags for potential swallowing problems such as aspiration.

Coma

The occurrence of coma, vegetative state, or minimal consciousness is a risk factor for swallowing problems. A positive relation exists between the severity of swallowing problems and the duration of coma. Specifically, Lazarus and Logemann (1987) found that survivors who experienced coma for more than 24 hours had (a) increased oral transit times, (b) longer delays in initiating the swallowing reflex, and (c) more severe aspiration than people who were comatose for shorter periods. In addition, individuals with initial scores below 6 on the Glasgow Coma Scale and below Rancho Level III are at greater risk for swallowing problems than people with initial scores above those levels (Mackay et al., 1999).

Tracheostomy/Mechanical Ventilation

The presence of a tracheostomy tube or mechanical ventilation is also a risk factor for swallowing problems. People who require use of a tracheostomy tube or mechanical ventilation for a period greater than 2 weeks are significantly more likely to exhibit swallowing problems than those without such a history (Mackay et al., 1999). Using videofluoroscopy, Schurr and colleagues (1999) found that 22 of 31 survivors of severe TBI (71%) had problems with penetration, aspiration, or both after removal from a mechanical ventilation device.

Impaired Cognitive Functioning

Decreased arousal, attention, and cognition often present as the basis for many swallowing problems among individuals with diffuse axonal injuries such as that associated with TBI (Rowe, 1999). Individuals with low initial Rancho Levels (Hagen, 2000; see Appendix 5.B) are at greater risk for swallowing problems than individuals with high initial ratings (Mackay et al., 1999). Therefore, having information about an individual's initial Rancho Level as well as his or her current level is important.

Individuals functioning at Rancho Level I are in coma or vegetative states, and swallowing assessments are not appropriate. Individuals at Rancho Levels II and III demonstrate some responsiveness to environmental events, but their decreased arousal and inconsistent awareness of surroundings continue to make oral feeding trials inappropriate. Many people at these stages have a combination of motor and cognitive impairments that contribute to the presence of swallowing disorders. Decreased muscle coordination, range of motion, and strength negatively affect the swallowing process.

Swallowing status varies widely across individuals functioning at Rancho Level IV. Key characteristics of this level are confusion and agitation. Behaviors are often unpredictable and impulsive, survivors at this level cannot sustain attention even in highly structured situations, and primitive oral reflexes (i.e., rooting reflex, sucking reflex) are exhibited. Because of these characteristics, nutritional needs of many survivors are met exclusively through alternative feeding methods. With one-on-one monitoring by a speech–language pathologist, a select few can attempt controlled food trials. Depending on how the individual manages with these trials, the speech–language pathologist may determine that a formal assessment (such as a modified barium swallow [MBS] study or fiberoptic endoscopic evaluation of swallowing [FEES] is appropriate to rule out aspiration.

In addition to any remaining physiologic components, cognitive impairments affect the safety of swallowing among survivors of TBI (Cherney & Halper, 1996). For individuals functioning at Rancho Levels V to VII, agitation is no longer a primary concern; however, impaired cognitive functioning manifested as decreased alertness, attention, memory, and self-regulation may contribute to unsafe swallowing. As a result, close supervision during meals may be necessary. Other survivors may not need any swallowing intervention; however, the speech–language pathologist should complete a bedside exam, or at least an informal observation, on anyone admitted with a diagnosis of TBI. Whenever aspiration is suspected, a formal evaluation (a modified barium swallow study or FEES) should be performed to confirm or rule out this possibility.

Specific Procedures for Survivors with Impaired Consciousness

Swallowing assessment procedures vary with a survivor's level of cognitive functioning. Individuals functioning at Rancho Levels I and II are not appropriate for any swallowing assessment; however, informal assessment of prefeeding skills can be performed with individuals functioning at Rancho Level III. This includes evaluating the presence of (a) abnormal sensation, (b) absent or delayed swallows, and (c) primitive oral reflexes. See Figure 9.5, Panel 3 for questions to ask in evaluating the swallowing reflexes in a person with impaired consciousness.

Abnormal Sensation

Sensory impairments commonly occur with damage to the brain stem (Rowe, 1999). Two forms of abnormal sensation—hypersensitivity and hyposensitivity—may be present in survivors of TBI. Both can be assessed by gently stroking the cheek, lips, or tongue with an oral swab or toothette. *Hypersensitivity* is present when increased tone results. This presents as a retraction or pursing of the lips, a clenching of the jaw, tongue protrusion or retraction, or hyperextension or turning of the head away from the stimulus (Ylvisaker & Logemann, 1985). *Hyposensitivity*, in contrast, appears as reduced or absent sensitivity to touch. This prevents the individual from feeling and manipulating a bolus effectively.

Absent or Delayed Swallow Response

Absent or delayed swallows are very common following TBI (Lazarus & Logemann, 1987). Assessment involves observation and performance of Logemann's (1983) Four Finger Test. For this test, the speech–language pathologist places his or her index finger under the survivor's chin to assess tongue base movement and places his or her middle finger on the hyoid bone to assess elevation of the hyoid. Simultaneously, the ring and pinky fingers are placed above and below the thyroid cartilage to assess thyroid movement during swallowing. This enables the speech–language pathologist to estimate oral transit time. Typically, the elapsed time between the initiation of tongue movement and the triggering of a swallow reflex is approximately 1 second. Longer oral transit times may indicate a pharyngeal stage swallowing disorder. If a cough response occurs, aspiration is the likely cause.

Presence of Primitive Oral Reflexes

During the early stages of recovery from TBI, the rooting, sucking, biting, and chewing reflexes (see Appendix 5.A in Chapter 5) commonly reappear because a loss of cortical control allows for the disinhibition of subcortical functions. These reflexes occur both spontaneously and in response to stimulation. During stimulation of the lips, gums, tongue, or face, the speech–language pathologist should assess how long (in seconds) the survivor can tolerate stimulation before a reflex occurs. As medical status improves and cortical control becomes reestablished, primitive oral reflexes decrease in frequency and duration.

Specific Procedures for Survivors with Regained Consciousness

Even after a survivor of TBI regains full consciousness, cognitive and motor impairments continue to impact swallowing function. In Figure 9.5, Panels 5 and 7 list appropriate assessments for this stage of recovery. Hence, while speech–language pathologists perform assessment procedures such as bedside evaluations, MBS studies, and FEES, they need to take into account cognitive and behavioral issues. For example, survivors functioning at Rancho Level IV, and sometimes Level V, are particularly prone to problems associated with agitation and distractibility. Because of this, assessments should occur in environments free of visual and auditory distractions; all unnecessary noise should be eliminated, and lighting should be dimmed to promote a calm atmosphere. At Rancho Levels V to VI, impulsivity and ongoing deficits in attention and concentration negatively affect swallowing function during assessment procedures. A rapid rate of eating and drinking—that is, "shoveling" food and "chugging" drinks—and difficulty focusing on specific assessment tasks increase the likelihood of choking and aspirating material. Some survivors may develop a behavior of biting the utensil when eating. If this situation arises, use of rubber-coated utensils is recommended. Speech–language pathologists must make modifications and accommodations for these cognitive and behavioral issues when performing the specific assessment procedures described below.

Bedside Swallow Evaluation

A bedside evaluation is often the first formal assessment of a survivor's swallowing ability. The purpose of the evaluation is to identify food and liquid consistencies that the person can tolerate safely with or without the use of compensatory techniques. Bedside evaluations are performed both with individuals who are NPO (i.e., who take nothing by month) and individuals for whom questions exist about the appropriateness of their present diet.

The first step in a bedside swallowing evaluation is to perform a comprehensive oral–motor examination. This includes assessments of (a) muscular strength, range of motion, and sensitivity of the lips, cheek, and tongue; (b) velopharyngeal competence; and (c) the presence of primitive oral reflexes. Arvedson (1993) makes specific recommendations for assessing the oral–motor skills of infants and children. For infants, the examination should focus on (a) efficiency and rhythm of lip, tongue, and jaw movements during sucking, and (b) posture, tone, reflexes (i.e., rooting), and motor control of oral and facial structures. For children, the exam should begin with an observation of head and trunk control in a typical seated position; body alignment, head and mouth position, the presence of primitive reflexes, and abnormal tone should be the primary concerns.

The next step is observing how well food is tolerated. The procedures vary greatly when assessing infants as opposed to children and adults. If the infant is tolerating per oral (PO) intake, the speech–language pathologist should observe the infant feeding for approximately 15 to 20 minutes (Arvedson, 1993). A typically developing infant's sucking sequence is made of bursts of 10 to 30 successive sucks (Arvedson, 1993; Weiss, 1988). Initially, strength and coordination of this successive pattern may appear within normal limits; however, as fatigue occurs, impairments may become evident. The speech–language pathologist should be alert to the following: changes in cardiac and respiratory rates and patterns, gagging, spitting, tongue thrusting, squirming, withdrawal from the feeding source, arching of the back and neck, and decreased arousal.

For children and adults, a variety of food and liquid consistencies are presented. Typically this includes regular dry foods (e.g., crackers), soft foods (e.g., banana), purees (e.g., applesauce), and, sometimes, mixed textures (e.g., cereal with milk). Liquid consistencies include thin liquids (e.g., water) and two types of thickened liquids: nectars which are slightly more viscous than water (e.g., apricot or pear juice) and honey-consistency liquids which are more viscous than nectar (e.g., those created by adding thickeners to any liquid the individual desires). For all foods and liquids, the therapist should initially present small amounts and gradually progress to larger bites or sips. To protect against aspiration while assessing mastication, the examiner can wrap a bite-sized piece of meat in gauze. The survivor chews the wrapped bolus while the examiner holds the end of the gauze to prevent swallowing.

What is the best order for presenting foods and liquids during a bedside evaluation?

Foods and liquids of differing consistencies should be presented in order from the least to the most difficult to manage. For foods, the recommended progression is pudding, applesauce, banana, bread, dry cracker, cereal and milk; for liquids, the recommended progression is honey-thick, nectar, thin liquid. The amount of food or liquid presented should progress from a small bite or sip (approximately ½ teaspoon) to a slightly larger bite or sip (approximately 1 teaspoon) to a large bite or sip (heaping teaspoon); for liquids, demonstration of management of multiple sips and use of a straw should follow single sips.

Visual inspection of the meat allows for determination of efficiency and extent of mastication.

A final step of bedside evaluations for children and adults involves observing the survivor feeding him- or herself. This provides an opportunity to determine whether the survivor selects an appropriate amount of food or liquid, adequately paces eating, or pockets food. Sometimes, difficulty is not apparent until the meal is nearly complete and fatigue or agitation sets in. The evaluation should be terminated when the individual is no longer safely managing the foods or liquids presented.

Throughout the evaluation, the clinician is looking for signs and symptoms indicative of a disorder of the oral preparatory, oral, and pharyngeal swallowing phases. Once a problem arises, some speech–language pathologists advocate the immediate introduction of compensatory techniques and body or head positioning to alleviate the swallowing problem. Others may be more conservative, however, and recommend additional assessment—such as a modified barium swallow procedure—before introducing compensatory strategies.

Although the bedside swallow evaluation provides valuable insight about current swallowing status, limitations exist. Several warning signs may be evident during a bedside evaluation, but actual penetration and aspiration of food and liquid cannot be directly observed. For example, consider the fact that more than 50% of people who aspirate regularly during modified barium swallow studies are not identified as aspirating during bedside evaluations (Logemann, 1998). The clinician must decide whether the bedside evaluation provides adequate information to make a safe judgment about current swallowing status or whether further assessment procedures are warranted. Anytime penetration or aspiration is suspected, further assessment is needed.

Modified Barium Swallow

A modified barium swallow (MBS; Figure 9.5, Panel 7)—also referred to as videofluoroscopy—is a radiographic procedure to examine the effects of bolus size, bolus texture, head and body positioning, and compensatory strategies on swallowing status (American Speech-Language-Hearing Association, 1992). Its purpose is to identify whether aspiration of any liquid or food is ocurring and, if so, to determine the cause or causes (Logemann, 1983). Arvedson and colleagues (1994) referred to the MBS as "the procedure of choice for children to delineate the pharyngeal and upper esophageal phases of the swallow that can only be inferred by bedside clinical assessment" (p. 173).

Procedures for performing MBS studies vary from facility to facility. Typically, a radiologist and speech–language pathologist work together. The radiologist's knowledge of structural abnormalities combined with the speech–

What is barium?

Barium is a metallic, alkaline element that, when combined with foods or liquids, makes them visible on radiographic studies. It comes in liquid, powder, paste, and pill forms. The liquid or powder forms can be mixed with liquids and puree-consistency foods. The paste form is applied to solids, such as a cookie or cracker. The pill form is used to simulate the individual's ability to swallow medications in pill form. The liquid form of barium can affect the consistency of solids and liquids with which it is mixed, and, hence, powdered thickener must sometimes also be added to obtain the desired consistency.

language pathologist's expertise in oral and pharyngeal patterns results in optimum diagnosis and management decisions (Logemann, 1983). In all instances, the procedures should be videotaped for later analysis.

The same variety of food and liquid consistencies used during bedside evaluations are presented during MBS studies; however, during an MBS study, all foods and liquids are combined with barium so they are visible in the fluoroscopic image. Different philosophies exist about how best to present food trials during MBS studies. Some clinicians recommend beginning with the most difficult consistency to determine the presence of aspiration, while others prefer starting with the food consistency best tolerated during the bedside evaluation. In either case, because fatigue is a frequent problem following TBI and can contribute to swallowing problems, MBS studies with survivors of TBI need to be extensive. Although no signs of aspiration may appear in the early part of a MBS study, aspiration may occur as fatigue sets in.

By performing MBS studies on 22 adult survivors of severe TBI, Mackay et al. (1999) found that aspiration occurred during the swallow in 71% of cases, before the swallow in 41% of cases, and after the swallow in 18% of cases; more than one time of aspiration (i.e., before, during, or after the swallow) occurred in 36% of cases. In a similar study, Lazarus and Logemann (1987) found that 20 of 53 survivors of TBI (38%) aspirated during MBS studies, with the primary cause being the absence of swallowing responses.

Arvedson et al. (1994) completed MBS studies with 186 children with neurologically based dysphagia to detect disorders of the pharyngeal stage and presence of aspiration. Aspiration was detected in 48 of the 186 participants (26%). For 58% of cases, aspiration occurred before or during the swallow; for 42% of cases, aspiration occurred after the swallow. Of the 48 participants who aspirated, only 8% were diagnosed as having postnatal central nervous system injuries.

Fiberoptic Endoscopic Examination of Swallowing

A fiberoptic endoscopic examination of swallowing (FEES; Figure 9.5, Panel 7) is another procedure used to determine the presence or absence of aspiration. During this procedure, a flexible fiberoptic endoscope is connected to a small video camera lens. The endoscope is inserted transnasally and held in the oropharyngeal cavity to provide a view of the pharynx projected onto a color monitor. Unlike MBS studies, FEES does not allow observation of the actual swallow; elevation of the pharynx and posterior contraction of the tongue base push the endoscope aside resulting in a moment called "white-out" (Langmore, 1996). However, the FEES procedure is actually more comprehensive than MBS in that assessment of the vocal folds can occur as well as assessment of premature spillage, pooling in the valleculae or pyriform sinuses, residue after swallowing, and penetration or aspiration (American Speech-Language-Hearing Association [ASHA], 1992).

The types of professionals involved in FEES procedures vary depending on state and facility regulations. Although ASHA guidelines indicate that performing FEES is within the speech–language pathologist's scope of practice, some facilities insist that a physician—usually an otolaryngologist—be present.

Langmore (1996) recommends assessing the function of all anatomical structures involved in swallowing immediately following insertion of the endoscope. Table 9.3 describes assessment tasks and the focus for evaluating the (a) velum, (b) hypopharynx and larynx at rest, (c) handling of secretions and frequency of swallows, (d) tongue base, (e) respiration, (f) airway protection, (g) phonation, and (h) pharyngeal musculature. Any abnormalities may be indicative of potential swallowing problems, and additional attention can be directed to these structures during the swallowing portion of the FEES procedure.

The next step in the FEES procedure requires presentation of the same consistencies and progression of food and liquid amounts as used in bedside evaluations and MBS studies. For FEES, all foods and liquids are combined with food coloring, usually green, to allow for better visibility during swallowing. Although the actual swallow cannot be observed, a residual trail of food coloring in the pharynx or below the level of the vocal folds is indicative of penetration or aspiration. If a small amount of aspiration occurs, presentation of the same consistency and amount should be repeated with implementation of compensatory strategies and changes in positioning. If aspiration occurs twice or is severe, that consistency and amount should be discontinued and a denser consistency tried.

Table 9.3
Procedures for Anatomic and Physiologic Assessment During FEES

Structure	Task	What to observe
Velum	Have person swallow or phonate oral and nasal sounds	Velopharyngeal closure
Hypopharynx and larynx	Scan the area with the scope	Abnormal color, symmetry, or structures (nodules)
Secretions and swallow frequency	View with scope, enhancing view with a drop of green food coloring if needed	Amount and location of secretions (in lateral channels, laryngeal vestibule, subglottal area) over 2- to 5-minute period
		Frequency of dry swallows during 2-minute period
Tongue base	Have person repeat /kʌkʌkʌ/	Extent and symmetry of movement
Respiration	Have person sniff or inhale deeply	Symmetry and rate of movement of structures at rest
		Extent of vocal fold abduction during inhalation
Airway protection	Have person cough	Movement and symmetry of true and false vocal folds
	Have person hold breath lightly, hold breath as tightly as possible, and hold breath for 7 seconds	
Phonation	Have person sustain /i/	Overall laryngeal functioning
	Have person repeat /hi/ 5 to 7 times	
	Have person count from 1 to 10	
	Have person produce vowel sound and glide upward in pitch	
Pharyngeal musculature	Have person hold breath and blow cheeks out forcefully	Depth and symmetry of pyriform sinuses
	Have person strain voice and grunt or say /i/ in high, loud voice	Symmetry and extent of contraction of middle and inferior constrictors

Note. Adapted from *FEES Examination Protocol,* by S. Langmore, 1996, November, paper presented at FEES Workshop, San Diego Rehabilitation Institute. Copyright 1996 by Susan Langmore. Adapted with permission.

Survivors of TBI who are confused or agitated—such as those functioning at Rancho Level IV and perhaps some individuals at Level V—may not tolerate the FEES procedure because of the invasive nature of the transnasally inserted endoscope. In addition, survivors who cannot sustain attention for an extended period of time may have difficulty tolerating the length of the FEES procedure. However, because the person is not exposed to radiation, performance of FEES allows for assessment of a greater variety and amount of food than performance of a MBS study. Table 9.4 provides a comparison of the relative advantages and disadvantages of the FEES and MBS study procedures.

Hoppers and Holm (1999) performed FEES procedures with survivors of TBI and found that premature spillage and delayed swallow reflexes were the two most common impairments. Leder (1999) used FEES procedures to assess the swallowing status of 47 survivors of TBI in surgical or intensive care units. He found that 30 of the 47 survivors could safely tolerate some form of oral diet, but aspiration occurred in the remaining 17 (36%). Approximately half (9 of 17) of the people who aspirated displayed silent aspiration.

Leder and Karas (2000) investigated the use of FEES among 30 pediatric patients (ages 11 days to 20 years). The researchers assessed 7 patients first via MBS study, followed by FEES, and compared the findings. The remaining 23 patients underwent FEES only. Findings indicated 100% agreement between the two assessment procedures. Of the 23 individuals, 10 demonstrated

Table 9.4
Considerations for Performing MBS Versus FEES Procedures

Consideration	MBS	FEES
All phases of swallow visible	Yes	No
Video recording capabilities	Yes	Yes
Voice-over capabilities	Yes	Yes
Radiation exposure	Yes	No
Can be performed at bedside	Yes	Yes
Special chair required	Yes	No
Invasive procedure	No	Yes
Speech–language pathologist can perform procedure	Yes	No[a]
Physician must be present	Yes	No[a]
Can assess vocal fold function	No	Yes
Person can view procedure as it occurs	No	Yes

[a]States regulate whether a physician must be present during performance of FEES procedures.

dysphagia; for 3 of them, the cause of injury was TBI. Oral dysphagia was present in 4 patients; pharyngeal dysphagia was present in 7 patients; and aspiration was present in 5 patients (3 with silent aspiration).

Additional Assessment Tools Used with Infants and Children

Other procedures are also recommended for assessing dysphagia among infants and children. These include upper gastrointestinal studies (UGI), ultrasonography, radionuclide imaging, and cervical auscultation (Arvedson & Christensen, 1993; Lefton-Grief & Loughlin, 1996; Logan & Bosma, 1967; Siktberg & Bantz, 1999). Readers interested in learning more about these procedures are referred to textbooks that focus on dysphagia in infants and children, such as *Pediatric Swallowing and Feeding: Assessment and Management* (Arvedson, 2002).

Treatment

Researchers have documented that swallowing treatment facilitates the return to oral intake of food and liquid by survivors of TBI. Specifically, Schurr and colleagues (1999) found that, even among adults who sustained severe TBIs and who required mechanical ventilation at some point during their recovery, over 83% (20 of 24) progressed to the point of tolerating food and liquid presented orally after swallowing treatment. Of course, to achieve this outcome, treatment must be individualized and take into consideration a survivor's cognitive status and motor functioning.

Although feeding and swallowing disorders appear to be similar between adults and children, limited research exists documenting treatment outcomes among infants and children (Arvedson, 1993). Additional considerations exist when treating children with TBI. The following sections provide (a) treatment guidelines and compensatory strategies appropriate for all survivors at different levels of cognitive functioning as measured by the Rancho scale and (b) additional considerations for treating children.

Treatment Guidelines and Compensatory Strategies

Rancho Levels I to III

At early stages of recovery from TBI, no oral feeding occurs; rather, the focus of swallowing treatment is on decreasing abnormal sensation, increasing the consistency and speed of swallow initiation, and inhibiting the presence of primitive reflexes. Because of survivors' inconsistent awareness of external events, all treatment sessions should include verbal explanations about what is happening.

Abnormal Sensation. As described earlier, abnormal sensation may be in the form of hypersensitivity or hyposensitivity. If hypersensitivity is present, the goal is desensitization, so the survivor can tolerate stimulation for longer periods of time before reflexes or increases in tone occur. Desensitization should begin with the face and progress to the oral cavity. Ylvisaker and Logemann (1985) suggest applying firm pressure to the face using a warm washcloth or fingers, being careful not to trigger oral reflexes by getting too close to the lips. Once the survivor tolerates facial stimulation, oral stimulation can begin. For this, a glycerin swab or slightly moist toothette (a small stick with a sponge on the end of it) may be used to stroke the survivor's lips lightly. As tolerance increases and sensitivity decreases, the stimulation should proceed to include the survivor's gums, tongue, cheeks, and palate.

Hyposensitivity is treated by gently exercising the facial and oral muscles. Ylvisaker and Logemann (1985) suggest stimulation of muscles by tapping them firmly with fingers, brushing them rapidly with a washcloth, or applying ice to them followed by soft rubbing with a dry towel. Following these procedures, the muscles can be exercised through massage and passive range of motion exercises.

Absent or Delayed Swallow Response. Sometimes, no swallow response occurs following stimulation, or a swallow may be present but only after a lengthy delay. In these situations, the goal is to increase the frequency of swallowing and decrease the delay of response. Because survivors at Rancho Levels I to III display no responses or inconsistent alertness, eliciting and improving the speed and consistency of swallowing is best done with external rather than intraoral stimulation. One method is to place two or three fingers externally at the base of the tongue (i.e., under the survivor's chin and above the thyroid cartilage), apply firm pressure, and stroke in an anterior-to-posterior motion. This prompts initiation of lingual movement in some survivors, and a swallow response may follow.

Presence of Primitive Oral Reflexes. Primitive oral reflexes (see Appendix 5.A in Chapter 5) are usually inhibited naturally as neurological recovery occurs; however, with some survivors of severe TBI, neurological recovery may be limited, and these reflexes may persist indefinitely. No direct treatment exists to inhibit primitive oral reflexes in survivors of TBI. Rather, speech–language pathologists should monitor the types of stimulation that elicit reflexes and focus on desensitization of the associated structures.

Rancho Levels IV to X

Many survivors of TBI functioning at Rancho Levels IV to X can tolerate at least some food and liquid orally; however, not all can meet nutritional needs through oral intake. Depending on swallowing status, treatment may take several forms. For those tolerating PO intake, a portion of swallowing treatment may occur during meals to allow for assessment and training in the use of compensatory techniques. Because of limitations in memory and self-regulatory skills, some survivors may not implement compensatory techniques effectively or at all, and supervision during meals may be necessary to ensure follow-through. At other times and for other survivors, sessions may focus on executing oral motor and pharyngeal exercises and applying thermal stimulation. Survivors functioning at Rancho Level IV have a particular problem with agitation that can impact swallowing treatment. If a survivor becomes agitated, stop the current activity and give the survivor an opportunity to calm down. Once the agitation has dissipated, intervention can resume; however, if agitation recurs, the focus of the session should shift from swallowing to another area, perhaps relating to cognition or language. Overall, treatment strategies for survivors functioning at Rancho Levels IV to X include training in compensatory techniques, implementing strengthening exercises, using thermal stimulation, and making diet modifications as needed.

Compensatory Techniques. Compensatory techniques serve to minimize an individual's risk of aspiration. The implementation of postural strategies and swallowing maneuvers can sometimes eliminate the need for diet modifications. However, if the strategies fail to eliminate aspiration, changes in food and liquid consistencies may be necessary and appropriate. Many of these techniques may be effective for individuals functioning at Rancho Levels IV, V, and VI. However, because posttraumatic amnesia has not yet resolved, these individuals will not use these techniques independently, and direct supervision during meals will be needed to ensure appropriate implementation.

Postural strategies involve manipulating the position of the head or body. Commonly used techniques include tucking the chin, turning the head to the weaker side of the body, tilting the head to the stronger side of the mouth and pharynx, and, in rare instances, tilting the chin or head backward. As outlined in Table 9.5, selection and implementation of each of these strategies are dependent on the source of a survivor's swallowing problem.

Swallowing maneuvers involve skillful modification of steps within the swallow process itself. The techniques used most frequently include (a) double swallows, (b) effortful swallows, (c) supraglottic swallows, (d) the Mendelsohn maneuver, and (e) alternation of food and liquid. Each should be trained first without foods or liquids until the individual demonstrates consistent perfor-

Table 9.5
Swallowing Problems Addressed by Various Postural Strategies

Swallowing strategy	Source of swallowing problem
Chin tuck	Delayed trigger of the swallow response
	Reduced airway closure
Head turn to weaker side of body	Unilateral pharyngeal/laryngeal weakness or paralysis
	Reduced laryngeal elevation
	Reduced cricopharyngeal opening
Head tilt to stronger side of mouth	Unilateral pharyngeal weakness
	Unilateral oral weakness
Chin/head tilt backward	Delayed oral transit time but normal pharyngeal and laryngeal control

mance and understanding. Table 9.6 summarizes the procedures for performing each technique and indicates the type of swallowing problems for which each is appropriate.

Strengthening Exercises and Thermal Stimulation. Strengthening exercises and thermal stimulation are forms of indirect therapy that may improve swallowing function. They are appropriate both for individuals who cannot tolerate any PO intake and for individuals on modified diets.

Oral–motor exercises targeting the tongue, lips, cheeks, and larynx should relate directly to identified swallowing disorders. A typical regimen requires 10 repetitions of each exercise three times daily. Lists of sample exercises are provided in most swallowing texts.

Thermal stimulation is often implemented with individuals having absent or delayed swallow responses. It involves holding a laryngeal mirror in a cup of ice or ice-cold water for approximately 10 seconds, followed by quick, gentle strokes along the faucial arches from top to bottom about four to five times on each side. Immediately following this stimulation, the individual should attempt to swallow either saliva or a small amount of cold liquid, depending on his or her oral intake status.

Research documenting the efficacy of thermal stimulation is inconclusive. Some researchers found no increase in the facilitation of swallow responses following thermal stimulation (Ali, Laundl, Wallace, deCarle, & Cook, 1996; Knauer, Castell, Dalton, Nowak, & Castell, 1990; Selinger, Prescott, & Hoffman, 1994), but others found that thermal stimulation resulted in a greater

Table 9.6
Procedures for Implementing Various Swallowing Maneuvers

Swallowing maneuver	Source of problem	Procedure
Double swallow (dry swallow)	Residue in pharynx	Follow initial swallow with two or three additional dry swallows
Effortful swallow	Residue in pharynx	Squeeze hard during swallowing or imagine swallowing a golf ball
Supraglottic swallow	Reduced airway closure	1. Inhale and hold breath
		2. While holding breath, swallow
		3. Cough to clear any residual material left in the pyriform sinuses or vallecula
Mendelsohn maneuver	Reduced laryngeal elevation Reduced opening of the cricopharyngeal sphincter	1. Swallow several times to increase awareness of laryngeal elevation
		2. Elevate larynx and maintain this position for several seconds during the swallow
Alternating foods and liquids	Residue in oral, pharyngeal, or laryngeal cavity	Take a sip of fluid after each bite of solid food

number of swallows, a decrease in the delay of triggering swallow responses, or both (Kaatzke-McDonald, Post, & Davis, 1996; Lazzara, Lazarus, & Logemann, 1986; Rosenbek, Robbins, Fishback, & Levine, 1996).

Diet Modifications. Diet modifications are appropriate only when other strategies prove ineffective (Logemann, 1993). To be effective, everyone interacting with a survivor must be aware of current diet modifications to ensure swallowing safety across all situations.

With respect to food, diets include regular, chopped, mechanical soft, and pureed. The difference between a regular diet and a chopped diet is that for a chopped diet, all foods are cut into small, bite-sized pieces. A mechanical soft diet is moist, and the meats are ground; foods such as dry crackers and hard vegetables are excluded. A pureed diet includes only smooth textures such as mashed potatoes, squash, or food blended to this consistency.

For liquids, three consistencies exist: thin, nectar, and honey-thick. Thin liquids include those such as water and fruit juices. Nectars are slightly more viscous such as tomato juice and some blended fruit drinks. Honey-thick liquids are quite dense and should pour slowly. Prethickened nectar and honey-thick consistencies can be purchased from food manufacturing and distribution companies or can be made by adding powdered thickener—available at local pharmacies—to various liquids. Anytime a person is restricted to drinking nectar or honey-thick liquids, hydration levels should be closely monitored, because people tend to consume smaller amounts of these than thin liquids.

Additional Considerations for Treating Children

In addition to the treatment guidelines stated above, Arvedson (1993) recommends that treatment with children focus on proper body positioning, method of food presentation, nipple feeding, and food textures. For example, children who have difficulty with anterior–posterior transit may benefit from a semi-reclined position that uses gravity to facilitate propulsion of the bolus (Ylvisaker & Weinstein, 1989). For children who are spoon-feeding, the parent or caregiver should place the spoon midtongue to leave the bolus in a central position for facilitating a timely swallow. Adding slight downward pressure of the spoon on the tongue aides with lip closure. Specific placement of the parent's or caregiver's hands may be necessary to maintain adequate jaw control or lip closure. To encourage sucking and facilitate oral stimulation needed for adequate nipple feeding, Arvedson (1996) recommends using a pacifier or gloved finger to stroke the infant's or child's tongue at a rate of one stroke per second. Slight downward pressure should be used while stroking from the middle of the tongue toward the tip. Presenting foods having specific textures or temperatures may also positively enhance swallowing. For more comprehensive treatment strategies specific to children, readers are referred to textbooks dedicated entirely to dysphagia such as *Pediatric Swallowing and Feeding: Assessment and Management* (Arvedson, 2002) and *Pediatric Dysphagia Resource Guide* (Hall, 2001).

Ethical Considerations

All speech–language pathologists must comply with ASHA guidelines, state guidelines, and the policies and procedures of the facility in which they are employed. On occasion, a situation may arise in which a client or family member does not agree with the speech–language pathologist's professional recommendations and is therefore noncompliant. Any survivor of TBI, or the person acting as power of attorney for the survivor, has a right to refuse treatment. However, the primary speech–language pathologist must be confident that the person making this decision is cognitively able to do so and understands all of the associated consequences of not following the recommendations.

Family members tend to focus on the survivor's resumption of eating as a major achievement in the recovery process. As a result, family members sometimes persistently try to persuade the therapist to begin oral feedings before the survivor is ready. Occasionally, family members secretly try to feed the survivor food or liquid that cannot be safely tolerated. If this situation arises, the speech–language pathologist should first review all medical documentation with the survivor and/or caregiver, such as the MBS or FEES video, to reiterate the existing problem and associated consequences if diet recommendations are not followed. Then, the speech–language pathologist should discuss the situation with the primary physician who may assist by reinforcing the recommendations with the family. The speech–language pathologist should document in the medical records all recommendations and the associated consequences if recommendations are not adhered to, the survivor or caregiver's resistance to the recommendations, and any other measures taken to reiterate the diet recommendations and the related risks. If the survivor or caregiver still refuses to adhere to the recommendations, some departments or facilities may ask that a waiver be signed.

A waiver is one way a professional can protect his or her license should anything negative result from the survivor's or caregiver's reluctance to follow the recommendations. The form should include information pertaining to the current recommended diet even if the recommendation is NPO. It should also include a statement indicating that the person signing the waiver has been thoroughly educated on the associated risks of aspiration and possible pneumonia if recommendations are not followed. A sample waiver is shown in Figure 9.6.

Summary

Swallowing problems associated with traumatic brain injury sometimes appear as temporary conditions and sometimes appear as permanent disabilities. Implementation of swallowing treatment, such as teaching compensatory strategies and making diet modifications, often enables survivors to tolerate oral intake safely and avoid the need for an alternate method of feeding (Schurr et al., 1999). Any attempt to ameliorate swallowing problems requires ongoing

Patient Name: _____   Physician: _____

Diagnosis: _____   Date: _____

The purpose of this document is to verify completion of training by the speech–language pathologist with the patient and family regarding safety, risks, strategies, and education pertaining to swallowing and modified food consistencies. The patient, family, physician, and speech–language pathologist are core members of the rehabilitation team. Decisions are made by the team to ensure optimal safety of the patient. In compliance with our code of ethics, the speech–language pathologist is responsible for designing the therapeutic intervention for remediation of swallowing problems and determining an appropriate diet that best prevents risks for aspiration.

I/we have been educated on the current
swallowing status of _____
                                              (Patient's Name)

The following materials and recommendations have been reviewed with me/us.

Food consistency _____   Positioning _____

Liquid consistency _____   Cueing _____

Swallowing strategies_____   Amount of supervision _____

1. Patient/family received literature on dysphagia on_____(date).
2. Viewed MBS/FEES video on _____(date).
3. Reviewed anatomy and physiology of a normal and abnormal swallow
    on_____(date).
4. Therapist reviewed swallowing strategies and positioning on_____(date).
5. Patient/family reverse-demonstrated swallowing strategies on _____(date).

I/We DO/DO NOT agree with the above recommendations and DO/DO NOT
choose to follow these recommendations.

Additional comments:_____

_____

_____

_____

_____   _____
Speech–Language Pathologist   **Date**

_____   _____
Patient   **Date**

_____   _____
Family Member   **Date**

Figure 9.6. Sample waiver form.

assessment, a dynamic treatment plan, and a team approach. Swallowing function cannot be assessed and treated as a separate entity from the person. Rather, a survivor's current abilities and impairments as a whole—particularly those related to cognition—have a direct impact on the approaches implemented throughout the assessment and treatment process.

 Case Example: Long-Term Status

About 2 years after Chad was discharged from swallowing therapy, he reported being able to drink thin liquids again. His continued performance of oral–motor exercises at home—sometimes with the help of his family— finally enabled him to tolerate foods and liquids of all consistencies safely. Even now, however, he requires additional time to eat and must maintain an upright posture whenever eating or drinking.

References

Adamovich, B. B. (1990). Treatment of communication and swallowing disorders. In M. Rosenthal, E. R. Griffith, M. R. Bond, & J. D. Miller (Eds.), *Rehabilitation of the adult and child with traumatic brain injury* (2nd ed., pp. 374–392). Philadelphia: Davis.

Ali, G. N., Laundl, T. M., Wallace, K. L., deCarle, D. J., & Cook, I. J. (1996). Influence of cold stimulation on the normal pharyngeal swallow response. *Dysphagia, 11,* 2–8.

American Speech-Language-Hearing Association. (1992, March). Instrumental diagnostic procedures for swallowing. *Asha, 34*(Suppl. 7), 25–33.

Annoni, J., Vuagnat, H., Frischknecht, R., & Uebelhart, D. (1998). Percutaneous endoscopic gastrostomy in neurological rehabilitation: A report of six cases. *Disability and Rehabilitation, 20,* 308–314.

Arvedson, J. C. (1993). Management of swallowing problems. In J. C. Arvedson & L. Brodsky (Eds.), *Pediatric swallowing and feeding: Assessment and management* (pp. 327–387). San Diego: Singular.

Arvedson, J. C. (1996). Dysphagia in pediatric patients with neurologic damage. *Seminars in Neurology, 16,* 371–386.

Arvedson, J. C. (2002). *Pediatric swallowing and feeding: Assessment and management* (2nd ed.). San Diego: Singular.

Arvedson, J. C., & Christensen, S. (1993). Instrumental evaluation. In J. C. Arvedson & L. Brodsky (Eds.), *Pediatric swallowing and feeding: Assessment and management* (pp. 293–326). San Diego: Singular.

Arvedson, J., Rogers, B., Buck, G., Smart, P., & Msall, M. (1994). Silent aspiration prominent in children with dysphagia. *International Journal of Pediatric Otorhinolaryngology, 28,* 173–181.

Cherney, L. R., & Halper, A. S. (1996). Swallowing problems in adults with traumatic brain injury. *Seminars in Neurology, 16*, 349–353.

Field, L. H., & Weiss, C. J. (1989). Dysphagia with head injury. *Brain Injury, 3*, 19–26.

Gross, H., Kling, A., Henry, G., Herndon, C., & Lavretsky, H. (1996). Local cerebral glucose metabolism in patients with long-term behavioral and cognitive deficits following mild traumatic brain injury. *Journal of Neuropsychiatry, 8*, 324–334.

Hagen, C. (2000, February). *Rancho Los Amigos Levels of Cognitive Functioning–Revised.* Presentation at TBI rehabilitation in a managed care environment: An interdisciplinary approach to rehabilitation, Continuing Education Programs of America, San Antonio, TX.

Hall, K. (2001). *Pediatric dysphagia resource guide.* Albany, NY: Delmar.

Hoppers, P., & Holm, S. E. (1999). The role of fiberoptic endoscopy in dysphagia rehabilitation. *Journal of Head Trauma Rehabilitation, 14*, 475–485.

Kaatzke-McDonald, M. N., Post, E., & Davis, P. J. (1996). The effects of cold, touch, and chemical stimulation of the anterior faucial pillar on human swallowing. *Dysphagia, 11*, 198–206.

Knauer, C. M., Castell, J. A., Dalton, C. B., Nowak, L., & Castell, D. O. (1990). Pharyngeal/upper esophageal sphincter pressure dynamics in humans: Effects of pharmacologic agents and thermal stimulation. *American Journal of Digestive Diseases and Sciences, 35*, 774–780.

Kramer, S. S., & Eicher, P. M. (1993). The evaluation of pediatric feeding abnormalities. *Dysphagia, 8*, 215–224.

Langmore, S. E. (1996, November). *FEES Examination Protocol.* Paper presented at FEES Workshop, San Diego Rehabilitation Institute, San Diego, CA.

Lazarus, C., & Logemann, J. A. (1987). Swallowing disorders in closed head trauma patients. *Archives of Physical Medicine and Rehabilitation, 68*, 79–84.

Lazzara, G., Lazarus, C., & Logemann, J. A. (1986). Impact of thermal stimulation on the triggering of the swallow reflex. *Dysphagia, 1*, 73–77.

Leder, S. B. (1999). Fiberoptic endoscopic evaluation of swallowing in patients with acute brain injury. *Journal of Head Trauma Rehabilitation, 14*, 448–453.

Leder, S. B., & Karas, D. E. (2000). Fiberoptic endoscopic evaluation of swallowing in the pediatric population. *The Laryngoscope, 110*, 1132–1136.

Lefton-Grief, M. A., & Loughlin, G. M. (1996). Specialized studies in pediatric dysphagia. *Seminars in Speech and Language, 17*, 311–329.

Logan, W. J., & Bosma, J. F. (1967). Oral and pharyngeal dysphagia in infancy. *Pediatric Clinics of North America, 14*, 47–61.

Logemann, J. A. (1983). *Evaluation and treatment of swallowing disorders.* Austin, TX: PRO-ED.

Logemann, J. A. (1993). *Manual for the videoflouroscopic study of swallowing* (2nd ed.). Austin, TX: PRO-ED.

Logemann, J. A. (1998). *Evaluation and treatment of swallowing disorders* (2nd ed.). Austin, TX: PRO-ED.

Logemann, J. A., & Ylvisaker, M. (1998). Therapy for feeding and swallowing disorders after TBI. In M. Ylvisaker (Ed.), *Traumatic brain injury rehabilitation: Children and adolescents* (2nd ed., pp. 85–89). Boston: Butterworth-Heinemann.

Mackay, L. E., Morgan, A. S., & Bernstein, B. (1999). Swallowing disorders in severe brain injury: Risk factors affecting return to oral intake. *Archives of Physical Medicine and Rehabilitation, 80*, 365–371.

NovaCare Rehabilitation. (1991). *Neurogenic dysphagia: Patient identification, evaluation, treatment.* King of Prussia, PA: Author.

Petersen, S. R., Jeevanandam, M., & Harrington, T. (1993). Is the metabolic response to injury different with or without severe head injury? Significance of plasma glutamine levels. *The Journal of Trauma, 34,* 653–661.

Rosenbek, J. C., Robbins, J., Fishback, B., & Levine, R. L. (1996). Effects of thermal application on dysphagia after stroke. *Journal of Speech and Hearing Research, 34,* 1257–1268.

Rowe, L. A. (1999). Case studies in dysphagia after pediatric brain injury. *Journal of Head Trauma Rehabilitation, 14,* 497–504.

Schurr, M. J., Ebner, K. A., Maser, A. L., Sperling, K. B., Helgerson, R. B., & Harms, B. (1999). Formal swallowing evaluation and therapy after traumatic brain injury improved dysphagia outcomes. *Journal of Trauma: Injury, Infection, and Critical Care, 46,* 817–823.

Selinger, M., Prescott, T. E., & Hoffman, I. (1994). Temperature acceleration in cold oral stimulation. *Dysphagia, 9,* 83–87.

Shellito, P. C., & Malt, R. A. (1985). Tube gastrostomy: Techniques and complications. *Annals of Surgery, 201,* 180–185.

Siktberg, L. L., & Bantz, D. L. (1999). Management of children with swallowing disorders. *Journal of Pediatric Healthcare, 13,* 223–229.

Tanaguchi, M. H., & Moyer, R. S. (1994). Assessment of risk factors for pneumonia in dysphagic children: Significance of videofluoroscopic swallowing evaluation. *Developmental Medicine and Child Neurology, 36,* 495–502.

Weiss, M. H. (1988). Dysphagia in infants and children. *Otolaryngology Clinics of North America, 21,* 727–735.

Ylvisaker, M. A., & Logemann, J. (1985) Therapy for feeding and swallowing disorders following head injury. In M. Ylvisaker (Ed.), *Head injury rehabilitation: Children and adolescents* (pp. 195–215). San Diego, CA: College-Hill Press.

Ylvisaker, M. A., & Weinstein, M. (1989). Recovery of oral feeding after pediatric head injury. *Journal of Head Trauma Rehabilitation, 4,* 51–63.

Yorkston, K. M., Honsinger, M. J., Mitsuda, P. M., & Hammen, V. (1989). The relationship between speech and swallowing disorders in head-injured patients. *Journal of Head Trauma Rehabilitation, 4,* 1–16.

Young, C. (1993). Nutrition. In J. C. Arvedson & L. Brodsky (Eds.), *Pediatric swallowing and feeding: Assessment and management* (pp. 157–208). San Diego: Singular.

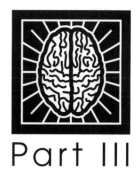

Part III

Understanding Reintegration

Psychosocial Recovery of Youth and Adolescents with Traumatic Brain Injury
Nature of the Problem and Intervention Approaches

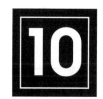

William J. Warzak and Karla Anhalt

Approximately 4% of youth will experience some form of head trauma by the time they graduate from high school (Savage, 1991). The full extent of a young child's injury may not be apparent for several years because its effect may not be evident until a later point in the child's development (Rutter, Chadwick, & Shaffer, 1983). The child's passage through adolescence may be particularly complicated by the sequelae of brain injury. Many students with TBI require special education services and accommodation (Savage, 1991). Even those with apparently mild injuries and no loss of consciousness may have impaired attention, memory, and emotional control (Binder, 1986; Levin, Benton, & Grossman, 1982). Furthermore, TBI can exacerbate preexisting cognitive deficits (Dean, 1985). Even subtle deficits may affect social, familial, and academic functioning (Eisenberg, 1989; Levin et al., 1982; Rosenthal, 1983).

Obstacles to psychosocial adjustment vary as a function of the injury's type and severity, but many commonalities across injuries also merit discussion. This chapter addresses, from a behavioral perspective, the many psychosocial issues that arise from TBI. Interventions that focus on an adolescent's social environment—including parents, peers, and teachers as primary agents of change—are emphasized. The cognitive and behavioral sequelae that complicate psychosocial functioning are reviewed, along with behavioral principles and procedures that may be effective in helping youth and adolescents adjust to TBI. Adjustment issues related to interactions within a family, with peers, and at school receive particular emphasis. Issues related to sexuality and the potential for abuse also are addressed. Finally, the implications of TBI on potential psychiatric and affective disturbance are discussed.

Sequelae of Traumatic Brain Injury

Many factors influence the sequelae of TBI in children. Among these are the nature of an injury, such as a closed-head versus penetrating wound; its location; and its severity. TBIs are typically described as *mild*, *moderate*, or *severe*, with each level of injury yielding differing levels of residual impairment. Up to

50% of patients who sustain mild head injuries (e.g., minimal cerebral bruising, swelling, or tissue strain) report symptoms months later (Rimel, Giordani, Barth, Boll, & Jane, 1981; Rutherford, 1989; see Chapter 4). Headaches and impaired memory may be ongoing concerns and may disrupt family functioning even 1 year postinjury (Evans, Evans, & Sharp, 1994; Hu, Wesson, Kenney, Chipman, & Spence, 1993). Parents and school staff may interpret subsequent challenging behavior as lack of motivation, noncompliance, or defiance, not recognizing the role TBI may play in influencing behavior (Warzak, Allan, Ford, & Stefans, 1995).

People with moderate brain injuries may make good recoveries, but they frequently report persistent headaches, memory deficits, and difficulties performing activities of daily living (Rimel et al., 1981). Children with this level of injury often recover some academic skills and abilities—especially during the first year postinjury; however, many children with moderate TBI plateau during the second year of recovery, with skills and abilities remaining substantially below their preinjury status and below that of uninjured peers (Jaffe, Polissar, Fay, & Liao, 1995; Koskiniemi, Kyykka, Nybo, & Jarho, 1995). The continued residual impairment experienced by these students results in difficulties at home as well as at school. Adolescents who at one time performed well academically, socially, or athletically may have lost these advantages. Further complicating matters, many such students clearly recall their preinjury abilities and are aware of their new limitations. ⟵ very important

Children with severe injuries may experience significant deficits across wide areas of functioning including attention, concentration, memory, reasoning, impulse control, and speech and language skills (Levin et al., 1982). Chronic motor, behavioral, and affective impairments are common (Mitiguy, Thompson, & Wasco, 1990). Many of these children do not regain independent function and require much day-to-day care. The level of care required by survivors of severe TBI greatly affects the quality of life and daily routine of all family members.

Psychosocial Adaptation

Family Issues

Nature of the Problem

Brain injuries often occur suddenly. Parents must learn to adapt to a child who is different from the person they knew preinjury. A postinjury adolescent may present with significant limitations, a different social repertoire, and affective and behavioral deficits (Cooley & Singer, 1991; Warzak, Allan, et al., 1995).

Everyday activities ranging from dressing and hygiene to simple household chores, school responsibilities, and homework may be affected. For example, assisting youth who can no longer dress independently requires a change in daily routine for parents or siblings. Memory deficits may make it difficult to complete simple household chores or individual tasks. Previous conversations may be forgotten or jokes may be told repeatedly to the annoyance of family members. Once-active adolescents may now spend far greater portions of their time at home, reducing the privacy or activities of other family members. Parents may resume the role of primary caregiver for adolescents who were once relatively independent. These new parental responsibilities often come in addition to other, more routine, parental expectations and obligations. Over time, parents themselves may become socially isolated, resentful, or depressed (Jacobs, 1988; Lezak, 1978).

The greater the deficits and the chronicity of impairment, the greater the demands placed on the family system and the more likely that characteristics of the family—positive or negative—will affect rehabilitation and psychosocial outcomes. Family disorganization and dysfunction are likely to be exacerbated by the presence of a family member with chronic impairment. Because rehabilitation outcomes tend to be positively associated with effective family functioning (Maitz & Sachs, 1995), family variables need to be assessed as part of any rehabilitation plan.

Interventions

Families may benefit from the guidance of a professional who is familiar with the cognitive, behavioral, and affective consequences of TBI. Not only can such a professional provide realistic expectations, coping strategies, and support to the injured individual, they may also help family members deal with feelings of grief, resentment, anger, or depression.

Given the neuropsychological status and behavioral repertoire of some adolescents with TBI, previously effective parenting strategies now may be ineffective, and parents may benefit from new strategies to help their child develop a more adaptive and appropriate repertoire. One such approach that has been effective across a wide variety of children and problem behaviors is behavioral parent training. The focus is on changing the behavior of parents and significant others to effect changes in an adolescent's behavior (Anderson & Warzak, 2000; Warzak & Anderson, 2001). For example, the simple verbal delivery of requests or commands may no longer be sufficient if a youth's response to auditory stimuli, understanding of spoken language, or retention of commands over time has deteriorated. Similarly, the adolescent may respond with frustration to situations previously mastered but now beyond his or her capability. Parents can use a combination of approaches to address these issues. Alternative cueing strategies may be required, task analyses conducted, or functional assessments performed. Extrinsic incentives (e.g., points redeemable for various rewards) may help to shape, increase, and maintain newly acquired skills or to motivate the adolescent to complete previously mastered tasks, keeping in mind that conditions that previously served to reinforce behavior may no longer be effective because of changes in cognitive functioning (e.g., changes in perceptual, sensory, or motor skills).

Peer Interactions

Nature of the Problem

A variety of conditions may prevent an adolescent from participating in familiar activities post-TBI. For example, the person may have motor deficits that render previous activities impossible. Even students who have made good recoveries may have residual deficits. For example, one student athlete with a good recovery from an auto accident resulting in mild-to-moderate TBI had great difficulty returning to varsity basketball competition. Although his motor skills had recovered to a great degree, he could not attend sufficiently to instructions while in the tense and boisterous ambiance of basketball games. In addition, he often could not remember recently reviewed play strategies, crowd noises were a distraction, and his memory for plays was impaired enough to impede his performance.

Some survivors of TBI present with specific social skills deficits such as poor conversational skills, poor turn-taking, and interrupting. Poor monitoring of social cues and difficulty regulating one's own behavior complicate these situations (Borod & Koff, 1990; Hopewell, Burke, Weslowski, & Zawlocki, 1990); in turn, these limitations can lead to other dysfunctional behavior. Adolescents with TBI may experience difficulty maintaining old friendships and developing new ones when their social repertoire is impaired. Behavior that once served to encourage the presence of peers (e.g., telling contextually appropriate jokes, engaging in conversational reciprocity) may no longer be present, and new behaviors may appear that are inappropriate and that discourage social contact by others. Finally, some former friends simply may be uncomfortable with or embarrassed by injured peers and, therefore, may avoid social interactions with them.

Interventions

The issue of social reintegration is an important one for adolescents with TBI because many of them demonstrate difficulty interacting with others. Driving, dating, and other activities associated with independence may need to be postponed indefinitely, functionally isolating an adolescent (Warzak, Allan, et al., 1995). Because social isolation virtually precludes adequate psychosocial adjustment and is a risk factor for depression, parents must be taught the importance of fostering their child's social contacts, perhaps by encouraging or arranging activities for them and ensuring that they have the appropriate repertoire to engage in those activities. Some social skills may need to be relearned, and, much like for other rehabilitation goals, performing task analyses of necessary skills may be helpful. Adolescents with skill deficits need training to teach them the specific social skills they are lacking and need opportunities to practice newly learned skills.

If the goal is to reintegrate an adolescent into a school setting, target behavior might focus on riding the school bus, initiating conversations, or giving and receiving compliments. The behavior to meet each objective should be operationally defined to permit accurate measurement of performance and to facilitate the delivery of appropriate consequences contingent upon the adolescent's behavior. Careful consideration of the components of each task helps to ensure that goals remain within the range of a youth's current behavioral competency. Limitations caused by the TBI that render a youth less responsive to cues and consequences that were effective preinjury require special consideration (Warzak & Kilburn, 1990).

A common complaint among people with TBI is difficulty following conversations and making contributions to them. This is especially the case in social settings with multiple sources of distraction (e.g., in classrooms, in cafeterias, or on school buses). Difficulty screening out extraneous stimuli may result in reduced levels of appropriate interaction with peers. Instruction about how to position oneself to minimize distractions or about ways to request that conversations be moved to another location is beneficial. Providing opportunities to practice these requests in instructional settings allows for the teaching and reinforcement of appropriate skills prior to a youth's attempt to implement them in the natural environment.

The sequence of teaching social interactions for the above situation could be as follows. First, the adult models the appropriate behavior, and the adolescent practices in the presence of the adult, who provides supportive feedback and reinforces approximations to the desired end result. Second, the adolescent practices with a peer or confederate (e.g., brother or sister) who has been instructed to reinforce the correct response (e.g., "Sure, that would be fine") and then change position or location to minimize distractions. Third, the adolescent with TBI could practice the interaction in a natural setting such as the cafeteria, library, or playground. Eventually, programmed training could be withdrawn to allow more natural consequences—such as positive peer interaction—to maintain the response.

School

Nature of the Problem

Effective return to the classroom setting is among the most challenging and important rehabilitation goals because of the confluence of issues related to functioning in cognitive, motoric, and interpersonal domains. The classroom is the locus of much learning and psychosocial skills building and, as such, provides the building blocks for the development of effective social and vocational repertoires. Failure to return successfully to school is often a poor prognostic indicator, implying at best practical limitations for the student, and at worst serious cognitive, motor, and/or psychosocial deficits. Students and family members may be especially concerned about the return to school and may push for a premature return to the classroom that may not be in the best interest of the student.

The initial concern is a student's ability to cope with basic classroom conditions, ranging from the level of stimulation to the pace of academic instruction. If youth return to school too soon after injury, they may be unprepared to deal with traditional classroom expectations (Ylvisaker, Hartwick, & Stevens, 1991). Therefore, the rate at which they work, process information, and acquire and retain new information must be evaluated. Educators must also ascertain the extent to which students can work independently and how much assistance, if any, they require. Prior to the student's return to school, professionals should ensure that a student with TBI has functional classroom skills including communication skills, the ability to stay on task, the ability to function in a small group environment, and the ability to follow simple instructions (Cohen, 1991). Settings geared primarily to students with developmental delays may have the greatest resources but may be inappropriate for students with TBI given that some survivors have areas of relatively normal cognitive and social functioning.

Intervention

As addressed in the next chapter, dealing effectively with school reintegration requires an Individualized Education Program (IEP) that integrates various data into an educational plan while keeping in mind that the cognitive and behavioral functioning of recently injured students is not static. The IEP must be flexible, contain short-term goals, and be reviewed frequently to detect changes in the student's status (Cohen, 1991; Savage, 1991). Modification of the regular education schedule is often appropriate; this might involve a lighter course load, half-day scheduling, use of a resource room, special tutorial sessions, or brief breaks throughout the day to combat fatigue. Goals and objectives that focus on cognitive processes, learning-to-learn strategies, problem solving, and adaptive behavior may be among the most appropriate for students with significant deficits. A comprehensive evaluation of these children may require neuropsychological and behavioral assessment to determine the cognitive and environmental events that affect daily performance. For example, students may require extra time for traveling between classes, perhaps at a time when the school halls contain few students. Students who experience visual–spatial deficits or otherwise have difficulty remaining oriented may require a school "buddy" to assist between classes, help with notes, assemble materials, and perform other various tasks (Warzak, Mayfield, & McAllister, 1998).

Coordinating school programming with rehabilitation efforts in the home requires close communication among all relevant parties. One common method of school-to-home communication is through notes; these notes can provide frequent feedback to the student during the course of the school day and a quantifiable summary of the adolescent's behavior to his or her parents or guardians at the day's end. Parents then present appropriate consequences, contingent upon the nature of the daily report, thus extending their influence from the home to the school. For example, a target behavior for a student with TBI might be "being prepared when class begins." This could be defined as having appropriate books and a pencil on the desk and being seated when the bell rings. Another target behavior might be "participating in class," with the definition that the student will raise his or her hand and ask two relevant questions or make two relevant points during each class period. Defining target behaviors in objective and measurable terms is important so that the student, teachers, and parents share an understanding of the expectations. At the end of each class, the teacher would record a "plus" or a "minus" to indicate whether the student met the behavioral expectations. At home, having more pluses than minuses would earn a privilege or special reward tailored to the student's interests.

Finally, many students with TBI have a strong desire to graduate with their class. School staff should permit participation in graduation exercises if at all possible. Many students who complete high school the summer after graduation—or even later—gain substantial social and psychological benefit from being with their class during graduation exercises.

Sexuality

Nature of the Problem

The development of sexuality and sexual adjustment may be altered by TBI. The relevant effects of TBI vary as a function of the age at which the injury occurred. For example, a congenital injury with residual impairment will be integrated into ongoing sexual development, and the experience of disability will shape maturation and sexual adjustment. TBI that occurs in childhood or adolescence, however, may affect long-held beliefs and expectations regarding sexuality, the role of the youth in social–sexual situations, and sexual functioning itself. Other factors such as the level of residual cognitive and motor impairment, the conspicuousness of impairment, if any, and mobility limitations also may affect long-term sexual adjustment and outcome (Kewman, Warschausky, Engel, & Warzak, 1997).

Youth with TBI have difficulty acquiring information and skills related to the development of social relationships and sexual behavior (Baugh, 1984; Cole, 1981, 1988; Tharinger, Horton, & Millea, 1990; D. N. Williams, 1987). Circumstances as varied as limited mobility and a lack of appropriate materials for individuals with sensory or cognitive deficits affect the availability of relevant information. Also, cognitive deficits may limit understanding of community standards and consequences of sexual behavior (Freeman, Goetz, Richards & Groenveld, 1991; Giami, 1987; J. K. Williams, 1983). In addition, particular patterns of impairment interfere with the detection of subtle social cues—such as facial expressions or voice intonation—that provide information relevant to the social appropriateness of sexual behavior (Schuster, 1986; Warzak, Evans, & Ford, 1992; Warzak & Kilburn, 1990). Additionally, certain injuries result in disinhibition, thus prompting sexual behavior inappropriate to the time, place, or person with whom it is initiated (Zencius, Wesolowski, Burke, & Hough, 1990).

Youth with TBI also may be at risk for sexual exploitation. They may not perceive or accurately attend to cues that might otherwise warn them of dangerous situations. On the other hand, they may be aware of these cues, but their disability may prevent them from leaving threatening situations independently (Freeman et al., 1991). They may have difficulty ascertaining the intentions of others or may be unaware of inadvertent cues their behavior may provide to those with whom they interact. Difficulty anticipating consequences combined with impaired problem-solving skills may result in adolescents with TBI placing themselves in exploitative situations with fewer alternatives to remove themselves safely than are available to their unimpaired peers (Warzak, Kuhn, & Nolten, 1995).

Intervention

Along with normalization and community integration comes a responsibility to educate youth about sexuality and sexual functioning, to assist youth in developing safe and responsible sexual behavior, and to promote sexual adjustment (Baugh, 1984). Issues ranging from the level and type of disability to the cultural heritage of participants will affect strategies and procedures developed to promote sexual adjustment (Schwartzbaum, 1992). Given that no single socially approved standard of sexual behavior exists (Kempton, 1988), parents and providers must agree on a common set of goals that focus on a specific adolescent's sexual adjustment.

The social acceptability of programs related to sexual adjustment, including the interest of students and staff in participating in them, has not been evaluated. Programs that do not have interested participants and dedicated staff are bound to be ineffective. Further, sex education programs must be tailored to accommodate individual limitations, including general developmental level and cognitive, sensory, and social skills deficits. An assessment of individual needs must include an evaluation of existing sexual knowledge and current behavioral repertoire. Contraceptive methods requiring planning and judgment may not be suitable for individuals whose cognitive processes are very immediate and concrete.

Having recognized the risks faced by adolescents with TBI, professionals can take steps to protect them from sexual exploitation by peers or others. Because no single behavioral profile indicates sexual abuse, those having regular contact with adolescents at risk need to attend to and investigate further any changes in behavior that may signify distress (Baladerian, 1991). With the exception of sexualized behavior and symptoms of posttraumatic stress disorder (PTSD), the short-term effects of sexual abuse are similar to what one sees in clinically referred populations in general (e.g., anxiety, fears, withdrawn behavior, school problems) (Beitchman, Zucker, Hood, daCosta, & Akman, 1991; Deblinger, McLeer, Atkins, Ralphe, & Foa, 1989; Kendall-Tackett, Williams, & Finkelhor, 1993). Most cases of abuse are identified through victim disclosure (Tharinger et al., 1990), making the student's assertiveness skills to report abusive episodes a practical and clinical concern (Kolko, 1988). Most assertiveness training programs in the area of sexuality have focused on unimpaired populations and have emphasized information, communication skills, and contraceptive issues (Burke, 1987; Committee on Adolescence, 1987; Flaherty, Marecek, Olsen, & Wilcove, 1983; Schinke, 1984; Shendell, 1992) rather than focusing on refusing unwanted sexual activity and reporting the occurrence of unwanted sexual contact. Few assertiveness training programs have been geared toward working with individuals with disabilities, and few have specifically targeted sexual refusal skills. Warzak and Page (1990) extrapolated refusal skills technology from the addictive behavior literature and successfully applied it to sexually active adolescents with disabilities including TBI. However, more work is needed in this area before effective sexual refusal strategies can be confidently developed for any population, including youth with TBI.

Anxiety and Depression

Nature of the Problem

Professionals and families need to be cognizant of the potential for anxiety and depression in survivors of TBI and the effects these disorders may have on behavior and psychosocial adjustment. Emotional and affective concerns are often less apparent than conduct problems and are less likely to be recognized and targeted for treatment by parents and school staff. Conduct problems (i.e., externalizing disorders) often disrupt school and family activities in a manner that requires immediate intervention (Albano, Chorpita, & Barlow, 1996), whereas internalizing problems (e.g., anxiety and depression) may not be seen as critical unless or until they precipitate a crisis. Left unattended, however, anxiety and depression can lead to very significant problems for adolescents with TBI and their family members.

Social anxiety and social avoidance may develop in adolescents with TBI for a variety of reasons. For example, individuals may have sustained injuries that they consider disfiguring, that impair their ability to ambulate independently or to speak clearly and effectively, or that in other ways separate them from their peers by appearance or function. These real or imagined limitations may contribute to social discomfort and awkwardness with peers who were previously friends and may curtail the development of new friendships. Furthermore, the reactions of others might be unpleasant, awkward, or otherwise aversive, leading the student with TBI to avoid certain social situations—even ones that were rewarding before the injury. Such situations may elicit social anxiety even if they did not previously evoke such a response. Social avoidance may be complicated by social skills deficits involving the loss of past skills or the difficulty acquiring new and developmentally appropriate skills. A combination of skills deficits and social anxiety can contribute to the social isolation of adolescents with TBI.

In addition to social avoidance and anxiety, people with TBI sometimes develop posttraumatic stress disorder (PTSD). In general, the more severe the head injury, the less likely that PTSD will develop (Cummings & Trimble, 1995) because patients with severe TBI are less likely to remember the details and psychological trauma of an accident. Among those who do experience PTSD, the disorder is often overlooked in light of other major cognitive and physical changes (Cummings & Trimble, 1995). Therefore, providers should be aware of PTSD symptoms, the three major characteristics of which are persistent reexperience of the traumatic event, persistent avoidance of stimuli associated with the trauma, and increased arousal not present before the PTSD event (American Psychiatric Association, 1994). To merit a diagnosis of PTSD, the symptoms should cause clinically significant impairment in social, occupational, or other significant areas of functioning (see Table 10.1).

However, even subclinical symptoms of anxiety may result in subjective discomfort, suggesting that individuals with TBI should be evaluated for the presence of anxiety-related dysfunction.

Given the potential everyday difficulties and long-term implications of TBI, it is not surprising that survivors are at risk for becoming depressed. To the extent that one's behavioral repertoire is compromised, an individual becomes less able to access activities that previously were enjoyable and sustaining and that previously contributed to a sense of well-being. School, social, and vocational activities may become more difficult or impossible, even with support. Thus, a loss of interest or motivation to participate in activities is not uncommon. Also, social isolation—a significant risk factor for depression—is common among those with significant deficits. Furthermore, individuals with TBI often are aware of their impairments in cognitive, social, and motor functioning, and comparisons to one's premorbid self may be especially difficult and

Table 10.1
Symptoms of Posttraumatic Stress Disorder

Symptom	Examples of manifestation
Reexperience of event	Complaints of thoughts about traumatic event
	Complaints of bad dreams or nightmares related to traumatic event
	Emotional recurrence of traumatic event (i.e., flashback episodes)
	Very upset when reminded of traumatic event
	Uncomfortable physical sensations when reminded of traumatic event
Avoidance	Avoidance of conversations associated with trauma
	Avoidance of people, places, or activities related to traumatic event
	Diminished interest in activities
	Restricted range of affect
Increased arousal	Difficulty falling or staying asleep
	Outbursts of anger
	Difficulty concentrating

Note. Adapted from the *Diagnostic and Statistical Manual of Mental Disorders–Fourth Edition,* by American Psychiatric Association, 1994, Washington, DC: Author. Copyright 1994 by the American Psychiatric Association. Adapted with permission.

disruptive to adjustment (Crooks & Baur, 1990; Kempton, 1988). The increased frequency of negative thoughts and affect may exacerbate symptoms of depression. Table 10.2 lists numerous symptoms that may indicate depression if several are present nearly every day over a 2-week period. For this reason, a suicide risk assessment in adolescents with TBI is necessary.

Depression is the psychological disorder most closely associated with suicidal behavior both in children and adults (Fremouw, de Perczel, & Ellis, 1990), and professionals should be cognizant of behaviors that suggest potential self-harm by adolescents with TBI. Feelings of hopelessness are especially indicative of suicide risk; such emotions and related cognitions may be manifest by reports of despair, lack of control, and pessimism about the future (Fremouw et al., 1990). Other general risk factors for child and adolescent suicide include repeated failures in school, limited peer social networks, major life stressors, and recent losses (Fremouw et al., 1990). These factors, consistent with the potential adverse psychosocial sequelae of TBI, place youth and adolescent survivors at increased risk for harming themselves or committing suicide.

Suicide risk increases if a youth has a specific, lethal method in mind (e.g., using a gun) and access to the method. The adolescent is at further risk if a history of previous suicide attempts exists. Parents or providers who suspect that an adolescent is at risk for self-harm should seek an immediate evaluation of the individual. Qualified mental health professionals in a person's work or school setting—such as school or clinical psychologists—may be the first

Table 10.2
Symptoms of Depression[a]

Reports feeling sad
Appears tearful
Significantly less interested in usual activities
Increased eating or loss of appetite
Weight gain or weight loss
Insomnia or hypersomnia
Observed psychomotor agitation or retardation
Reports feeling worthless or extremely guilty
Recurrent suicidal ideation

[a]The presence of several of these symptoms suggests a depressive episode if observed or reported nearly every day during a 2-week period.

Note. Adapted from the *Diagnostic and Statistical Manual of Mental Disorders–Fourth Edition,* by American Psychiatric Association, 1994, Washington, DC: Author. Copyright 1994 by the American Psychiatric Association. Adapted with permission.

people to contact. Alternatively, local mental health agencies typically have 24-hour crisis response lines that can help with the evaluation and hospitalization process if needed. A referral to an adolescent's pediatrician or to a child psychiatrist also may be warranted to rule out medical conditions that may present as anxiety or depression.

Intervention

A variety of treatment approaches for anxiety and depression exist, but behavioral procedures have been the most systematically studied. Procedures that have been helpful in treating anxiety include systematic desensitization, prolonged exposure, and modeling. To illustrate, systematic desensitization involves a three-step procedure that was developed by Wolpe (1958). Typically, during the first step individuals are taught deep muscle relaxation. The second step involves creating a hierarchy of anxiety-producing stimuli that initially contains situations producing little significant anxiety. Finally, adolescents expose themselves to these situations by approaching them—through their imagination or in vivo—while in a relaxed state (deep muscle relaxation is practiced immediately before and during exposure). The rationale for systematic desensitization involves two principles: (a) a relaxed emotional state is incompatible with feeling anxious; and (b) graduated exposure is likely to result in a successful outcome because the person experiences mastery of anxiety in a progressive manner. Detailed descriptions of other empirically validated interventions for anxiety in adolescents are available in the review by Barrios and O'Dell (1998).

With regard to the treatment of depression, cognitive–behavioral approaches have been the most widely studied (Kazdin & Marciano, 1998). Interventions proven to be helpful for adolescents include pleasant activity scheduling, social skills training, relaxation training, and communication skills training. *The Adolescent Coping with Depression Course* (Clarke, Lewinsohn, & Hops, 1990; Lewinsohn, Clarke, Rohde, Hops, & Seeley, 1996) teaches the previously mentioned skills and is a well-established program for the treatment of depression in adolescents. Again, empirical research has provided a well-grounded rationale for each of these techniques. For example, people with depression consistently have been found to engage in fewer activities that are rewarding for them. Thus, interventions that encourage adolescents to schedule and follow through with usual activities should help reestablish enjoyable events in their lives. In addition, older children with depression have been found to have greater social skills deficits than their nondepressed peers (e.g., Altmann & Gotlib, 1988; Kennedy, Spence, & Hensley, 1989). After an evaluation of an adolescent's skill deficits, an individualized program to teach social skills can be implemented. For example an adolescent may be taught assertiveness skills, ways to initiate a conversation with peers, and how to provide compliments to peers and adults. Providing structured opportunities in which to practice these skills is critical to success.

Behavioral Support Strategies

Nature of the Problem

Adolescents with TBI often experience behavior problems. Many times, these difficulties arise from defective contingencies established by well-intentioned adults. These contingencies—which may seem appropriate in the immediate context of an injury—may take the form of loosening the rules for the injured adolescent or reducing expectations relative to siblings and peers. Parents and school staff may have difficulty reinstating standard rules and procedures if and when a student's recovery permits him or her to function in a manner comparable to peers. While it is not uncommon for defective contingencies to lead to increasingly difficult-to-manage adolescents, inappropriate behavior resulting from the injury itself is also not uncommon. For example, behavioral excesses resulting from frontal lobe syndrome may be maintained by defective contingencies of reinforcement but also may be exacerbated by defective self-monitoring, self-regulation, and difficulty responding to changing environmental circumstances (i.e., difficulty learning from experience; Warzak et al., 1992). Similarly, some youth—particularly those with right hemisphere injuries—may not read social cues accurately and may demonstrate a lack of social awareness that results in inappropriate social behavior at home and elsewhere (Borod & Koff, 1990). These adolescents may possess appropriate social behavior but have difficulty interpreting social cues that dictate when such behavior should be exhibited. In both of these examples, a confluence of developmental, behavioral, and neuropsychological factors may obscure a clear etiology for behavioral dysfunction and complicate caregiver decisions.

Functional Assessment and Comprehensive Treatment Plans

If behavior problems are severe or persistent, a functional assessment should be conducted to guide treatment. A variety of direct and indirect functional assessment methodologies have been developed and can be adapted for parental use (Anderson & Warzak, 2000). Indirect methodologies involve gathering information about target behaviors via interview with parents and professionals who work with the student. Various interview formats are designed to assess adaptive behaviors and also may identify potential incentives for behavior change. Direct methods of functional assessment involve observing an individual's behavior in the context in which it occurs and recording over time each occurrence of the target behavior as well as antecedent and consequent events. This involves identifying who was present, the location, and what occurred before the target behavior was exhibited (e.g., mom asked the child to clean up, the child was playing alone). Also, what happened following the behavior would be noted in terms of who responded and specifically what they did (e.g., mother prompted the child to move, sister moved away from the child).

Once several instances of a behavior have been observed, patterns may emerge. For example, many individuals with moderate to severe TBI have difficulty coping with complex social stimuli (Alexander, 1984; Goethe & Levin, 1984; Lezak, 1988). If challenging behavior often occurs when the child is in large, noisy groups, efforts could be made to minimize the amount of time the child spends in such settings or to allow the individual to leave the situation when needed. A functional assessment may reveal that problems are more likely to occur at the end of the child's school day, perhaps as a result of fatigue (Warzak, Allan, et al., 1995). A schedule that allows for daily, structured rest time may be valuable in reducing incidents of problem behavior as well as facilitating performance in school and elsewhere (Cohen, 1991). Thus, environmental changes may preclude challenging behavior from occurring or escalating.

Based on the results of the functional assessment, a comprehensive treatment plan can be developed to teach the adolescent the necessary skills to access a reinforcer that he or she has previously received only as a contingent consequence of challenging behavior (e.g., staff termination of an undesirable activity contingent upon the disruptive or aggressive behavior of the student). Intervention typically includes three key components: (a) ecological changes, (b) skill building, and (c) differential consequences that follow problem behavior and appropriate behavior (Anderson & Warzak, 2000). For example, if findings from the functional assessment suggest that a high school student is throwing classroom materials to escape difficult academic tasks, educators can teach the student an appropriate way to ask for a break from these tasks. These alternative skills—in this case asking for a break—become part of an adolescent's repertoire only when their use is rewarded immediately and consistently. If positive consequences are provided consistently for these adaptive behaviors, the rates of these behaviors tend to settle at acceptable levels rather than to be overused or abused (Anderson, Freeman, & Scotti, 1999).

The final component of a comprehensive treatment plan involves identifying consequences for both challenging and appropriate behavior. Again, consequences should be identified based on the results of the functional assessment. For example, if the functional assessment suggests that challenging behavior is maintained by peer attention, such attention must not be provided upon the occurrence of challenging behavior; on the other hand, the adolescent should receive frequent staff and peer attention when he or she behaves appropriately. This may require teaching peers to respond in specific ways to the student's behavior and arranging consequences to motivate unimpaired peers to comply with the treatment plan. Some adolescents may benefit from reinforcers such as access to preferred activities or items that are contingent on exhibition of appropriate behavior. Such items could be withdrawn temporarily if the adolescent exhibits problem behavior.

The selection of consequences to motivate an adolescent's performance needs to be done carefully. Unlike unimpaired youth, people with TBI may have experienced physical or neuropsychological changes that render them unable to perceive or to respond to previously effective consequences. Potential reinforcers may be identified through discussion with the adolescent, completion of reinforcer survey schedules (e.g., Clement & Richard, 1976; Elliot, 1993), and observing an adolescent's everyday preferred activities.

Person-Centered Planning

Person-centered planning (PCP) makes rehabilitation and educational efforts a cooperative venture between the student, parents, and school staff. PCP focuses on developing achievable goals for people with disabilities by using specific procedures to identify and pursue those goals within the context of what a person wants and needs (Kincaid, 1996). For people with disabilities—including adolescents with TBI—this type of planning values (a) participating in community life, (b) making lasting friendships, (c) favoring individual preferences, (d) gaining respect and dignity in the community, and (e) supporting the development of personal competencies (Kincaid, 1996).

The use of PCP tools also helps parents and staff attain a broad understanding of a person's history, strengths, and needs. The following paragraphs and the case example on person-centered planning describe team-based assessment and intervention, PCP tools that help team members gain an in-depth understanding of the focus person, and PCP tools that can be used to improve an individual's current and future quality of life and psychosocial functioning.

Team-Based Assessment

The tools of PCP are likely to be most effective when important people in a person's life (e.g., school staff, family members, friends, and the survivor) work together as a team. Team-based assessment and intervention offer several advantages. First, the meeting's content (e.g., the person's social history) can be

Case Example: Person-Centered Planning

Shortly before school started, a team met to talk about Tammy's transition to 10th grade. Tammy had sustained a moderate-to-severe TBI in an automobile accident when she was 12 years old. Her subsequent deficits challenged a school staff that had little to no experience working with severely injured students with limited communication skills. Of particular concern was her long-standing history of physical aggression, typically in response to staff demands. School staff who attended this meeting included the principal, the 10th-grade regular and special education teachers, a speech–language pathologist, and the 9th-grade special education teacher. Tammy and Tammy's family—her older brother, her mother, and her father—also were at the meeting.

Two team members served as facilitators: one served to direct and elicit appropriate content from team members and the other summarized the content by drawing pictures and writing key words on large sheets of paper that could be seen by all participants. This provided a multimodal presentation of the proceedings and captured details that may have been overlooked in a simple written summary of the proceedings. By the end of the meeting, Tammy's 10th-grade school staff had noted her tendency to hit teachers in order to escape tasks that were boring to her, such as coloring by herself. They noted that Tammy had not hit anyone in regular education classrooms or when she was working individually with a staff member. They also noted that Tammy enjoyed playing outside and working on puzzles. In response to the meeting, Tammy's school staff planned to have a variety of puzzles available to Tammy, to do activities outside as much as possible, and to integrate Tammy in regular education activities to the maximum extent possible. In addition, they decided to teach Tammy an effective and appropriate means to communicate that she wanted a break from classroom activities.

accessed by all members. Second, group meetings are good contexts to discuss new ways for the adolescent to access typical community resources, to achieve short-term goals related to meaningful life outcomes, and to obtain team members' commitment to achieving these goals. Finally, PCP focuses on creating an environment in which members are both teachers and learners (Kincaid, 1996). No one person is considered the expert on the team, so staff, family members, and the injured adolescent can all contribute to and learn from team activities.

Several tools exist to provide a team with a comprehensive understanding of an adolescent's preinjury history and current needs and interests. One example is the Making Action Plans tool (MAPS; Falvey, Forest, Pearpoint, & Rosenberg, 1997). MAPS provides a semistructured method for reviewing a person's history, fears, strengths, and needs. In discussing a survivor's history, for example, critical life events are discussed; this may include a discussion of the time and severity of injury as well as the impact of TBI on the family's life. A review of the person's strengths highlights skill recovery, areas of improvement in behavioral or emotional functioning, and positive qualities. The team can decide the extent and the scope of the information needed and focus on the adolescent's quality of life at home, at school, or in the community, as needed.

Other PCP tools help the team to develop workable goals and objectives related to quality of life issues as reported by the person with TBI. A discussion of these tools is beyond the scope of the present chapter, but the interested reader is directed to the work of Falvey, Forest, Pearpoint, and Rosenberg (1997) and Kincaid (1996) for further discussion of these issues.

Conclusion

Many obstacles to psychosocial adjustment confront youth and adolescents with TBI. Not the least of these is the wide variety of cognitive and psychosocial problems and impairment levels presented by these individuals. This chapter addressed the many psychosocial issues that confront survivors of TBI from a behavioral and environmental perspective. If the relevant environmental variables are adroitly manipulated, the social environment can shape and maintain appropriate and adaptive repertoires for those with TBI. Adjustment issues related to interactions within the family, with peers, and at school require exploration, because these are the arenas in which adolescents' primary social interaction occurs.

Despite the focus of this chapter on the psychosocial difficulties that often result as emotional, cognitive, or behavioral sequelae of TBI, professionals should not assume that survivors of TBI will automatically have significant problems adjusting. Many at-risk youth—including some survivors of TBI—cope effectively with life stressors (Mash & Dozois, 1996). In addition, many adolescents with TBI experience difficulties in psychosocial adjustment due to factors other than TBI. Adolescence is a developmental stage during which individuation and separation issues become salient; the issues are difficult and can present even in the absence of injury, often to the confusion of parents and school staff (Kewman et al., 1997; Warzak, Allan, et al., 1995).

Finally, parents and providers need to be attuned to similarities across youth rather than to focus on differences that result from TBI. Typically, many adolescents with TBI are just as interested in music, movies, current fashion, and being accepted as their unimpaired peers. Families and professionals must foster opportunities for these individuals to participate in age-appropriate activities to the fullest extent possible. With successful facilitation of social reintegration, those with lasting impairment will experience minimal psychological distress and attain adequate psychosocial adjustment.

References

Albano, M. A., Chorpita, B. F., & Barlow, D. H. (1996). Childhood anxiety disorders. In E. J. Mash & R. A. Barkley (Eds.), *Child psychopathology* (pp. 196–241). New York: Guilford Press.

Alexander, M. P. (1984). Neurobehavioral consequences of closed head injury. *Neurology and Neurosurgery: Update Series, 5(#20).*

Altmann, E. O., & Gotlib, I. H. (1988). The social behavior of depressed children: An observational study. *Journal of Abnormal Child Psychology, 16,* 29–44.

American Psychiatric Association. (1994). *Diagnostic and statistical manual of mental disorders* (4th ed.). Washington, DC: Author.

Anderson, C. M., Freeman, K. A., & Scotti, J. R. (1999). Evaluation of the generalizability (reliability and validity) of analog assessment methodology. *Behavior Therapy, 30,* 31–50.

Anderson, C. M., & Warzak, W. J. (2000). Using positive behavior support to facilitate the classroom adaptation of children with brain injuries. *Proven Practice, 2,* 72–82.

Baladerian, N. J. (1991). Sexual abuse of people with developmental disabilities. *Sexuality and Disability, 9,* 323–335.

Barrios, B. A., & O'Dell, S. L. (1998). Fears and anxieties. In E. J. Mash & R. A. Barkley (Eds.), *Treatment of childhood disorders* (2nd ed., pp. 249–337). New York: Guilford Press.

Baugh, R. (1984). Sexuality education for the visually and hearing impaired child in the regular classroom. *Journal of School Health, 54,* 407–409.

Beitchman, J. H., Zucker, K. J., Hood, J. E., daCosta, G. A., & Akman, D. (1991). A review of the short-term effects of child sexual abuse. *Child Abuse and Neglect, 15,* 537–556.

Binder, L. M. (1986). Persisting symptoms after mild head injury: A review of the postconcussive syndrome. *Journal of Clinical and Experimental Neuropsychology, 8,* 323–346.

Borod, J. C., & Koff, E. (1990). Lateralization for facial emotional behavior: A methodological perspective. *International Journal of Psychology, 25,* 157–177.

Burke, P. J. (1987). Adolescents' motivation for sexual activity and pregnancy prevention. *Pediatric Nursing, 10,* 161–171.

Clarke, G. N., Lewinsohn, P. M., & Hops, H. (1990). *Adolescent coping with depression course: Leader's manual for adolescent groups.* Eugene, OR: Castalia.

Clement, P. W., & Richard, R. C. (1976). Identifying reinforcers for children: A children's reinforcement survey. In E. J. Mash & L. G. Terdal (Eds.), *Behavior therapy assessment: Diagnosis, design, and evaluation* (pp. 207–216). New York: Springer.

Cohen, S. B. (1991). Adapting educational programs for students with head injuries. *Journal of Head Trauma Rehabilitation, 6*(1), 47–55.

Cole, S. (1981). Disability/ability the importance of sexual health in adolescence: Issues and concerns of the professional. *SIECUS Report, 9*(5–6), 3–4.

Cole, S. (1988). Women, sexuality, and disabilities. *Women and Therapy, 7,* 277–294.

Committee on Adolescence. (1987). Role of the pediatrician in management of sexually transmitted diseases in children and adolescents. *Pediatrics, 79,* 454–456.

Cooley, E., & Singer, G. (1991). On serving students with head injuries: Are we reinventing a wheel that doesn't roll? *Journal of Head Trauma Rehabilitation, 6*(1), 47–55.

Crooks, R., & Baur, K. (1990). *Our sexuality.* New York: Benjamin/Cummings.

Cummings, J. L., & Trimble, M. R. (1995). *Concise guide to neuropsychiatry behavioral neurology.* Washington, DC: American Psychiatric Press.

Dean, R. S. (1985). Foundation and rationale for neuropsychological bases of individual differences. In L. Hartledge & K. Telzrow (Eds.), *Neuropsychology of individual differences* (pp. 7–39). New York: Plenum.

Deblinger, E., McLeer, S. V., Atkins, M. S., Ralphe, D., & Foa, E. (1989). Post-traumatic distress in sexually abused, physically abused, and nonabused children. *Child Abuse and Neglect, 13,* 403–408.

Eisenberg, M. G. (1989). Introduction: Special issue on traumatic brain injury rehabilitation. *Rehabilitation Psychology, 34*(2), 67.

Elliot, S. (1993). *Preferred behavioral inventory and intervention planner.* Madison: University of Wisconsin Press.

Evans, R. W., Evans, R. I., & Sharp, M. J. (1994). The physician survey on the post-concussion and whiplash syndromes. *Headache, 34,* 268–274.

Falvey, M. A., Forest, M., Pearpoint, J., & Rosenberg, R. L. (1997). *All my life's a circle: Using the tools Circles, MAPS, & PATHS.* Toronto: Inclusion Press.

Flaherty, E. W., Marecek, J., Olsen, K., & Wilcove, G. (1983). Preventing adolescent pregnancy: An interpersonal problem solving approach. *Innovations in Prevention, 2,* 49–63.

Freeman, R., Goetz, E., Richards, D., & Groenveld, M. (1991). Defiers of negative prediction: A 14-year follow-up study of legally blind children. *Journal of Visual Impairment and Blindness, 85,* 365–370.

Fremouw, W. J., de Perczel, M., & Ellis, T. E. (1990). *Suicide risk: Assessment and response guidelines.* New York: Pergamon.

Giami, A. (1987). Coping with the sexuality of the disabled: A comparison of the physically disabled and the mentally retarded. *International Journal of Rehabilitation Research, 10*(1), 41–48.

Goethe, K. E., & Levin, H. S. (1984). Behavioral manifestations during the early and long-term stages of recovery after closed head injury. *Psychiatric Annals, 14,* 540–546.

Hopewell, C. A., Burke, W. H., Weslowski, M., & Zawlocki, R. (1990). Behavioral learning therapies for the traumatically brain-injured patient. In R. L. Wood & I. Fussey (Eds.), *Brain damage, behavior & cognition: Cognitive rehabilitation in perspective* (pp. 229–245). New York: Taylor & Francis.

Hu, X., Wesson, D. E., Kenney, B. D., Chipman, M. L., & Spence, L. J. (1993). Risk factors for extended disruption of family function after severe injury to a child. *Canadian Medical Association Journal, 149,* 421–427.

Jacobs, H. E. (1988). The Los Angeles Head Injury Survey: Procedures and initial findings. *Archives of Physical Medicine and Rehabilitation, 69,* 425–431.

Jaffe, K. M., Polissar, N. L., Fay, G. C., & Liao, S. (1995). Recovery trends over three years following pediatric traumatic brain injury. *Archives of Physical Medicine and Rehabilitation, 76,* 17–26.

Kazdin, A. E., & Marciano, P. L. (1998). Childhood and adolescent depression. In E. J. Mash & R. A. Barkley (Eds.), *Treatment of childhood disorders* (2nd ed., pp. 211–248). New York: Guilford.

Kempton, W. (1988). *Sex education for persons with disabilities that hinder learning: A teacher's guide.* Santa Monica, CA: James Stanfield.

Kendall-Tackett, K., Williams, L., & Finkelhor, D. (1993). Impact of sexual abuse on children: A review and synthesis of recent empirical studies. *Psychological Bulletin, 113,* 164–180.

Kennedy, E., Spence, S. H., & Hensley, R. (1989). An examination of the relationship between childhood depression and social competence amongst primary school children. *Journal of Child Psychology and Psychiatry, 30,* 561–573.

Kewman, D., Warschausky, S., Engel, L., & Warzak, W. J. (1997). The child and adolescent with disability or chronic illness. In M. L. Sipski & C. J. Alexander (Eds.), *Maintaining sexuality with disability and chronic illness: A practitioner's guide* (pp. 355–378) Gaithersburg, MD: Aspen.

Kincaid, D. (1996). Person-centered planning. In L. K. Koegel, R. L. Koegel, & G. Dunlap (Eds.), *Positive behavioral support: Including people with difficult behavior in the community* (pp. 439–465). Baltimore: Brookes.

Kolko, D. J. (1988). Educational programs to promote awareness and prevention of child sexual victimization: A review and methodological critique. *Clinical Psychology Review, 8,* 195–209.

Koskiniemi, M., Kyykka, T., Nybo, T., & Jarho, L. (1995). Long-term outcome after severe brain injury in preschoolers is worse than expected. *Archives of Pediatric and Adolescent Medicine, 149,* 249–254.

Levin, H. S., Benton, A. L., & Grossman, R. G. (1982). *Neurobehavioral consequences of closed head injury.* New York: Oxford University Press.

Lewinsohn, P. M., Clarke, G. N., Rohde, P., Hops, H., & Seeley, J. R. (1996). A course in coping: A cognitive–behavioral approach to the treatment of adolescent depression. In E. D. Hibbs & P. Jensen (Eds.), *Psychosocial treatments for child and adolescent disorders: Empirically based strategies for clinical practice* (pp. 109–135). Washington, DC: American Psychological Association.

Lezak, M. (1978). Living with the characterologically altered brain injured patient. *Journal of Clinical Psychiatry, 39,* 111–123.

Lezak, M. D. (1988). The walking wounded of head injury: When subtle deficits can be disabling. *Trends in Rehabilitation, 3,* 4–9.

Maitz, E. A., & Sachs, P. R. (1995). Treating families of individuals with traumatic brain injury from a family systems perspective. *Journal of Head Trauma Rehabilitation, 10*(2), 1–11.

Mash, E. J., & Dozois, D. J. A. (1996). Child psychopathology: A developmental-systems perspective. In E. J. Mash & R. A. Barkley (Eds.), *Child psychopathology* (pp. 3–60). New York: Guilford Press.

Mitiguy, J. S., Thompson, G., & Wasco, J. (1990). *Understanding brain injury: Acute hospitalization.* Lynn, MA: New Medico Head Injury System.

Rimel, R. W., Giordani, B., Barth, J. T., Boll, T. J., & Jane, J. A. (1981). Disability caused by minor head injury. *Neurosurgery, 9,* 221–228.

Rosenthal, M. (1983). Behavioral sequelae. In M. Rosenthal, E. R. Griffith, M. R. Bond, & J. D. Miller (Eds.), *Rehabilitation of the head injured adult* (pp. 197–208). Philadelphia: Davis.

Rutherford, W. H. (1989). Postconcussion symptoms: Relationship to acute neurologic indices, individual differences and circumstance. In H. S. Levin, H. M. Eisenberg, & A. L. Benton (Eds.), *Mild head injury* (pp. 217–228). New York: Oxford University Press.

Rutter, M., Chadwick, O., & Shaffer, D. (1983). Head injury. In M. Rutter (Ed.), *Developmental neuropsychiatry* (pp. 83–111). New York: Guilford Press.

Savage, R. C. (1991). Identification, classification, and placement issues for students with traumatic brain injuries. *Journal of Head Trauma Rehabilitation, 6*(1), 1–9.

Schinke, S. P. (1984). Preventing teenage pregnancy. In M. Hersen, R. M. Eisler, & P. M. Miller (Eds.), *Progress in behavior modification* (pp. 31–64). Orlando, FL: Academic Press.

Schuster, C. S. (1986). Sex education of the visually impaired child. *Journal of Visual Impairment and Blindness, 80,* 675–680.

Schwartzbaum, R. C. (1992). Social skills training: Ethical issues and guidelines. In I. G. Fodor (Ed.), *Adolescent assertiveness and social skills training* (pp. 67–81). New York: Springer.

Shendell, M. B. (1992). Communication training for adolescent girls in junior high school setting: Learning to take risks in self-expression. In I. G. Fodor (Ed.), *Adolescent assertiveness and social skills training* (pp. 28–42). New York: Springer.

Tharinger, D., Horton, C. B., & Millea, S. (1990). Sexual abuse and exploitation of children and adults with mental retardation and other handicaps. *Child Abuse and Neglect, 14,* 301–312.

Warzak, W. J., Allan, T. M., Ford, L. A., & Stefans, V. C. (1995). Common obstacles to the daily functioning of pediatric traumatically brain injured patients: Perceptions of caregivers and psychologists. *Children's Health Care, 24*(1), 133–141.

Warzak, W. J., & Anderson, C. M. (2001). Parenting children with brain injury: A behavioral perspective. In S. Lee & H. Fineman (Eds.), *Handbook of parent training* (pp. 253–276). New York: Academic Press.

Warzak, W. J., Evans, J., & Ford, L. (1992). Working with the traumatically brain injured patient: Implications for rehabilitation. *Journal of Comprehensive Mental Health Care, 2,* 115–130.

Warzak, W. J., & Kilburn, J. (1990). Behavioral approaches to activities of daily living. In D. E. Tupper & K. D. Cicerone (Eds.), *The neuropsychology of everyday life: Vol. 1. Assessment and basic competencies* (pp. 285–305). New York: Martinus Nijhoff.

Warzak, W. J., Kuhn, B. R., & Nolten, P. W. (1995). Obstacles to the sexual adjustment of children and adolescents with disabilities. In G. A. Rekkers (Ed.), *Handbook of child and adolescent sexual problems* (pp. 81–100). New York: Lexington.

Warzak, W. J., Mayfield, J. W., & McAllister, J. (1998). Central nervous system dysfunction: Brain injury, post-concussive syndrome, and seizure disorder. In T. S. Watson & F. Gresham (Eds.), *Handbook of child behavior therapy* (pp. 287–309). New York: Plenum Press.

Warzak, W. J., & Page, T. (1990). Teaching refusal skills to sexually active adolescents. *Journal of Behavior Therapy and Experimental Psychiatry, 21,* 133–140.

Williams, D. N. (1987). Becoming a woman: The girl who is mentally retarded. *Pediatric Nursing, 13,* 89–93.

Williams, J. K. (1983). Reproductive decisions: Adolescents with Down Syndrome. *Pediatric Nursing, 9,* 43.

Wolpe, J. (1958). *Psychotherapy by reciprocal inhibition.* Stanford, CA: Stanford University.

Ylvisaker, M., Hartwick, P., & Stevens, M. (1991). School reentry following head injury: Managing the transition from hospital to school. *Journal of Head Trauma Rehabilitation, 6*(1), 10–22.

Zencius, A., Wesolowski, M., Burke, W., & Hough, S. (1990). Managing hypersexual disorders in brain-injured clients. *Brain Injury, 4*(2), 175–181.

Transitioning to School
Educational Team Planning
for Students with Brain Injuries

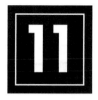

Pamela Brown

" *We looked to them for answers; they looked to us for answers.* "
—*Parent of an adolescent survivor of TBI*

According to federal legislation (Assistance to States, 1992), students are eligible for special education services when they experience brain injury due to an external physical force *and* the injury results in a functional disability or psychosocial impairment negatively affecting educational performance in cognition, language, sensation, perception, psychosocial behavior, or physical/motor functioning. The federal legislation does not specify assessment procedures or criteria. These are outlined in state regulations and differ among states.

Evolution of Team Rosters and Roles

When a young person receives inpatient hospitalization and rehabilitation, a medical team drives treatment planning, with a focus on the physical well-being and physical skills of the patient. Families usually do not play key roles in treatment decisions and, for shorter hospitalizations, community providers generally are not invited to participate in treatment team meetings; families may or may not attend meetings of the treatment teams. Generally, the family role is that of supporting and complementing medical treatment and rehabilitation. For instance, families are expected to respect recommendations for rest periods, follow instructions on physical assistance, and encourage their children's participation and effort in therapies that may be challenging and uncomfortable. As illustrated in the following case example on transitioning from hospital to school, the team is a medically oriented one.

Case Example: Transitioning from Hospital to School

When 14-year-old Seth Powers returned to school after his brain injury, his parents felt thrown into the roles of educational team leaders and brain injury consultants. Though Mr. and Mrs. Powers frantically searched for local team members who could provide expertise and guidance, what they found were capable educators who felt ineffectual, intimidated, and insecure. Everyone wanted someone else to lead.

From the time of Seth's injury until his discharge from rehabilitation, medical personnel led the way. Doctors called the shots on surgeries, medications, rehabilitation, and visitations. The parents' primary role was to nurture, support, and encourage their son. Opportunities to participate in team decision making were very limited. When options were presented to Mr. and Mrs. Powers, medical personnel guided their decisions by outlining pros and cons. Seth's family followed the lead of the neurologist, physiatrist, neuropsychologist, and a host of therapists. But, when Seth moved home, things were different.

Students with Short-Term Hospitalizations

Young people who are hospitalized for short time periods often move from the day-to-day, close oversight of a focused medical treatment team to the day-to-day oversight of well-intentioned—yet ill-prepared—family members and school personnel. Generally, transition is not well orchestrated. Local school administrators, teachers, and therapists may not have experience with the rehabilitation of youth with TBIs. They may assume that only medical and physical needs exist and warrant attention from the hospital-based medical team, school nurse, school principal, and family.

Accommodations at school may depend largely on a physician's recommendations—recommendations that generally focus on the student's physical well-being and healing. Sometimes, a school-based educational team is not even assembled because of the assumption that injuries will soon heal, and everything will be "fine." In such instances, accommodation planning is loose, uncoordinated, and insufficient.

As school personnel and family members recognize that challenges exist beyond the student's physical needs, team composition, focus, and roles change. The family or school personnel initiate a team expansion to include more educators, open more lines of communication, and generate more accommodations. The team may take on a formal structure as is typical of multidisciplinary, Individualized Education Program (IEP), or 504 teams. To address a range of concerns—such as behavior, peer relationships, and academic performance—the focus moves from "zoom" to "wide angle."

At this point, school personnel often look to the family for information and guidance, as if family members' immersion into the world of TBI elevated them, by default, to the status of brain injury experts. Simultaneously, the family may look to school personnel for help with academic issues—memorization strategies, ways to increase attentiveness during homework time, ideas for decreasing frustration with assignments that used to be easy, and much more. The team begins shaping new goals, but, without confidence in their knowledge and skills, team members may struggle to define roles clearly, establish leadership, communicate effectively, and plan and carry out an appropriate educational plan for the student. They may feel rudderless in a rocky, fast-moving stream.

On a more positive note, some locations have teams supported by local professionals—an area brain injury team, a brain injury consultant, staff or volunteers from a state brain injury association, therapists or educators who have experience working with youth with TBIs, or individuals who have at least some basic knowledge about TBI and related resources. When highly specialized teams are not

What are multidisciplinary, IEP, and 504 teams?

The Individuals with Disabilities Education Act (IDEA) (Assistance to States for the Education of Children with Disabilities, 1992) calls for multidisciplinary teams to determine a child's eligibility for special education and related services. A multidisciplinary team gathers and reviews information to assess whether an acquired brain injury has occurred, whether it has resulted in functional disabilities or psychosocial impairments, whether it has adversely affected learning, and whether a resulting need exists for special education and related services. When a multidisciplinary team finds a child eligible for special education and related services, an Individualized Education Program (IEP) team is put in place. The team composition may vary little from the multidisciplinary team, but the function is very different. The charge of the IEP team is to develop an educational plan to support the student's success. The plan will include a variety of elements, such as instructional settings, educational or developmental goals, strategies, timelines, types of appropriate assessments, consideration of assistive technologies, transition plans, and much more. In contrast to IEP teams, 504 teams emerged to meet the requirements of Section 504 of the Rehabilitation Act of 1973 (Department of Health, Education, and Welfare, 1977). Section 504 stipulates that "reasonable accommodations" be made for persons with disabilities. Under the Rehabilitation Act, criteria for determining who qualifies as disabled are less stringent than under IDEA; therefore, 504 plans may be used to accommodate students with special needs who do not meet the criteria outlined in IDEA. Multidisciplinary, IEP, and 504 teams all play very important roles in creating educational experiences that are appropriate and rewarding for students with TBI.

Build Your Brain Injury Team NOW!

Brain injury: No one expects it and, generally, no one prepares for it. But, the statistics on incidence suggest that professionals could encounter youth with TBIs several times over the course of their careers. It would behoove school districts to designate a cross-section of staff as their brain injury team and select from that a team leader—now! This group could design a professional development and education plan for themselves, expand their resources and networks related to TBI, and be prepared before the next brain injury occurs.

available locally, local team members can create networks of specialists through Internet connections, e-mail systems, telephones, and videoconferencing. They can access a wide range of experienced providers from inpatient rehabilitation settings, national associations, research centers, universities, and school districts. Even from remote locations, TBI specialists can help prevent complications and downward spirals for students and help maximize rehabilitation and education efforts. They can anticipate common problems and help teams avoid them; they can direct team members to helpful resources; and they can serve as short-term team leaders while local team members establish confidence in their own knowledge and skills.

Students with Long-Term Hospitalizations

When a child's inpatient rehabilitation extends for several months or more, team evolution may look quite different from that found in milder cases. With extended inpatient rehabilitation services, families and community providers are likely to develop knowledge about TBI and assume integral, active roles on the planning and intervention team prior to the student's return to home and school. During long inpatient stays, opportunities exist for learning about the implications of the student's brain injury and communicating that information to others. Additionally, inpatient rehabilitation staff will probably welcome and make use of information from teachers, therapists, family, and peers— such as the student's typical conversation topics, activity preferences, and curriculum expectations. Generally, the hospital-based rehabilitation team informally expands to include community providers and family during an extended stay; simultaneously, or shortly after the student's discharge, a formal, school-based team is likely to evolve. In these instances, team evolution may be relatively smooth, because team members have time to develop confidence in their roles and to develop the necessary understanding of the student's needs, potential obstacles, available resources, and helpful strategies.

Obstacles in Teaming

Teaming to support the rehabilitation, education, independence, and life quality of a student with TBI is a challenge. The teaming process often brings together strangers with different backgrounds, expectations, and philosophies to help ameliorate a situation they all wish had never occurred; even to develop appropriate goals is a respectable challenge. The problem-solving context in which they work is emotionally laden. After all, what they accomplish or fail to accomplish can have profound implications across the life of the child. As if the situation were not complex and intimidating enough, innumerable obstacles surface among team members to further complicate the process: miscommunications, turfism, inappropriate expectations for each other, ignorance, and so on. Many times, the most significant obstacles that teams face in their efforts to help students with TBIs involve conflicting goals, feelings of inadequacy, emotions, and time.

Conflicting Goals

Teaming to help students with TBIs means attempting to blend the goals of medical specialists, medically based rehabilitation therapists, educators, community-based therapists, family members, peers, and the student. Each team member may have different, yet valid, priorities. A variety of goals and perspectives is necessary to the rehabilitation and care of the whole child, but the differences certainly complicate planning, communication, and coordination. Differences in perspectives and goals may be influenced by many factors, one of which is how well each team member knew the student prior to injury. This knowledge colors perspectives and goals—for better or worse—and differences in this knowledge can create an undercurrent of conflicting goals among team members (see the following case example on conflicting goals).

Feelings of Inadequacy

Team members tend to come together in quite vulnerable positions: A special education teacher may feel insecure never having worked before with a student with TBI; a speech–language pathologist with a large caseload may be

Case Example: Conflicting Goals

Mike's team struggled to prioritize and compromise. It was the summer after his junior year in high school. Mike had acquired a TBI while skiing in March of that year. His recovery was progressing better than expected.

Prior to injury, college recruiters were scouting Mike for a basketball scholarship. That was his dream—then and now. However, Mike's neurologist was concerned about the young man's physical healing and risk of reinjury. He ordered restrictions on Mike's physical activity—no football, no basketball, no skiing, and no four-wheeling—for the remainder of his time in high school. The rehabilitation therapists knew of Mike's dream to play college ball. They were already working with him on ball skills and relearning plays. This seemed to be a motivating key to Mike's better-than-expected progress. Mike's teachers somewhat favored curtailing his activities, because they noticed greater fatigue on days he had physical education or worked with the occupational or physical therapist than on days with less exertion. Of course, Mike's peers wanted him back on the team, regularly reminding him that they could not do without him. Mike's parents were very afraid of the risks of reinjury, yet they were concerned that limiting Mike's activity would fuel a creeping depression. If you were on Mike's team, what would you suggest?

intimidated by the time and energy commitment associated with being assigned as team leader; parents may be overwhelmed by all that has occurred and feel emotionally unprepared to deal with the realities of their child's disabilities; an administrator may feel defensive, wondering about the adequacy of the district's service options. When a single team member feels inadequate, his or her expectations for others may increase; when the majority of a team feels inadequate, many members may hold high, unspoken, and inappropriate expectations for others. To a point, feelings of inadequacy can motivate team members to learn and to reach out for resources; however, feelings of inadequacy can also lead to helplessness, inaction, and team conflict.

Another scenario occurs when a conscientious, self-confident team member drives ahead with unrealistically high expectations for the student with TBI. If the student progresses slowly or not at all, the team member may become discouraged and experience sudden feelings of inadequacy. Team members need to recognize their own insecurities and vulnerabilities and mutually support and encourage one another. They can remind each other to draw upon their wide range of experiences with other youth; after all, some educational strategies used routinely with other students may be very effective for students with brain injuries (Hux & Hacksley, 1996). Team members need to focus on what they know and can do rather than contribute to team paralysis by focusing on obstacles, insecurities, and inadequacies.

Emotions

Sometimes team functioning is propelled forward by emotional energy, but other times the team can be destroyed by emotional fires. As mentioned previously, various vulnerabilities seem to come with membership on the team of a student with TBI. Add to that the kindling of a wide range of strong emotions, and a very volatile situation can arise. Families are experiencing an emotional shakedown, dealing with both the trauma and the host of complicating stressors that follow. Emotions related to the family's grieving process— often including the expression of denial or anger—color the teaming process. Furthermore, families may be uncomfortable with stigmas or unfamiliar aspects of school services for students with disabilities. They may mistrust other team members because their recent experiences may have shaken their faith—especially concerning professionals' ability to provide concrete answers and solutions. If the student or family experienced difficulties getting along with school staff before the accident, additional emotional baggage is hauled into team meetings and impacts objectivity, flexibility, and cooperation.

Time

When planning for and working with a student with TBI, relatively large initial investments of time are likely to yield substantial dividends. Initially, team members may need to commit substantial time to gathering information from the family and rehabilitation providers, getting to know the student, reading TBI materials, and sharing information with team members. Asking for administrative support for an up-front time commitment from staff is often helpful. This support might be in the form of altering work schedules for free periods, encouraging broad staff participation at team meetings, allowing for longer time for team meetings, or providing substitute teachers so staff can attend workshops. Although the initial time demands may seem overwhelming, adequate up-front time often minimizes time required later to address miscommunications, misunderstandings about the student's skills and needs, and inappropriate interventions.

"The Right Stuff": Ingredients for a Successful Brain Injury Team

Commitment to Learning About TBI

Team members do not need to be established TBI experts to be effective; they need only a commitment to learning about TBI and its unique implications. However, learning about TBI in general may not be enough; team members need to identify information that is pertinent to, and helpful for, their particular students. One way to start the learning process is to ask for recommendations about reading materials that others within the team or broader network have found to be particularly helpful. Another way to gain new insights into brain injury relatively quickly is to visit brain injury support groups. Individuals in support groups are generally heartened to have opportunities to teach others about TBI, strategies for coping, and the realities of resources. Visits with families and providers of other students with TBI can also provide fruitful learning experiences. Finally, though its use requires additional discernment, the World Wide Web has a seemingly infinite, ever-changing store of what you need to know, when you need to know it.

Communication

Team functioning can quickly deteriorate when communication is insufficient or inaccurate. Team members may assume that certain activities or supports have been in place, only to find out much later that this was not the case. Not only does this have a negative impact on the student; it can lead to frustration, mistrust, and resentment among team members. Unless the team communicates clearly who is responsible for what, important things go undone. Breakdowns in communication can also occur when providers use the jargon of their professions without providing explanation in layman's terms. Initially, enlisting the assistance of a school nurse to interpret and communicate medical reports accurately to the entire educational team may be helpful.

Team members need to develop a plan for ongoing communication among themselves and with key people outside the core team. Time should be set aside for regular, face-to-face meetings among team members. Appointments for phone conferencing during team meetings can allow for communication with people who otherwise could not participate. Recording and communicating information about the student through activity logs, journals, or some type of anecdotal records can be very helpful. Parents are particularly appreciative of such information. Journals can be sent home with students at the end of each week, though some parents and educators prefer daily communications regarding a student's activities.

Shared Goals

Team members sometimes have tunnel vision regarding their goals and roles with students with TBI. Each may provide a single piece, unaware of how that piece fits with those of other team members. Such fragmentation is counterproductive: If team members assume that they have independent roles to play, they may feel less need for communication and coordination with others, and they will be less likely to capitalize on opportunities for students to practice, review, and generalize team-identified priority skills across environments. Shared goals can result in more opportunities for distributed practice of important skills throughout a child's day (e.g., initiating communications, increasing time on task, practicing reading skills). Educators and therapists are also more likely to share strategies and progress updates when they know others are working on similar goals. Especially when a student has limited capacity for new learning, structuring opportunities to focus on priority objectives is important. Furthermore, shared goals can create enthusiasm and team momentum that fuel the drive for student recovery.

Effective Use of Available Resources

At least initially, teams often perceive that they have inadequate resources to provide services for students with TBI. They may immediately spend time and energy searching outside themselves for someone or some place with more resources rather than focusing on exploring, developing, and expanding internal resources. Sometimes administrators find it helpful to investigate the costs of residential services for students with TBI; after that, any issues related to the cost of developing or accessing local resources quickly dissipate. Other team members can assume responsibility for exploring services provided by people outside the local team: Can these services be provided locally? What additional resources would local provision require?

Teams need to identify what they can do well with their current resources of personnel, knowledge, skills, facilities, and materials. Identifying strong local staff (e.g., classroom teachers, special education teachers, therapists, and paraprofessionals) is of primary importance. Next, teams can identify areas in which their resources are marginal and develop a plan for quickly boosting these local resources through training, borrowing or purchasing materials, making facility accommodations, establishing agreements to utilize community facilities for work experiences, and visiting other schools to learn about their services for similar students. Such a plan may boost a team's confidence in its ability to do its job while simultaneously creating expectations and supports for continuously improving local resources for students with TBI.

Leadership

A local team leader may not always be the person who knows the most about TBI. Although specific knowledge is obviously helpful, a host of other qualities that contribute to effective team leadership also need consideration. Teams need someone to propel them forward, to challenge them to overcome apprehensions, to learn, to try new approaches, and to work together collectively to support student progress and quality of life. Team leaders need to be active listeners and active communicators while also being effective in facilitating communication among others. They need to be respectful of the fact that the team process—not the team leader—determines goals and roles for the student's education. Team leaders need to model a desire for learning about TBI, respect for the family and other team members, and actions that contribute to the student's achievement of identified goals.

Accommodation Planning

It may seem that the need for an accommodation plan or IEP would become obvious early in the TBI recovery process. In reality, most youngsters who acquire TBIs do not receive inpatient rehabilitation and do not return to school with written achievement or behavior plans. Although students may come to school with medical instructions for monitoring physical symptoms, they generally do not bring a plan for recognizing symptoms signaling changes in cognition, communication, or behavior. A plan for supports to minimize or prevent related frustrations and failures almost never exists.

Academic or behavior difficulties that appear after TBI are often attributed to other factors such as adolescence, a lack of motivation, poor parenting skills, attention-seeking behaviors, or preexisting difficulties such as attention-deficit/ hyperactivity disorder or learning problems. Interventions that focus on these problem areas by raising expectations without adding supports, requiring more homework, limiting leisure time (and rest), or restricting participation in extracurricular activities until grades improve may contribute to a downward spiral in student behavior and achievement. Plans for guiding observations, monitoring performance and behavior, preventing complications, and supporting success should be a part of every student's school reentry following TBI.

The Right Tool for the Right Job

Person-Centered Planning

A variety of educational planning tools are available for students with brain injuries. Each tool and each process has its own advantages. Person-centered planning (PCP) (Mount & Zwernik, 1988; Vandercook, York, & Forest, 1989) results in a relatively complete picture of the student. It is particularly effective in helping team members understand a student's aspirations and changes from preinjury to postinjury. The planning process for PCP initially requires more time than most other educational planning tools, but it supports the development of a unifying vision for the student and movement toward that vision, as well as compatible goals and shared ownership among team members.

Section 504 Plans

Section 504 plans (see detailed description in the preceding sidebar that answers the question, "What are multidisciplinary, IEP, and 504 teams?") may also be useful for guiding accommodations for students with TBI. Section 504 plans seem to be the tool of choice when the anticipated need for accommodations is short term due to the student's rapid pace of recovery. Section 504 plans are also useful when the team needs to assemble a plan quickly. Examples include situations in which a student returns to school relatively soon following injury or when a student is abruptly released from hospital-based rehabilitation and returns to school. In some instances, a 504 plan may serve as a stopgap until an IEP is in place. The 504 plan may also be preferred when the necessary accommodations are relatively simple—such as extensions on semester deadlines, rest periods during the day, testing modifications, or lower activity levels during physical education and recess.

Individualized Education Programs

When accommodations call for changes in the form or content of instruction (i.e., when they call for special education), an IEP will generally be used. The IEP has obvious advantages over a Section 504 plan as an accommodation planning tool for students with TBI: The IEP process encourages (a) identification of strengths, interests, and needs within the context of the regular curriculum; (b) collaboration with the student's family; (c) consideration of assistive technologies; (d) identification of related services to support educational goals; (e) systematic examination and response to behavior problems; and (f) transition planning. Generally, more educators participate in the IEP process than in 504 planning, hence supporting broader accommodation planning and implementation. Finally, because IEPs are required for all school-age students eligible for special education services, special education personnel are likely to be quite familiar with using the IEP as a planning tool. Educators may not be as familiar with 504 plans.

Individualized Family Service Plan

The Individualized Family Service Plan (IFSP) is considered the planning tool of choice for very young children (Zipper, Hinton, Weil, & Rounds, 1993). Compared with IEPs, IFSPs promote even stronger involvement of family, caregivers, and service providers. IFSP intervention planning views the child within the context of his or her family (a view, it must be said, that can be very beneficial for students with TBI of all ages). Another advantage of IFSPs over IEPs is that they assist in developing accommodations and supports in all of the child's natural environments rather than merely in the school setting. Especially when a child with TBI is relearning skills in several domains, identifying supports across life environments is important. Many students with TBI are relearning skills across domains; thus the IFSP format (although designed for very young children) can serve as a valuable model for students with TBI of any age.

You Cannot Eat a Pizza in One Bite

Planning formats such as the IEP offer a process for developing well-considered master plans. Even with such thorough plans, however, educators and therapists may wonder where to begin. Other planning tools exist to help educators prioritize, match learning opportunities with objectives and methods, and identify potential gaps or redundancies in instruction.

A *planning grid* is a tool that can assist in addressing these issues (Brown, 1999). To build a planning grid, team members prioritize learning objectives and list them vertically down the left column of a grid. Across the top row, the team lists various environments the child encounters throughout the day (e.g., riding to school, waiting on the school grounds before school, walking through the hallways, attending various classes, and eating lunch in the cafeteria). The team considers how each objective may or may not be addressed in each environment throughout the child's day.

After considering the entire planning grid, the team can decide whether the learning opportunities for priority objectives are sufficient or redundant. The grid enables the team to plan for skill practice, maintenance, and generalization. Moving through the grid may provide the team with a realistic picture of time constraints and ways to capitalize on previously unrecognized opportunities. It may move them to consider options "outside the box" of a child's typical school context. Matching learning objectives with educational environments also assists regular classroom teachers to better understand their roles when they have children with TBIs in their classrooms.

No matter the specific tools used to build the plan, the team must assume the plan will need to be changed fairly frequently. A student's physical healing and skill recovery may progress more quickly than expected. For other students, unforeseen complications may point to the need for additional supports. As educators, therapists, and family members develop a comprehensive understanding of a student's skills or interests, changes in the plan may be appropriate. Although IEPs are typically designed for implementation over the course of an entire year, teams may want to reconvene quarterly at least during the first year following the student's return to school. This schedule will allow for reviewing and updating the IEP so that it matches a student's needs.

Protocols for Return to School Following Injury

Avoiding "Too Little, Too Late"

Too often, complications that could be avoided with effective communication and planning arise when a student with TBI returns to school. In an ideal situation, schools would have contact people designated and procedures in place before a brain injury even occurs. Administrators would designate a person—such as the school nurse or counselor—to serve as the initial liaison among the school, the family, and the medical team. Local clinic and hospital staff and appropriate staff in regional hospitals or rehabilitation facilities would receive written notification and business cards indicating the designation of the liaison. This notification could include a written request that medical staff have parents inform the school liaison when a student is seen for TBI. In fact, with appropriate consent, medical personnel could contact school staff directly. Such procedures would streamline communication and prevent delays, disasters, and disappointments. Unfortunately, such procedural planning for students with TBI is the exception rather than the rule.

Injuries Without Hospitalization

The majority of TBIs are minor and do not result in hospitalization. Schools need monitoring and follow-up procedures for students who sustain such injuries (see the following case example on monitoring a mild TBI). Generally, students with mild TBI return to school with little or no guidance from school staff (Savage, 1991); school personnel may not even be aware that a student has sustained an injury, especially when it is mild and occurs over the summer months. Having monitoring and follow-up procedures in place, however, can prevent frustrations and complications for students. Furthermore, the school may have responsibilities and liability concerns related to safety if students are at an increased risk for reinjury.

Case Example: Monitoring a Mild TBI

Another long, grueling afternoon of football practice was nearing an end. Tyler had one more chance at Brett, and this time he was going to sack him! Crunch! Helmets smacked, and they were down. The sack was a success. Tyler grinned from ear to ear, crawled over Brett, pulled himself upward, and teetered back onto the turf. Boy, was he dizzy! And that ringing in his ears was obnoxious. Tyler shook his head, slowly pulled himself up, and, feeling nauseous, staggered over to the bench. What a ding! Tyler wondered how in the world that happened! On his way to the showers, Coach Warner caught Tyler out of the corner of his eye.

"What's the matter, Tyler? Did you let Brett get the best of you? You'd better not let that happen tomorrow! We're not going to let those Panthers get the best of us!"

After a poor night's sleep, an unending "killer" headache, and a very frustrating day, it was nearly game time.

Ending #1/No Protocol: One hit, two hits, six hits later, Tyler was down again. This time he didn't get up. Tyler moaned painfully as he was rolled onto the stretcher. He seemed to be mumbling something, softer and softer. Something was changing, something deep in his eyes. His body shaking, he began his trip to the emergency room. Vital signs checked, everyone calmed, the doctor assured everyone that Tyler's injury was "just a concussion." Back at school on Monday, still with an excruciating headache, Tyler struggled through his day. In fact, he struggled through all his days that quarter. Teacher conferences revealed that Tyler was having trouble finishing his assignments, paying attention in class, following instructions, and remembering facts for tests. Teachers wondered if he was depressed or if this was "just adolescence." Whichever the case, Tyler's current grades were destroying his chances of being admitted to college.

Ending #2/Local TBI Protocol: Oh, man! Why did he have to get Dr. Edwards to clear him to play? So what if he had a headache? He had played before when he did not feel well. Dr. Edwards asked a few questions, examined Tyler, and talked with him about the risks of play when he was still symptomatic (see Chapter 3, Table 3.4, for detailed return-to-play guidelines). He would not clear him for play and insisted on seeing him again the next week. Dr. Edwards provided Tyler's parents with a checklist, pamphlets on mild brain injury and concussion, and information to pass on to school personnel. School personnel met, established ongoing communication with the physician, and implemented some accommodative supports. Schoolwork was difficult for Tyler until a couple weeks had passed, the headaches subsided, and he got his energy back. In the meantime, he had extra study time instead of physical education class. Until cleared to start football practice again, he lifted weights and rode a stationary bike to keep in shape. Sure, he would rather have been playing football, but even he agreed it was not worth the risk.

Districts and their students benefit from systematic procedures for communicating between medical personnel and school staff when brain injuries occur. Quality examples of such protocols exist and are available in the TBI literature (e.g., Lash, Savage, & DePompei, 1998; Savage, 1997) or through organizations such as the Brain Injury Association of America. The following list provides steps for developing local procedures to identify and monitor students following TBI:

1. *Create a small, local planning team:* Include a school nurse, a school administrator, a local physician, a parent, and a teacher.
2. *Identify current procedures and written materials:* Identify steps usually taken by schools, families, and doctors when TBI affects school performance. Include information about local common practice, including written policies, procedures, forms, information sheets, and checklists; also identify resources from other states.
3. *Identify procedural gaps:* Locate the potential gaps or breakdowns in communication, information, and follow-through that could complicate the process of identifying, monitoring, and accommodating children with TBI.
4. *Codify local protocol for identifying, monitoring, and supporting students with TBI:* As a team, develop steps to support communication among parents, school personnel, and physicians. Examples include (a) having medical personnel provide parents with informational handouts about TBI, (b) establishing and regularly completing symptom checklists, and (c) developing a strategy sheet for families and educators to encourage the implementation of immediate, temporary accommodations when necessary.

Injuries with Extended Hospitalizations

When students experience lengthy hospitalizations, school personnel, other community-based service providers, and parents can do much to ease the student's return to school and home (Lash, 1992; Mira & Tyler, 1991; Ylvisaker et al., 1995). Longer hospitalizations suggest more severe injuries with multiple complications: considerable fatigue, continued outpatient treatment, medical follow-ups, issues related to physical accessibility, significant changes in appearance, supports needed for self-care, and so on. As illustrated in the following case example on transitioning from hospital to school, communication and planning need to begin early to ensure that necessary supports—such as additional paraprofessionals, home health services, accommodations at home and school for physical accessibility, training for staff—are in place.

Designating a team leader is critical in situations of moderate-to-severe TBI. Primary functions of this position include identifying a core team and

Case Example: Transitioning from Hospital to School

Sara's injury left her with nearly inaudible speech, limited use of her left forearm and hand, fatigue, and an intense desire to reconnect with her friends. Her best friend, Lyndsi, came to see her early after her injury. Shocked at what she saw, she never came back. Now, it was nearly time for Sara to go home. She had no idea what had been going on with her friends over the last 6 months. She was different now. Would they still like her? Could she keep up with them? Would friends get frustrated with her? Could she "hold her own" to help out with concessions, take her turn driving to youth group, manage her books at school? Would she need help from others? Would her friends be there to help her? The more questions she asked herself, the more nervous she got. Just then, there was a knock, and Cassie's smiling face peaked around the door. It was Lyndsi, Kerri, Jenna, Kelly, and Mrs. Jorgenson! For the next 2 hours they sat and laughed, got caught up on each other's lives, and made plans for Sara's return home: Sara would take the money at the concession stand, she would buy gas once in a while, and they would let Kyle (the wrestler) carry her books! She would rest in Mrs. Jorgenson's room during fifth period. The girls decided to touch base with Mrs. Jorgenson at the end of each day for a while, just to make sure things were going okay for Sara. Before the visitors left, they rolled out a huge poster signed by their classmates and hung it on the wall: "Welcome Home, Sara!"

other key players, establishing communication networks, coordinating services, updating others on the student's progress, encouraging TBI education among team members, and facilitating the student's reentry to school. Specific steps the liaison should perform are outlined in the checklist provided in Figure 11.1.

Skill Building

The Art: "I'll Care How Much the Teachers Know When I Know How Much They Care"

Effective instruction and learning do not occur in isolation; they occur within the context of innumerable influential life factors. For the student with a recent TBI, the influence of some variables is magnified. Although this is

(*text continues on page 279*)

1. **Contact student's parents**[1]

   _____ Obtain TBI Family Packets through state Brain Injury Association

   _____ Plan an initial, face-to-face visit with the following agenda:
   - Begin building a trusting relationship
   - Express the school staff's interest in planning for a successful reentry
   - Deliver Family Packet and other relevant local school information (e.g., special education and related services)
   - Create a mutual communication plan regarding student progress and educational and rehabilitation planning
   - Listen to parent concerns
   - Obtain written permission to communicate with other service providers (past and present)

2. **Gather and disseminate relevant information**

   _____ Obtain student information from family, medical and rehabilitation staff, current and past school staff, school files, peers, employers, etc.; the goal is to understand who the student was before injury and who he or she is now (personality, interests, skills, relationships, values, goals, etc.)

   _____ Obtain relevant information from rehabilitation facilities, brain injury organizations, the Internet, professional organizations, universities, etc., that may support team members' understanding of the child's injury, skills, and challenges

   _____ Plan a visit to the rehabilitation facility

   _____ Request video clips of the student throughout the course of a week

   _____ Develop an understanding of the child's unique brain injury

   _____ Find out about rehabilitation treatment and discharge plan (skills being addressed, rate of progress, projected discharge date)

   _____ Share relevant information with educational team, including parents

   _____ When appropriate, share relevant information (e.g., student's academic and behavioral history, educational expectations, local supports, etc.) with hospital and rehabilitation staff (allow parents to provide this information if they choose)

3. **Facilitate continued communication with family**

   _____ Obtain updates on student's progress and needs

   _____ Determine family concerns that the school can address (e.g., facilitating peer communication and education, supporting brothers and sisters)

   _____ Clarify the availability of school resources, the school's responsibilities, and the appropriate procedures for obtaining supportive educational services

   _____ Share information about other local and regional resources that may be of interest to family (e.g., home health, support groups, brain injury organizations, other families who have children with TBIs)

[1] Throughout this checklist, the term _parent_ is used to refer to the child's primary care provider. If a particular child is not in the care of a parent, substitute the term _guardian_.

(*continues*)

Figure 11.1. Tasks that facilitate school reentry: A liaison's checklist.

_____ Determine the parent's and the student's hopes, goals, and priorities for recovery

_____ Ask parents about the role they prefer to fill in the rehabilitation and educational process (e.g., leader, participant, follower)

4. **Initiate and coordinate team planning for school reentry**

_____ Frequently update information regarding the rehabilitation facility's discharge plan (it may change, resulting in short notice prior to child's return to school)

_____ Provide an inservice to staff regarding the child's needs, using the most effective route (e.g., video of student, video about reentry, written materials, informal consultation, group meeting)

_____ Establish a schedule for team meetings, including phone conferencing as needed (e.g., to include a representative from the rehabilitation facility or the student's doctor)

_____ Determine the child's strengths and challenges (understanding that they may be more successful in the structured, highly facilitated setting of the rehabilitation facility than in school, and that newly regained skills may not generalize easily)

_____ Develop a plan for further assessment of the child's strengths and challenges when this becomes necessary

_____ Determine potential school and community obstacles to the student's successful reentry and inclusion

_____ Generate strategies (e.g., peer education, hiring a paraprofessional, additional supervision) for overcoming challenges and obstacles

_____ Prioritize objectives and strategies

_____ Develop a timeline for reentry steps

_____ Delineate roles and responsibilities within the educational team

_____ Determine the student's eligibility for special education or other school services

_____ Generate an IEP, an IFSP, or a 504 Accommodation Plan, as appropriate, and map out the student's daily schedule

_____ Establish a team meeting time to review and revise the child's educational plan according to projected rate of progress (monthly at least)

_____ Revise the school–parent communication plan (e.g., to include new methods such as daily log, phone, weekly meetings)

5. **Monitor the student's success and the effectiveness of supports following school reentry**

_____ Determine the quality of the match between instruction and the child's skills

_____ Check the student's perception of his or her success (e.g., Does he or she feel that he or she is falling short relative to peers or compared to capabilities prior to injury?)

(continues)

Figure 11.1. *Continued.*

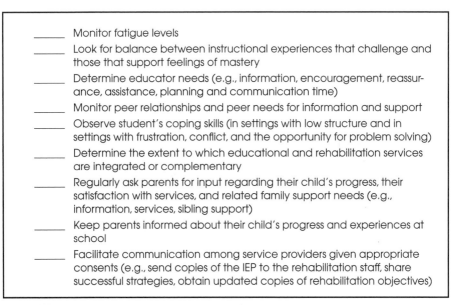

_____ Monitor fatigue levels

_____ Look for balance between instructional experiences that challenge and those that support feelings of mastery

_____ Determine educator needs (e.g., information, encouragement, reassurance, assistance, planning and communication time)

_____ Monitor peer relationships and peer needs for information and support

_____ Observe student's coping skills (in settings with low structure and in settings with frustration, conflict, and the opportunity for problem solving)

_____ Determine the extent to which educational and rehabilitation services are integrated or complementary

_____ Regularly ask parents for input regarding their child's progress, their satisfaction with services, and related family support needs (e.g., information, services, sibling support)

_____ Keep parents informed about their child's progress and experiences at school

_____ Facilitate communication among service providers given appropriate consents (e.g., send copies of the IEP to the rehabilitation staff, share successful strategies, obtain updated copies of rehabilitation objectives)

Figure 11.1. *Continued.*

somewhat unique to each child, factors that may color learning, classroom performance, and school relationships include trust, belonging, mastery, and self-management. Artful instruction weaves together approaches that target academic skills *and* issues related to healing, personal development, and reintegration following brain injury.

Educators may be reluctant to consider that such developmental issues warrant direct intervention; they may feel that specifically and proactively addressing such concerns is not their role. Educators need to realize, however, that students with TBI may not only lose skills related to math, self-care, and reading, but also lose strongly held personal understandings, beliefs, and coping skills that can influence what happens in the school setting. Students need assistance to relearn beliefs such as they are capable in many ways; effort makes a difference in what they accomplish; they have choices; the world (including school) is a safe place; they are loveable; and adults are available for support. All students' experiences shape their beliefs about others, themselves, and the future. For the student with TBI, these experiences and consequent beliefs may all be new. Designing instruction that shapes personal understandings and beliefs presents awesome responsibilities and incredible opportunities for educators.

Mastery/Competence

When a child returns to school following a TBI, much of the focus is on remediating disabilities. Therefore, during much of the day, the student confronts challenging tasks and faces frustration. He or she may be aware of pre-injury abilities or the things other students are accomplishing independently. Particularly with inclusionary models, educators need to provide adequate opportunities and supports for students to experience mastery. The required entry-level skills may be too much for newly returning students, and adults may find themselves wanting to push students to get them caught up with peers. The result for the student may be a downward spiral of frustration, dependence on others, discouragement, decreased motivation, and power struggles.

Educators and therapists need to plan purposefully for mastery experiences within a child's day. Adults should begin by listing skills the student can currently apply in designated contexts. Then, educators should select the skills most valued by the child, peers, and/or parents. Students should have opportunities built into their days to use these skills, preferably in cooperation with peers. However, if activities are too easy, the accomplishment may feel hollow and will not contribute to the student's sense of mastery. Applying a mastered skill to contexts that vary slightly from one another is one way to increase the challenge while maintaining the probability of success. Innumerable other techniques can spur feelings of competence: Visual charting of skill progress, videos that document and replay successes, and drawings and notes that highlight what a student does right (socially, academically, or otherwise) are just a few examples.

Self-Management

Students may need to relearn self-management skills following TBI. The child's injury may result in a diminished ability to manage him- or herself successfully in activities of daily living, academics, and peer interactions. The trauma of the injury, hospitalization, and rehabilitation experiences may contribute to self-management challenges, shaking a student's confidence and spurring feelings of helplessness. Inadvertently, adults' intentions to protect students from frustration or failure by doing things for them, restricting their activities, and allowing them to quit when tasks become difficult may squelch opportunities for self-management. The other extreme can easily occur as well: Students feel they are drowning and cannot manage because adults underestimate the extent of support needed.

Family and professionals can support the child's self-management in a variety of ways. Appropriate accommodations include reducing distractions, eliminating "triggers" for inappropriate behaviors, providing rest breaks for managing fatigue, utilizing visual schedules to support predictability, offering choices, "preparing" the student for schedule changes or less structured activities, and presenting checklists that the student can use to facilitate follow-through. Skills for self-management can also be taught directly. Adults can teach students how to use formats such as cause–effect drawings and "think sheets" to develop more independent problem-solving skills. Students can learn time management strategies such as estimating the amount of time needed for an activity, tracking the actual time elapsed, and comparing the estimate with the actual time needed. Using questioning strategies with students (e.g., "What do you need to do next? Do you need to look over the example again, or are you ready to do the first problem?") rather than telling them what to do is another means of encouraging independent thinking and self-management.

Trust

When a trauma or extremely negative event occurs, distrust and apprehensiveness are frequent by-products. With TBI, this distrust may target specific individuals or situations perceived as contributors to the injury (e.g., a driver, bike riding, sitting in bleachers, playing football), or it may be generalized to similar activities, other activities perceived as risky, or other people not directly known to be trustworthy. Sometimes, parents also have trust issues following a child's TBI; they may approach the first line of medical staff with apprehension, only to have it reinforced by doctors who do not answer their questions or who make inaccurate recovery predictions. By the time the family meets with school personnel, their mistrust, apprehension, and protective instincts may be quite potent. Children may pick up on the apprehension of parents and, consequently, feel insecure about their care and instruction at school.

School members need to build purposefully a sense of trust with students and family members following TBI. Families need assurance that providers have the student's best interests in mind. Educators can promote strong relationships by listening to families, hearing their stories, finding out what the student was like before injury, following through on commitments, admitting what they do not know and working to find additional information, setting up regular communication, being consistent, and meeting with families on their turf. With students, adults can provide predictability, opportunities for successes, a person to serve as a touchstone at the end of each day, and one-on-one interaction time.

Belonging

Particularly as students enter adolescence, peer relationships become the drawing force for school attendance and performance. Following a TBI, youths' greatest concerns are often the loss of friendships and alienation from peers. This alienation commonly intensifies over time. For teens, parents feel awkward in supporting peer interactions, because, prior to injury, parents did not participate in inviting their child's peers over or arranging group activities.

Furthermore, peers may be uncomfortable interacting with the student if significant changes have occurred in personality, awareness, communication skills, or mobility. Mutuality is important for building and maintaining relationships, but a student's ability to directly "give" in familiar ways may be drastically changed; the student may no longer be able to pick up the phone to call a friend, write notes, drive friends to school, or go shopping with a group of peers. The student's team should develop specific plans to address the student's need for belonging within the school setting and in the larger community.

Peer education is a good place to start in rebuilding relationships and belonging. Peer education can begin while a student is still hospitalized; peers can be prepared for what they will experience during hospital visits, facilitating interactions while in the hospital, and debriefing peers after hospital visits to answer questions, address concerns, and provide emotional support. If a student requires extended inpatient rehabilitation, the family, staff, and student may want to produce a video showing what the student can do, what skills they are working on, and what the rehabilitation facility is like. Such videos, assemblies with guest presenters, and small group discussions can support peer education prior to the student's return to school. When the student returns, purposeful planning for facilitated one-on-one or small group activities with peers (e.g., playing video games, making or putting up posters for upcoming school events, handing out programs at concerts or games) can foster feelings of belonging. Educators can encourage the student with TBI to take advantage of other opportunities—such as bringing treats to school and e-mailing cards to friends—so the student can contribute to peer relationships and prevent them from being one-sided.

The Science: "Success Precedes Motivation"

Particularly in the early stages of a student's recovery from TBI, therapists and educators should intentionally set the student up for successes. Success spurs motivation. Teachers must apply all they have learned about antecedent control, reinforcement, skill maintenance, and generalization. Baselines gathered in the rehabilitation setting may differ from those observed in the school or home settings because skills may not generalize to environments with different materials, cues, and reinforcements. Educators should obtain baseline measurements on specific priority skills in the settings in which they will be taught and applied. Teams need to identify and manage the antecedents—such as student groupings, verbal cues, schedule changes, time limits, or time of day—that contribute to skill application or breakdown. Reinforcement schedules may also need to be developed; these schedules should identify preferred reinforcers, the frequency of reinforcement, and methods for observing and recording performance. Teachers need to devise strategies for generalizing learning to new contexts and attaching new information to previously held knowledge.

Structured learning is particularly important for students with TBI. Students with TBI are likely to learn more easily when teachers identify objectives up front and structure activities to meet learning goals rather than expecting learning to occur through discovery. Instructional approaches that use concrete examples are also advantageous and contribute to learning success. In addition, the following paragraphs describe other factors that may contribute to student learning and success.

Who

Ideally, everyone who has regular contact with the student should play a part in teaching and reinforcing target skills. This includes teachers, administrators, kitchen staff, school secretaries, custodians, peers, paraprofessionals, parents, and caregivers. Global participation supports consistency in expectations, modeling, and cueing and helps ensure that inappropriate behaviors are not reinforced. Involving many people across multiple tasks and environments also supports the generalization and maintenance of skills. The core planning team should identify key players, share information on target skills and approaches, and touch base with others on the student's progress across environments.

What

Team agreement on instructional content for a student with TBI is a considerable challenge. Especially in planning for adolescents, differences of opinion often emerge concerning the amount of instruction that should focus on remediation or relearning of old skills (e.g., reading, writing, math facts and processes, and basic knowledge) versus the amount that should focus on mastering compensatory strategies and new learning. In the early stages of recovery, relatively large amounts of time are sometimes required for relearning previously known information and skills. This often takes the student out of the regular curriculum (at least temporarily), which is an issue for team members who would prefer to apply compensatory strategies immediately to support the student's continued participation in the regular curriculum. Examples of such compensatory methods include (a) the provision of partial outlines for following along and taking notes in class; (b) using word prediction software to speed written classroom work; (c) providing multiple-choice rather than free-recall tests; and (d) using lower reading level versions of literature for some classes.

Team members may also disagree about the provision of instruction on independent living skills versus academic skills. Students participating in regular classroom curriculum and learning activities focus largely on academics. If team members elect to shift the focus to independent living skills, the regular classroom may not provide the opportunities needed to build such skills (e.g., doing laundry, buying groceries, driving a car, keeping a record of purchases, addressing envelopes; see the next case example about accommodations across school and community). Students may also have unique strengths—such as auto servicing, performing data entry, or providing childcare—that team members would like to build on during the school day to foster future employment opportunities. In such cases, identifying long-term goals (e.g., employment, postsecondary education, independent living) and then working backward to identify present opportunities and needs is helpful.

Too often, teams pay little attention to reteaching skills for "learning how to learn" and for performing other cognitive tasks that determine what a student does with his or her knowledge. When intervention requires the relearning of cognitive skills—such as attention, organization, memorization, information retrieval, problem solving, and executive functioning—skill instruction can occur within the context of previously learned information, new learning, or combinations thereof. Instructional contexts can be endless: academic, self-care, leisure, work, socialization, and mobility, to name only a few. Cognitive interventions, then, can serve as the common thread among activities that promote relearning, new learning, and generalization of a wide range of skills and information (Ylvisaker, Szekeres, Hartwick, & Tworek, 1994).

When

Scheduling for the student with TBI can be a challenge. Due to fatigue, students may tolerate only a partial school day. Fatigue may persist for days, weeks, months, or even years postinjury. For some students, short rest periods throughout the day may enable them to participate in an entire day at school. Especially when students are in the early stages of recovery, continuous instruction over the summer months may be necessary. Aggressive summer instruction may be particularly important for students attempting to operate within the context of the regular classroom curriculum. Although some districts routinely offer summer programs, for others a request for summer services would be very unusual and would require substantial documentation of need.

Whatever the schedule, students with TBI commonly benefit from strategies that help them track their schedules. For students needing concrete scheduling supports, helpful interventions include posted picture schedules, verbal "2-minute warnings" from teachers to signal upcoming schedule changes, a simple written daily schedule, large sand or kitchen timers, watches with alarms, preprogrammed pager messages, or planners. Reminders from others are natural cues for students; such reminders might take the form of questions such as, "Don't you have something special going on after school today?" When particularly important events are scheduled, having a no-fail plan or safety net (e.g., a buddy system) is a good idea.

Where

Sometimes, a little thing can make a big difference. This certainly applies to the potential impact environmental factors have on students with TBI. Features that may go unnoticed by a teacher can be significant distractions for a student: a ticking clock, a furnace turning on and off, bright lights, classroom chatter, workspace clutter. Teachers and therapists need to keenly observe and respond to distracters with appropriate accommodations such as moving students into rows rather than having desks in clusters of four, teaching students to use quiet voices when working together, or providing quiet work areas that any student may opt to use.

School environments that require numerous transitions and frequent navigation from class to class can present additional challenges. Students may have difficulty keeping themselves spatially oriented, handling unstructured peer activity in the hallways, and tracking their own time. Transitions can be supported through methods such as pairing up students who have the same schedules, having the student's locker next to someone with the same schedule, placing teachers' pictures on the wall outside their classrooms, playing songs on the school intercom that end right before students are due in their next classes, or color coding hallways to rooms that are difficult to find.

Other environmental challenges may be present. Physical accessibility is often an issue for students with TBI. If major facility accommodations are needed, the student's team may need to develop temporary alternatives. The student's educational experiences may most appropriately occur across environments within the school setting and community, especially if the student's learning activities include work experiences. In such cases, the team must determine needs for environmental accommodations in settings such as the school office, cafeteria, or local businesses.

How

Learning objectives and accommodations are, of course, highly individualized. The methods for accomplishing objectives may range from nearly imperceptible (e.g., monitoring student progress, using raised line paper, reducing assignments, shortening tests, or color-coding instructions) to somewhat noticeably different (e.g., using slant boards, books on tape, alternate keyboards, different seating arrangements, talking calculators, or electronic spell check

Case Example: Accommodations Across School and Community

Thomas was an artist, a drifter, a loner. He was a quiet wanderer. In his past life, he had wandered into drugs and gangs and detention centers and now brain injury and life on a reservation. Though he lived with the effects of TBI—irritability, difficulty paying attention or sitting still in school, confusion, slow speech—life was actually better now. He was not particularly concerned about his future, but others certainly were. The latest issue was how to keep him in school. Thomas came and went as he pleased—or as he could tolerate. But now he had a new teacher and a new schedule and a new place to be. Mr. Terry would come over and make breakfast with Thomas. They would clean up together and do some laundry, then draw and paint. That was Thomas's favorite part of the day. The tribal office was the next stop to get assignments for lawn work, cleaning, or whatever else needed to be done. Then, Thomas and Mr. Terry would go to school. Thomas was on his own for lunch, a couple of classes, and the walk home. Thomas's new life was peaceful, safe, and productive—a better life, even after brain injury.

aids) to more complex (e.g., providing assistance with toileting and eating or using text-to-speech computer software, a full-time paraprofessional and several related service providers, or electronic augmentative communication devices). Innumerable resources are available to assist the educational team in brainstorming and deciding how to provide instruction and accommodations (Blosser & DePompei, 1994; Reed, 1998; Savage & Wolcott, 1995). Such tools may open the team to consideration of new possibilities and help them avoid unnecessary trial and error.

Summary

❝ Experience is not what happens to a man. It is what a man does with what happens to him. ❞
—Aldous Huxley (cited by L. J. Peter, 1977, p. 185)

A child's brain injury changes lives beyond his or her own. Effects ripple throughout a community to family members, friends, educators, therapists, and even people the child does not know. Just as people experience a child's cry differently, each person experiences a child's brain injury in a different way. Others' experience of and reactions to the TBI will affect the child's experience either in positive or negative ways: Do people reach out? Take the initiative? Ignore? Look to someone else? Hope the problem will go away? Ask for help? Make a plan? Feel like they do not have time to deal with it? Ask the child what he or she needs? Wait until it is too late and things have fallen apart? Support the parents? Following a child's TBI, people make choices among the many ways they may experience and react to the child's brain injury. The choices ripple back—powerful, erratic, inveterate, imperceptible—altering the experience of the child and making a difference, for better or worse.

When TBI happens to children, big "make-a-difference" opportunities emerge: There is the opportunity to lead a team, know a child, know a family, surf the Internet, burn some midnight oil, learn more, and teach others. But now—before TBI affects someone near you—is the time to prepare for that opportunity to make a difference. Odds are that, at some point, TBI will touch every educator or clinician. If that big "make-a-difference" opportunity has come and gone, keep Mark Twain's words in mind: "Although the past may not repeat itself, it does rhyme" (cited by Kurtz & Ketcham, 1992, p. 153). Be prepared; some child is—or will be—counting on you to make a difference.

What About Graduation Requirements?

For academically competitive high school students, partial school days following TBI can complicate a student's efforts to meet graduation requirements. This issue should be specifically addressed early on in post-TBI educational planning. Required classes may not be offered during the portion of the day the student is in attendance, and policies may state that students must complete a minimum number of courses prior to graduating. These factors can delay graduation, and such delays can be very discouraging to students. When injuries occur during or near the senior year of high school, students are sometimes allowed to participate in graduation ceremonies with their class despite the ongoing work required to complete assignments missed during hospitalization and recovery.

Options to help students meet graduation requirements include summer courses via small groups, one-on-one time with instructors or tutors, or Internet courses. The IEP can be a useful tool to tailor graduation requirements. Via the IEP, planning teams can make provisions for earning credit toward graduation in alternate activities: work experiences, special projects, or course substitutions. Sometimes, as in cases in which a student needs to delay graduation to meet local requirements, the young person or some team members may be tempted to opt for a GED rather than a diploma. This decision needs careful consideration, because a diploma is now frequently a minimum employment standard accepted by industries and employers. The planning team needs to look far ahead even when the student's short-term goal is to graduate with classmates.

References

Assistance to States for the Education of Children with Disabilities Program and Preschool Grants for Children with Disabilities, 57 Fed. Reg. 44794–44852 (Sept. 29, 1992).

Blosser, J. L., & DePompei, R. (1994). *Pediatric traumatic brain injury: Proactive intervention.* San Diego: Singular.

Brown, P. (1999). *TBI tip sheet series.* Cozad, NE: Dawson County Productions.

Department of Health, Education, and Welfare: Nondiscrimination on the Basis of Handicap, 42 Fed. Reg. 22675–22702 (May 4, 1977).

Hux, K., & Hacksley, C. (1996). Mild traumatic brain injury: Facilitating school success. *Intervention in School and Clinic, 31*(3), 158–165.

Kurtz, E., & Ketcham, K. (1992). *The spirituality of imperfection.* New York: Bantum.

Lash, M. (1992). *When your child goes to school after an injury.* Boston: Exceptional Parent.

Lash, M., Savage, R., & DePompei, R. (1998). *Back to school after a mild brain injury or concussion.* Wolfeboro, NH: L & A.

Mira, M., & Tyler, J. (1991). *Students with traumatic brain injury: Making the transition from hospital to school.* Denver, CO: Love.

Mount, B., & Zwernik, K. (1988). *It's never too early. It's never too late. A booklet about personal futures planning* (Publication #421-88-109). St. Paul, MN: Governor's Planning Council of Developmental Disabilities.

Peter, L. J. (1977). *Peter's quotations.* New York: Morrow.

Reed, P. (Ed.). (1998). *Assessing students' needs for assistive technology: A resource manual for school district teams.* Amherst: Wisconsin Assistive Technology Initiative.

Savage, R. C. (1991). Identification, classification, and placement issues for students with traumatic brain injuries. *Journal of Head Trauma Rehabilitation, 6*(1), 1–9.

Savage, R. (1997). *Bing, bang, bong: When your child has a concussion.* Wolfeboro, NH: L & A.

Savage, R., & Wolcott, G. (Eds.). (1995). *An educator's manual: What educators need to know about students with brain injury.* Washington, DC: Brain Injury Association.

Vandercook., T., York, J., & Forest, M. (1989). The McGill Action Planning System (MAPS): A strategy for building the vision. *The Journal of the Association for Persons with Severe Handicaps, 14*, 205–215.

Ylvisaker, M., Feeny, T., Maher-Maxwell, N., Meserve, N., Geary, P. J., & DeLorenzo, J. P. (1995). School reentry following severe traumatic brain injury: Guidelines for educational planning and a proposed hospital to school protocol. *Journal of Head Trauma Rehabilitation, 10*(6), 25–41.

Ylvisaker, M., Szekeres, S., Hartwick, P., & Tworek, P. (1994). Cognitive intervention. In R. Savage & G. Wolcott (Eds.), *Educational dimensions of acquired brain injury* (pp. 121–184). Austin, TX: PRO-ED.

Zipper, I., Hinton, C., Weil, M., & Rounds, K. (1993). *Family-centered service coordination: A manual for parents.* Cambridge, MA: Brookline Books.

Transitioning to Work

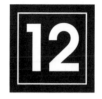

Pamela Brown

Employment of people with brain injuries: It is not a pretty picture. Rates of employment following TBI range from a meager 18% to an unbelievably high 88% (O'Neill et al., 1988). If individuals are not employed 6 months post-injury, they are not likely to become employed (O'Neill et al., 1998). Those who do return to work do not necessarily sustain employment; maintaining employment is even more challenging for individuals with brain injuries than obtaining employment (Prigatano, 1993).

Why does it matter so much whether individuals with TBI work? Work for survivors of TBI is important for the same reasons that work is important for other people: It promotes self-respect, it brings satisfaction, it provides a reason to get up in the morning, it fosters belonging, it provides security and income, and it contributes to identity. Furthermore, for individuals with TBI, the goal of returning to work often provides a reason for participating in rehabilitation. It furnishes incentive to endure unyielding pain, motivation for putting "mind over matter" to combat fatigue, and confirmation of the survivor's abilities after months or years of conflicting evidence. Work puts people back in give-and-take relationships. It puts them in the community. In short, service providers have very important work to do: ensuring that individuals with brain injuries have important work to do.

Redefining Work

The Social Context of Employment

U.S. culture places a high value on independence and individual rights. Although U.S. law supports equity in services to and opportunities for persons with disabilities, popular culture encourages some erroneous thinking among members of the community at large. For example, many people believe that (a) accomplishing a goal alone is of more value than accomplishing a goal through a group effort; (b) people with disabilities have more to gain from their inclusion in work settings than people without disabilities; (c) inclusion

289

requires more of nondisabled people than they get in return; and (d) family variables are not priority elements for consideration when planning vocational rehabilitation services. Such perspectives complicate efforts to establish inclusion, mutuality, community, and real-world interdependence for survivors of TBI. Fortunately, attitudes about fiercely defending independence as a primary goal may be changing.

Over the decade of the 1990s, the government's adoption and support of vocational models that value interdependence and individuals' social contexts have grown. The movement has been toward more natural, typically occurring supports rather than reliance on formal, specialized supports for persons with disabilities. As a result, family members frequently participate actively in vocational assessment and service planning (Hosack & Malkmus, 1992), coworkers serve as job mentors rather than having this role assumed by job coaches from programs outside a business, and community volunteer opportunities serve as contexts for practicing job skills rather than as settings in which all participants are persons with disabilities. More and more frequently, a team of people significant in the life of a person with TBI—rather than hired professionals and support staff—assists with planning and provides support to achieve work and life goals (Nisbet, 1992).

Other social trends are also bolstering the movement toward incorporation of natural or universal supports. These include federal legislation aiming to reduce barriers and disincentives to work and a tight employee pool spurring employer willingness to accommodate and support special needs. For example, the Workforce Investment Act promotes the integration of a range of training and employment services to improve accessibility, choice, and employment outcomes for potential workers (Employment and Training Administration, 1998). This may kindle an expanded pool of job opportunities and job training and support options for all individuals, including those with brain injuries.

> ❝ It's kind of fun to tell them I'm a sure bet. For every 1 dollar they invest in me, they'll save the public 14 dollars in public assistance. How could they say no to that?! ❞
> —40-year-old survivor of TBI

Another legislative encouragement to work is the Work Incentives Improvement Act of 1999. This act attempts to ensure adequate income and quality health care coverage for individuals with disabilities who become employed. In the past, many individuals with disabilities have been reluctant to become employed if the trade-off meant living in poverty or losing access to necessary, government-funded health care. Through this act, employees with TBI can increasingly retain access to government income subsidies, government health care, and other necessary government services.

Competition for employees, tax incentives for employers, and changes in the insurance industry have also resulted in increased access to health care plans offered by employers. Businesses find it feasible and necessary to offer quality health care coverage as part of employee benefit packages. Developments such as these are finally making employment a practical option for many individuals with TBI.

Endless Possibilities: The Array of Work Options

Work may need to be redefined for some individuals with brain injuries. Typically, *work* is thought to be synonymous with *employment*. However, by definition, work is any sustained physical or mental effort performed to overcome obstacles and achieve an objective or result. If individuals with TBI cannot be successful in employment, a wide range of other work options exists in which they can engage to find meaning, develop relationships, network, and improve skills (see the following case example on work options). These experiences may also be important in building toward future employment. Or, for individuals who can succeed in competitive employment following TBI, additional work experiences may serve to provide contexts for meeting other personal

---

 Case Example: Work Options

Dan had struggled for a long time after his TBI, feeling that life just did not have much meaning anymore. At 32, he wanted to work; he wanted to contribute. The right opportunity finally surfaced: One of Dan's old high school friends was working on safety education with his students and asked Dan if he would tell his story to kids. Dan was reluctant but did it for his old friend. Not only did the students get the safety message, Dan got the message that he did, indeed, have unique gifts and could make important contributions. He found a niche. He found meaning. He found self-respect. A teacher at the school where Dan spoke commented, "Here he was, talking with a gymnasium full of middle school kids and you could have heard a pin drop. He really got through to them like no one else has. Now, that's what I call a gift."

Selecting from the Work Array: Now What?

Even when work opportunities are selected for the development of "soft skills" or for personal satisfaction, certain elements must be considered thoughtfully. Discussing and planning for the following may prevent conflicts, disappointments, and frustrations:

- role(s) in the work situation

- work that *needs* to be done

- work that worker or coworkers *want* to have done

- who does what work

- plans for getting work done

- identification of natural supports

- accommodations needed for carrying out work responsibilities

- accommodations needed for full participation (e.g., social conversation, lunch, restroom facilities, etc.)

- what to do if plans are not working

goals such as job advancement, community involvement, personal satisfaction, or relationship development.

Table 12.1, Work Options Array, outlines a wide range of work opportunities—from household tasks to community service to telecommuting to traditional competitive employment. Survivors, family members, and some professionals often fail to consider fully the variety of options available when planning rehabilitation, work, and community reintegration. The Work Options Array may offer ideas for ways to match more appropriately work experiences with an individual's skills and goals.

Redefining Work-Related Dreams, Values, and Goals

Any discussion centering around planning for a life of work after TBI must begin with dreams. Identifying life dreams and work's role in realizing those dreams can direct the development of employment goals. Work experiences that are compatible with life dreams are more motivating than other experiences—a feature that is especially important early on in the recovery process for individuals with TBI who are facing significant losses in their work life or who have already experienced work failures (see the later case example on making employment work).

Individuals may have had strong dreams for their lives and work prior to injury; they may have even been living out those dreams. Unfortunately, the dreams often remain unchanged following TBI, even when an individual's life circumstances, skills, personality, and knowledge change tremendously. Working toward these dreams can encourage recovery, or it can seriously complicate one's ability to gain satisfaction from work experiences that are within the realm

Table 12.1
Work Options Array

Work option	Description
Citizen of the household	Carrying out one's responsibilities for interdependent home life (e.g., grocery shopping, cleaning, handling conflicts, paying bills, taking care of pets, caring for children, participating in healthy conversation, doing laundry)
Member of a neighborhood	Establishing mutually beneficial roles with one's neighbors (e.g., watering lawns, baking, visiting elders, monitoring children's group play, unloading groceries, mowing, walking a neighbor's dog)
Volunteerism	Identifying opportunities to contribute within one's community (e.g., tending flowers in parks, singing in church choir, serving benefit meals, assisting with scouts, fundraising, taking tickets at local productions or sports events)
Hobbyist	Developing an interest or skill that provides personal satisfaction and avenues for sharing interests with others (e.g., gardening, computer graphics, collections, woodworking, reading, following community sports, Internet-surfing, photography, dance)
Team/group membership	Practicing cooperation and give-and-take as part of a small group (e.g., local intramural sports teams, card club, Special Olympics, parent–teacher association, service organization, golf foursome, support group)
Job shadowing	Observing others in various job roles in actual work situations (e.g., receptionist, bricklayer, nurse's aide, physical therapist, realtor, salesperson, mechanic, childcare provider, teacher, telemarketer)
School-based jobs	Assisting with work others need to have done in the school setting (e.g., copying, delivering messages, handling money in the cafeteria, serving as a teacher's aide, cleaning or servicing vehicles, checking out library materials, landscaping)
Simulated work experiences	Work experience for students outside of school, usually combined with extracurricular activities, student organizations, and supervised work experiences (e.g., farming experiences through Future Farmers of America; leadership opportunities through Family, Career, and Community Leaders of America; advocacy through Students Against Drunk Driving)

(continues)

Table 12.1 *Continued.*

Work option	Description
School-based enterprises	Integrated entrepreneurship and academics, usually for high school credit (e.g., print shops, childcare centers, auto detailing, construction, restaurants)
Work centers	Work associated with structured settings, usually with close supervision and reduced complexity of tasks (e.g., packaging, assembly, house or office cleaning, lawn care, delivery service, auto detailing, seasonal crafts, jewelry construction)
Supported employment	Competitive employment with supports—such as a job coach, transportation, supervision, job restructuring—that are not time-limited (e.g., one-to-one coaching on bagging groceries and stocking shelves at a grocery store, intermittent oversight of production speed and quality, facilitation of work of small cleaning crew or telemarketing department)
Mentorships	In leisure or work contexts, model, coach, and encourage workers on skills needed for job success (e.g., getting along with coworkers, completing paperwork, handling phone calls, managing job frustrations, being on time, appearing professional)
Transitional employment	Temporary work for the purpose of assessing and strengthening readiness for more advanced or demanding placements
Freelancing	Independent contracting on a competitive basis; usually part-time but may be full-time (e.g., writing, accounting, altering clothing, performing carpentry, making presentations, publishing organization newsletters, providing computer training, servicing automobiles, catering)
Temporary services	Short-term, competitive employment that provides a temporary work opportunity, references, and a "foot in the door" for possible future employment
Part-time employment	Competitive employment that meets the needs of individuals challenged with fatigue, stress management, or health complications
Job sharing	Two compatible, part-time employees sharing responsibility for one job

(continues)

Table 12.1 *Continued.*

Work option	Description
Apprenticeships	On-the-job training opportunities that generally co-occur with learning through courses or workshops and that lead to certification, licensure, or other job-specific credentials
Internships	Employment experiences that typically follow a series of courses and last from several weeks to several months
Traditional competitive employment	Full- or part-time, nonsubsidized, paid employment in jobs with accommodations as warranted
Telecommuting	Working at home, or at a satellite office site via technology (telemarketing, Web site development, credit services, research, phone answering service, responding to customers via e-mail and Web visits)
Career tracks	Employment in companies or jobs that present obvious opportunities for ongoing skill development and job advancement
Entrepreneurs	Self-employment following a business development plan; may also lead to the hiring and supervision of employees

of one's current capabilities but not consistent with old dreams. When new skill levels do not coincide with long-held dreams, individuals may need considerable time and support to give up old dreams and replace them with new ones.

To strive toward achievable dreams, survivors of TBI need a "dream team." A dream team is just what one would imagine: It is a small group of people who care deeply about the core member; who actively encourage an individual to identify and express dreams; who provide guidance, enthusiasm, and practical feedback on steps in pursuit of dreams; who lend support when steps falter, dreams fade, or things just fall apart; and who work together to build new dreams when old ones no longer fit. A dream team may be only a few people who are close to a survivor—parents, a spouse, a best friend—or it may be part of a more or less organized circle of support involving neighbors, distant relatives, and mentors. These are people whose involvement is driven by relationships, not by roles (see the case example on creating a dream team).

Service providers may or may not be part of a survivor's inner circle, but they would be wise to encourage individuals with TBI to identify and continually

Case Example: Making Employment Work

"It took 11 years, but here I am!"

Looking down at his shoes and shaking his head, Jerry softly confessed, "There were times I just about didn't make it. I just kept thinking, 'It's got to get better.' My family tried to encourage me for a long time. They would bake me a cake to celebrate my new job; I think they must have baked 17 cakes. I'd get fired, or quit, and there'd be tears. . . . Lots of them. Then, I think they just got tired of it all. They didn't exactly give up on me. I think they just tried to remove themselves from the pain and the mess of it all. Then I met Doug. His nephew had cerebral palsy, so he sort of knew what it was like trying to get along, trying to fit in. Doug needed another driver for his route. He drove with me himself for 3½ weeks and a couple of times each week after that, just for awhile. Things aren't perfect, but we work it out. I've been working for Doug for 5 years now. Yeah, that's why they made me this really big cake."

tap into their dream teams. No service provider can provide all of the support necessary to help all clients identify, cope with, and accomplish their dreams. When clients do not have a circle of support, or dream team, providers may spend valuable time and energy unsuccessfully attempting to fill that void. Many individuals with TBI feel alienated and struggle to identify people to form a dream team. Providers can help them reach out to others through brain injury support groups, Centers for Independent Living, houses of worship, or Internet-linked peer support networks.

Dream team processes vary from informal one-on-one conversations between friends to scheduled meetings among relative strangers. No matter what process is used, it should begin with the individual identifying dreams, writing them down, and sharing them with at least one other person. Examples of well-developed processes for involving others in identifying and planning toward an individual's dreams include circles of support (Forest & Pierpoint, 1992) and Person-Centered Planning (Nisbet, 1992). These facilitated group processes also engage the whole team in supporting an individual's steps toward dreams and goals.

Dream-mapping can also be supported through a wide range of available materials (ACT & National Career Development Association, 1994; Research

Creating a Dream Team

Survivors of TBI often need assistance in identifying key people for their dream teams. Providers can begin with questions such as Who spends the most time with you? Whom would you like to see more often? Who makes you feel good when you are around them? Who cares the most about you? Who have you known the longest? Who has influenced you the most? Who listens to your secrets? Who has always been nice to you? Who cheers you up when you feel down? Who will always be there for you?

and Development Team, 1998; Swanson, 1991). Most materials are effective both in one-on-one and small group situations. These materials break the process of future planning into concrete steps. For instance, if individuals cannot identify abstract dreams, they can use a multiple-choice format to identify preferences or values. Such activities help connect skills, interests, values, dreams, goals, and strategies. Other activities—such as completing a matrix for comparing secondary education options or making a chart to compare jobs related to interest areas—assist in evaluating choices. Clusters of activities lead individuals through a process of evaluating dreams and choices through tasks such as identifying a dream job, imagining what it would be like, interviewing others who hold such a job, visiting a site where this type of work is done, recording observations on a brief worksheet, and comparing expectations with realities discovered about the dream job.

Matchmaking: The Worker and the Workplace

Assessing Readiness: The Worker and the Workplace

❝ We were preparing for her return at the same time she was preparing to come back. We went through a sort of rehabilitation of our own. ❞
—Jon, owner and manager of an auto parts store

Readiness To Work

Determining work readiness is, of course, a highly individualized process that considers a variety of factors such as the client's individual skills, goals, mobility, health, job requirements, job accommodations, housing, and supports for independent living. In some ways, readiness to work is a bit like readiness to date: No one ever feels fully prepared; mistakes are made; the unexpected is bound to happen; mismatches occur; expectations are adjusted; and, eventually, things get more comfortable.

Researchers have identified several factors that influence readiness to work following TBI. These include the severity of injury, duration of coma, length of hospitalization, scores on admission or discharge functional independence scales and neuropsychological tests, history of alcohol abuse, amount of education, and age (Sander, Kreutzer, Rosenthal, Delmonico, & Young, 1996). However, these factors are not predictive of the stability of employment. Estimates of employment success vary widely depending not only on the previously mentioned factors, but also on factors such as the nature of the workplace, employer attitudes, stability of housing and transportation, the definition of employment (e.g., part time, full time, academic study, supported employment), and the timelines used to define successful employment (Corthell, 1993).

Sources for Assessing Readiness

Readiness applies both to the individual with TBI and the potential work environment. Both need to be assessed prior to placements.

A lot of information about work readiness comes from assessments routinely performed with individuals with TBI: medical evaluations, neuropsychological workups, communication assessments, health history reports, interviews, self-reports, and assistive technology consultations. Other information is more specific to planning work experiences and includes interest inventories, job analyses, and situational assessments.

Interest inventories often consist of multiple-choice questions or rankings that ask for the identification of preferences among types of activities. These inventories assist individuals in identifying their strongest preferences, such as working with people, independence, or physical activity. The information is organized into preferred work clusters, such as data, things, ideas, and people (ACT & National Career Development Association, 1994). Once the clusters are sorted, individuals can explore occupations that fall within their preferred clusters, eventually narrowing vocational goals. Interest inventories are available in texts, on software, and on the Internet. Identification of a specific work goal or a narrow grouping of related jobs is a major step toward worker readiness.

Job analyses are time consuming but important for understanding work demands, obstacles to success, and potential accommodations. Jobs may be analyzed by reviewing job descriptions and related print materials, interviewing employees, and making observations at the work site. Job analyses provide information about essential versus related job functions, potential safety concerns, and "soft skills" needed for success on the job. Without a job analysis, individuals with brain injuries are likely to encounter many unexpected demands and confusion about roles. Job analyses increase the probability of success by clarifying expectations and identifying appropriate accommodations.

Situational assessments provide a means of evaluating worker performance in a job similar to one being sought. The assessment occurs over time and may include a mentor or job coach. During situational assessments, professionals gather information not only on the individual with TBI but also on the environment, tasks, procedures, and social supports needed for success. Situational assessments also allow for testing various accommodations and determining whether a job is a good match for an individual.

Time Frame for Assessing Readiness

Assessing work readiness only prior to an initial job placement is insufficient. Instead, assessments must be ongoing. Not only do worker characteristics such as skills, medical conditions, and motivations change, but workplace variables relating to time constraints, changes in team composition, and promotions change as well. As a result, a long-term commitment is needed to make the match work.

Matchmaking Realities and Tips

Workplace accommodation strategies for individuals with brain injuries can involve a myriad of variables, for example, social relationships, physical demands, scheduling, distractions, and learning pace. Fortunately, many individuals have assistance from service providers—such as vocational rehabilitation counselors—to comb through the seemingly infinite number of factors that could make or break a work experience. These providers can help identify and implement necessary accommodations. However, many individuals with even mild brain injuries struggle on their own to do job matchmaking and accommodation planning. The following information may be especially helpful in such situations to provide a basis for thinking about the who, what, when, where, and how of work site accommodation planning.

Who

For employment success, employers and other key company representatives (e.g., human resource personnel, foremen, team leaders, and supervisors) must be supportive of necessary accommodations. Accommodations may require changes—for example, changes in procedures, equipment, and schedules that require "upper level" approval. Mid-level managers have the power to facilitate or block these changes. Approaching employers with information on the benefits of such accommodations for several employees is generally advantageous.

To accommodate an individual with TBI successfully, relationships with coworkers need to be considered. A coworker mismatch can doom a job placement. Particularly with placement into a new job, persons with brain injuries may not cope well with relationship challenges. Efforts should be made to identify a coworker who can serve as the ambassador or mentor for the new employee. The role of this key coworker is to encourage, observe, model work strategies and expectations, offer tips, and provide other supports for the new employee's success.

What

The specific skills required for a particular job may not be fully known even to an employer or supervisor. Gathering information on job requirements from those who work very closely with the person in the position or others who hold or have recently held the position is important. When gathering information, consider which job tasks are essential and which are preferred. Finding out what other positions require is also helpful; sometimes two or three positions can be reorganized to better suit company and individual needs. To provide adequate support for job maintenance and advancement, a service provider should explore any foreseeable changes in company services, organization, job changes, and supports.

Private job-placement services or agencies such as Vocational Rehabilitation may provide job analysis services. Staff may perform observations within a job setting and may interview workers to identify the skills necessary for a particular job. Such an analysis clarifies expectations for both the employee and the employer, points out necessary supports, and helps prevent mismatches in job placements. The analysis may also help professionals design a system with a continuum of skill development and job responsibilities—an apprenticeship, for example. Such an analysis can be particularly helpful for job reentry, because it allows an employee to begin in a fairly simple position with few complex skill demands and gradually work toward a more advanced and complex position.

When

Although traditional work schedules are effective for some individuals with TBI, they present huge obstacles for many survivors. Due to fatigue, an 8-hour workday or several consecutive workdays may not be feasible and may compromise job success and health. Health-related complications—such as sleep disorders, the need for frequent medical appointments, or periods of depression—may disrupt regular work schedules as well. Some individuals can provide the equivalent of a 40-hour workweek if job tasks are spread out with split shifts or are completed over the course of a 6- to 7-day workweek.

Many individuals with TBI are successful with part-time jobs. For some, this is sufficient, particularly if another family member works and contributes income to the household or if the survivor receives financial assistance from family, roommates, or government programs, such as subsidized income, housing, or health benefits. In some situations, however, the income and benefits received from employment need to cover living expenses and to provide access to necessary care, such as health insurance and attendant services.

Where

Factors in the physical work environment can strongly influence work performance. Noise can distract and agitate people with TBI, even when the noise is nearly imperceptible (e.g., a ticking clock) or calming (e.g., music) to others. Excessive activity (e.g., phones ringing continuously, people walking by frequently, many people working in the same area at one time) can also disrupt work flow. If sensory disruptions to vision or hearing occur as a result of brain injury, special attention may need to be given to appropriate lighting, acoustics, and the position of work areas. Obviously, employees with significant physical disabilities may need adaptations in their work environments such as ramps and height adjustments for work surfaces, shelving, and machinery.

Transportation to work may be a barrier for some individuals with TBI. Many do not have a license to drive, at least temporarily, following injury. Especially in a tight labor pool, a driver's license can be an important asset, giving one applicant an edge over another. Without a license, individuals may need to carpool, use public transportation, or relocate closer to the business. For those individuals in need of transportation for employment, limited financial support may be available through state agencies.

Home or satellite offices may be a helpful possibility. Home offices can provide several advantages—such as a place for rest if fatigue sets in, fewer transitions, and an emotionally comfortable environment. For individuals who need more structure or guidance, a home office may not be successful unless a work partner is present. In these cases, a satellite office may offer a work site with supervision, equipment, and supplies located closer to the individual's home than the main office. These may be long-term, established satellite sites or temporary, cooperative satellites. Cooperative satellites are particularly useful when a survivor transitioning from school to employment engages in work for a business through a supervised work site at school or when a clubhouse or organization contracts with businesses for specific services (e.g., packaging, mailings, assembly). Fortunately, advances in technology and communications are opening doors to home and satellite office options.

How

Endless accommodation possibilities exist for how jobs are done. With new technologies, the options are ever-increasing. Keys to successful job accommodating center around an individual's awareness of personal strengths and challenges, the willingness of others to provide accommodations, the willingness of survivors to accept and utilize accommodations, and creativity and commitment on the part of employers, coworkers, and survivors. Table 12.2 provides

Table 12.2

Sampler of Accommodation Possibilities: Changing How Jobs Are Done

Skill	Accommodation possibilities
Reading/ writing	Provide drawings to supplement written instructions
	Provide manuals on CD for computers with text-to-speech functions
	Use portable electronic readers with voice output
	Use portable keyboards for making job notes
	Assign coworkers as reporters or note-takers
	Provide books on tape
Math/ measurement	Use pocket calculators
	Use electronic measurement devices
	Use color-coded measuring cups
	Provide laminated "cheat sheets" with measurement formulas
	Use bookkeeping software with automatic calculation functions
	Use talking calculators

(continues)

Table 12.2 *Continued.*

Skill	Accommodation possibilities
Organization	Use color-coded forms
	Use labeled storage containers
	Provide consistent job routines
	Have team leaders perform daily job setups
	Make daily progress reports
	Use checklists
	Use visual timers
	Use maps
	Have hallways color-coded
	Use paper planners
Memory	Use pagers for reminders
	Use electronic memory aids
	Use pocket recorders
	Use written instructions
	Use "to do" lists
	Use watch alarms with recorded voice reminders
	Use electronic planners with alarms
Social communication	Provide coaching on unwritten social rules for conversation
	Provide staggered break times to set up pleasant coworker interactions
	Provide coworkers with strategies for successful social interactions
	Define off-limit topics, words, or phrases
Problem solving	Provide time-outs to allow a person to calm down
	Assign a team leader or coworker to facilitate problem solving
	Arrange mediated discussions after work
	Provide multiple-choice options to solve dilemmas
	List the pros and cons of a situation
	Write out or draw options for solving problems

suggestions on ways of making accommodations to promote survivors' success and achievement.

Matchmaking Regulations: The Americans with Disabilities Act (ADA) and Employment of Persons with TBI

Accommodating workers with brain injuries is not just a good idea: It is the law. However, workers and service providers need to understand that the Americans with Disabilities Act of 1990 (ADA) simultaneously protects the opportunities of individuals with disabilities and the interests of employers. It attempts to balance the rights and responsibilities of both the employee and the employer. The following sections highlight some key stipulations of ADA.

Reasonable Accommodations: What Are They?

ADA requires employers to make reasonable accommodations for qualified individuals with known physical or mental disabilities. *Reasonable accommodations* are those job-related adjustments that enable a person with a disability to successfully carry out the essential functions of a job. Such accommodations vary widely, including such steps as reassignment to another position, a part-time or modified work schedule, provision of assistive technologies, or reorganized work teams.

Qualified individuals are those who satisfy job requirements and who can perform the essential functions of the position with or without accommodations. *Essential functions* are those duties that must be performed to meet the requirements of a job description; they are duties that cannot be transferred to another position without fundamentally changing the nature of the position. While an employer need not create a new job for an individual with TBI, the employer may be required to reallocate nonessential job functions to other employees. This is referred to as *job restructuring*.

Reasonable Accommodations: What About Employer Hardship?

The ADA does not require employers to make accommodations that pose undue hardships for their businesses. An *undue hardship* is a change that is significantly difficult or expensive. It is determined by assessing several factors, such as the nature and cost of an accommodation, the financial resources of the business, and the impact of an accommodation on business operation. Typically, requested accommodations cost little or nothing (BruySre, 1999). To reduce employer costs for accommodations that might otherwise present a hardship, tax credits are available to businesses that reduce architectural barriers, target jobs for individuals with disabilities, provide assistive technologies, or utilize interpreters.

Reasonable Accommodations: What About Safety?

Employers may be reluctant to hire an individual with TBI because of safety concerns. These concerns may relate to coordination, seizures, judgment, temper control, difficulties sustaining attention, fatigue, or a number of other factors. According to ADA, such concerns are founded only if there is clear, documented evidence that the individual poses a "direct threat" to him- or herself or others due to the nature of the job and the specific characteristics of the individual's disability. This safety-related evidence is generally obtained from medical and psychological reports, but it may also be supported through sources such as interviews and reports about recent work experiences. When safety is a concern, the hiring process should include consideration of accommodations to eliminate the direct threat or reduce it to an acceptable level.

Reasonable Accommodations: What About Employee Misconduct?

Under ADA, employers may hold individuals with TBI to the same performance and conduct standards as other employees. Even when an employee engages in misconduct related to his or her disability, if the misconduct warrants discipline according to the business policy, the employer may discipline the employee. A preferred alternative is to prevent problems of misconduct before they occur by providing related, reasonable accommodations (e.g., an extended lunch hour or break time for rest; the option to leave the work area to briefly "cool down" when frustration is high; flexible scheduling to avoid issues of tardiness). In instances when reasonable accommodations will prevent problems of misconduct, the employer is responsible to make them. With issues of misconduct, establishing a balance between providing accommodations to support an individual with TBI and not imposing undue hardship on the business is difficult.

Continuing Education: Lifelong Learning

> ❝ *I was afraid that once rehabilitation ended, so did my learning. For once, I'm glad I was wrong!* ❞
> —*Cindy, a survivor of TBI who just earned her credentials to be a certified nursing assistant*

Today's economy and jobs are in continual flux. Many businesses are in an ongoing process of recreating themselves to improve quality and gain a competitive advantage. Because of this, individuals would be wise to assume that the skills required for their jobs today may not be the skills they need for the same employment in the future. Regarding TBI, employers who hire survivors may ask them to take on new responsibilities without realizing the difficulties associated with a new role and with learning and applying new skills. Or people with TBI may need to take on additional, but familiar, responsibilities because of a promotion, only to discover that they cannot integrate and manage additional tasks. In such instances, individuals with TBI who required little job training or few accommodations when they entered their jobs may need more training and accommodation as the employment situation evolves. Although a variety of educational avenues are available for learning new skills, they cluster into two major categories: work-based learning and postsecondary education.

Work-Based Learning

To support continuous business development and improvement, employee training is a high priority of successful businesses (Senge, Kleiner, Roberts, Ross, & Smith, 1994). Businesses are increasingly likely to have internal processes and resources for employee training and increasingly likely to arrange for and to financially support on-site employee education. Although this push for continuous learning can be a significant obstacle for some individuals with TBI, for others it offers a workplace culture that accepts and actively supports ongoing reeducation.

Coupled with business support of ongoing education has been a renewed interest in work-based learning for students in transition from school to work. This includes experiences such as apprenticeships, paid work experiences, cooperative education, job shadowing, business and industry mentoring, simulated work experiences through student vocational organizations, service learning, and school-based enterprises. The result is an increased number of partnerships between schools and businesses and more work-based learning opportunities for both youth and adults than were previously available.

The following is a short list of the ever-expanding opportunities for apprenticeships. These occupations are learned through supervised, on-the-job training and related classroom instruction. Requirements range from 1 to 5 years of on-the-job training and the equivalent of 3 to 4 weeks of classroom training. As apprentices move through training requirements, they generally receive higher compensation. Some apprenticeships result in certification or licensure in the chosen profession.

Animal care	Auto body	Auto mechanic
Barber	Building maintenance	Carpenter
Computer network manager	Cook	Cosmetologist
Counter clerk	Dental assistant	Dispatcher
Drafter	Electrician	Farm worker
Floral designer	Food service manager	Furniture finisher
Game warden	Graphic designer	Groundskeeper
Illustrator	Interior designer	Lab technician
Locksmith	Nursing assistant	Painter
Paperhanger	Phone installation	Phone operator
Photographer	Postal clerk	Retail sales
Roofer	Secretary	Small engine repair

For many people with TBI, businesses offer some of the finest educational opportunities through work-based learning. On-the-job training offers contextualized learning situations in which employees can learn work skills within work environments. Such training is multimodal; provides a rich variety of cues; offers ongoing, concrete practice for skill acquisition and maintenance; reduces generalization problems; and provides fairly immediate feedback for skill improvement. These features may be particularly supportive of job skill development for individuals with TBI who have difficulty with abstraction, initiation, new learning, generalization, long-term memory, self-awareness, strategic thinking, and integration.

Work-based learning experiences need to be individualized and designed for success. Although many formats are available for evaluating and providing feedback on worker performance in work-based learning situations (Paris & Mason, 1995), relatively few guides are available for designing individualized work-based learning situations. In conjunction with the information provided in Tables 12.1 and 12.2, the work-based learning outline shown in Table 12.3 may serve as a framework for planning work-based learning situations for individuals with TBI. Additional resources (e.g., Marshall, Martin, Maxson, & Jerman, 1995; Parent, Kregel, & Wehman, 1992; Wehman & Sherron, 1995) are helpful and should be consulted.

Table 12.3
Work-Based Learning: Planning Considerations

Individual characteristics	Workplace characteristics
Interests, preferences	Entry-level opportunities
Values	Opportunities for continued, advanced work
Motivations to work	Coworker mentoring/coaching experience
Dislikes	Motivators, support for accommodations
Fears, worries	History of accommodations
Skills, talents	Knowledge of typical accommodations
Social behavior	Work schedules
Skill challenges	Safety concerns
Medical needs	Legal considerations
Work experience	Coworker relationships
Strategies	Means for solving problems
Support system	Means for communicating progress or concerns
Transportation	Physical environment
Related issues (substance abuse, depression, family issues)	Related issues (family members who work at the same site, dress codes, conversation topics, etc.)

Postsecondary Education

    ❝ *I guess she did it because she's always dreamed of doing it. To tell you the truth, we weren't sure if college was a good idea for Kristen. There are so many pressures, so many deadlines, so many distractions. Her first semester was awful. She almost threw in the towel. But, you know, then she realized that it was okay to go part time and take a little longer to finish. Lots of people do it that way now. It took her 6 years, some summer classes, and lots of ups and downs, but she did it. Kristen didn't have people beating down the doors to hire her after college, but over time, she has worked her way up the ladder, so to speak. Now she's helping plan recreational therapies and events for elderly people, through senior*

centers and nursing homes. She loves it. I think she's really discovering her gifts. That's something she might not have done without that college diploma. Sometimes it really is a ticket to work. I'm usually not thankful that Kristen is stubborn, but this is one time I can say I am really thankful that she was determined. It was the only way she could be to make all of this happen. 🙷
— *Kurt, Kristen's proud and thankful dad*

Realities and Tips

Postsecondary education options and experiences for individuals with TBI vary wildly. Occasionally, individuals with brain injuries succeed in traditional programs without much unique planning or accommodation. Other survivors cannot even navigate the application process. Some strategies, however, seem to be relevant for the majority of individuals with TBI who consider postsecondary education. The suggestions listed in Table 12.4 may smooth the transition to postsecondary education for both transition-age students and clients who have already graduated from high school.

Regulations and Tips

The Rehabilitation Act of 1973 prohibits discrimination on the basis of physical or mental disability. Section 504 applies to all recipients of funding from the U.S. Department of Education—including colleges, universities, postsecondary vocational education, and adult education programs. Section 504 stipulates that

> a recipient . . . shall take such steps as are necessary to ensure that no handicapped student is denied the benefits of, excluded from participation in, or otherwise subjected to discrimination under the education program or activity operated by the recipient because of the absence of educational auxiliary aids for students with impaired sensory, manual, or speaking skills. (Office of Civil Rights [OCR], 1998, p. 1)

Auxiliary aids might include books on tape, electronic readers, computers with speech-to-text functions, or a range of other devices that support accessibility.

Title II of the ADA prohibits state and local governments from discriminating on the basis of disability and is enforced in public postsecondary training institutions. Similarly to Section 504 of the Rehabilitation Act of 1973, the nondiscrimination provisions of the Title II regulations generally include the

(*text continues on page 313*)

Table 12.4

Tips for Postsecondary Planning with Transition-Age Students with TBI

Tip	Explanation
Begin postsecondary planning by age 14	Postsecondary plans may affect course selection, even in the middle school years.
Build a competitive edge	Encourage participation in carefully chosen extra-curricular activities, community service, and work experiences to give students with TBI a more competitive edge for college entrance and scholarships.
Try backward chaining to plan courses	To identify the courses and experiences needed, first identify the vocational goal and necessary post-secondary training, including specific courses likely to be required. Then, identify high school courses to support success in the postsecondary courses. (This process also provides a reality check on whether a student is willing and able to meet the challenges necessary for the vocational goal.)
Consider taking summer courses	Because many postsecondary institutions have challenging entry and scholarship requirements (several years of high school math and science, foreign language proficiency, minimum grade point averages), students with TBI may need to take fewer classes per semester to complete courses successfully and maintain a competitive grade point average. This may necessitate taking summer courses during high school.
Identify the pros and cons of postponing graduation	Although students and parents generally do not consider this a desirable alternative, the advantages often outweigh the disadvantages. Postponing graduation enables a student to take a reduced load each semester, thus minimizing fatigue and school demands. It also provides students with additional recovery and rehabilitation time while living at home and receiving public school services. Some students continue in the high school environment through age 21 to gain work experiences or to participate in programs combining postsecondary coursework, high school classes, and work experiences.

(continues)

Table 12.4 *Continued.*

Tip	Explanation
Visit some postsecondary classes and ask about course requirements	This provides concrete information for students who do not have a realistic frame of reference about the rigor of postsecondary courses. Students who visit several classes and examine course syllabi first-hand have a basis for comparing various courses of study.
Learn and practice self-advocacy	While in high school, students with TBI need to learn self-advocacy skills so they can use them in other situations. Students need to be able to identify and communicate their strengths, challenges, needs, and preferences. Allowing students to guide their own IEP processes is one way to teach and practice such self-advocacy.
Clarify vocational goals	Students with TBI should enter postsecondary training with a specific vocational goal in mind. Vocational uncertainty is likely to jeopardize financial support. This uncertainty could also result in the frustration of taking unnecessary courses. Having a specific end goal in mind can also help students with TBI cope with challenges encountered along the way.
Determine whether the individual needs a degree, certification, or a small number of specific classes	Individuals often assume they must attend a 4-year institution to achieve employment goals. This is not always true. People with TBI may need assistance examining training options. They may be able to enter jobs with an associate's degree, engage in apprenticeships that lead to licensure, take specialized certificate programs, or take specific courses through adult education, continuing education, private businesses, distance education, or online.
Identify and compare ways to receive comparable training	Several ways may be available to complete educational requirements: beginning at a 2-year college and transferring credits to a 4-year program; taking evening or weekend classes; taking summer courses; attending a college in which students take only one course at a time, yet complete several courses during a year; taking tests to pass out of general studies requirements. Exploring options may reveal large variations in travel requirements, cost, length of time necessary to complete requirements, and links to job opportunities.

(continues)

Table 12.4 *Continued.*

Tip	Explanation
Identify accommodations or supports likely to be needed	List accommodations or services a student with TBI is likely to need such as tutors, books on tape, note-takers, organizational support, extended testing or work time, access to a computer with voice-to-text and text-to-speech technology, quiet places for study, morning classes, and accessible building and campus facilities. This will facilitate comparison of available accommodations at different postsecondary institutions.
Visit the campus to get first-hand accounts and tips on accommodations	Visits with students, faculty, and student services personnel provide more information than is available from college brochures. Students can obtain first-hand reports about managing classes and gaining accommodations. They also can get information about instructors who are accommodating, tutors who are helpful, ways to avoid penalties for missing classes because of physical ailments, classes to avoid, and ways of approaching faculty or administrators when problems arise.
Find out how to access accommodations and services	Clarify the types of information the institution needs (e.g., a copy of most recent IEP, a letter from doctor, assessment results) for a student to be eligible for accommodations or support services. Ask about cost and funding for accommodations and services. Make sure everyone understands responsibilities and timelines.
Find out how many courses constitute full-time attendance	In some instances, being a full-time versus a part-time student affects scholarship opportunities. Also, some insurance companies require that dependents be full-time students to maintain coverage through their parents' policies.
Ask about social opportunities	Social interaction is important for fun, emotional support, assistance, and job networking. Knowing whether an institution is a "suitcase college" in which students leave town on weekends and during summers or whether opportunities exist for year-round, productive social activities is helpful. Because many students with TBI are older than traditional students and may have children, knowing the types of social opportunities available for them is important.

(continues)

Table 12.4 *Continued.*

Tip	Explanation
Make sure other necessary supports are accessible	Some students with TBI need to know about the availability and costs of services for transportation or personal care. Others may need access to medical specialists, support groups, rehabilitation therapists, or other services.
Identify possible funding sources	Some people with TBI use vocational rehabilitation services to assist with postsecondary planning and funding. Others access typical financial aid sources through postsecondary institutions or private lenders. Individuals should check into the wide range of scholarships, fellowships, loans, grants, and awards available specifically for people with disabilities.
Map out timelines	Many individuals with TBI need assistance identifying and meeting deadlines for activities such as submitting applications, requesting accommodations, and applying for special housing. Establishing a broader timeline that includes other steps—such as visiting campuses and researching scholarship opportunities—is often helpful.

provision of auxiliary aids and services by institutions of higher education: "A public entity shall furnish appropriate auxiliary aids and services where necessary to afford an individual with a disability an equal opportunity to participate in, and enjoy the benefits of, a service, program, or activity conducted by a public entity" (OCR, 1998, p. 2). In addition to auxiliary aids, services might include such accommodations as tutors, readers, or note-takers.

When postsecondary students with TBI need auxiliary aids and services, they must provide adequate notice about the nature of their disabilities and must assist in identifying appropriate aids and services. The appropriate postsecondary representative to notify varies depending on the institution and the nature of the needed accommodation. A student generally begins the process with an academic adviser. Students may have to provide documentation of the need for auxiliary aids and services, or the institution may have its own process to verify such needs.

When an accommodation is necessary for postsecondary participation, the institution must make it available unless provision of the aid or service would cause an undue burden. (The determination of "undue burden" is made on a case-by-case basis.) The institution may not place an arbitrary limit on what it is willing to spend for auxiliary aids or services. It may not refuse to provide auxiliary aids because it believes that other providers of the services exist. Also, it may not make provision contingent upon the availability of funds. However, the institution may meet its obligations by assisting the student in obtaining outside funding for the aid or service, such as through vocational rehabilitation or a charitable organization. Ultimately, provision of the aid is the institution's responsibility (OCR, 1998).

Summary

Work is much more than employment. It is an expression of what we value, a giving back to our community, an avenue for friendships, and a reason to venture forth into each new day. It is a means of challenging ourselves, discovering our talents, and realizing our limitations. Our work—whether at home, in school, or in the community—helps define who we are as individuals and as part of society. Work is an imperative rehabilitation and life goal for individuals with TBI, regardless of whether they ever become competitively employed. Tom's story in the following case example sort of says it all.

 Case Example: Achieving Life Goals

You know, before Tom's brain injury he was one of 12 students, worldwide, selected to study music at this conservatory in Europe. While he was there, he played with big names, legends. He was becoming one of THE guys—like a Kenny G. Nine months before Tom left Europe, he married his high school sweetheart, Sara. Three months before he left Europe, he finished a huge CD—solos, duets with the "big dogs," some of his own compositions, the works. One month before he left Europe, Tom contracted an illness that put him in a coma for 8 months. Tom and his new bride came home to tears, not cheers; to a critical care hospital wing, not a couple's first home; to only remnants of dreams through CDs and photos.

It has been 7 years now. Tom can't talk. He can hardly hold a spoon. He certainly can't play his sax. And Sara, she pretty much takes care of Tom full time. Tell me, how does he find a purpose in life after all this? Sometimes he just seems so sad. And Sara seems so tired. You know, they

(continues)

Case Example: Achieving Life Goals *Continued.*

both love Italian food, gardening, cooking, taking pictures, music. I just wish they could find some outlet for their interests, something to take them out of the pain of every day, some type of fulfilling work to do. Like their own Internet site or something. Maybe a kind of virtual travelogue—photos and information on European destinations, musical selections, a place for travelers to share favorite pictures and Italian recipes, gardening ideas, travel tips. You know, this really isn't a bad idea! I just never thought about it before. I guess we all quit letting ourselves dream of something better, maybe because we thought it would never be good enough or like it was before. But that's long past now and Tom's so unhappy. I'd say its time to start dreaming again, wouldn't you?! We never would have thought that Tom's dreams took him as far as they did before; who knows where they could take him now? Yeah, it's time to start over. It's time to dream again.

References

ACT & National Career Development Association. (1994). *Realizing the dream: Career planning for the 21st century.* Iowa City: ACT Publications Department.

Americans with Disabilities Act of 1990, 42 U.S.C. § 12101 *et seq.*

BruySre, S. M. (Ed.). (1999). *Employment and disability series.* Ithaca, NY: Cornell University, ILR Program on Employment and Disability.

Corthell, D. W. (Ed.). (1993). *Employment outcomes for persons with acquired brain injury.* Menomonie: Research and Training Center, University of Wisconsin–Stout.

Employment and Training Administration. (1998). *Implementing the Workforce Investment Act of 1998.* Washington DC: U.S. Department of Labor.

Forest, M., & Pierpoint, J. (1992). Families, friends, and circles. In J. Nisbet (Ed.), *Natural supports in school, at work, and in the community for people with severe disabilities* (pp. 65–86). Baltimore: Brookes.

Hosack, K., & Malkmus, D. (1992). Vocational rehabilitation of persons with disabilities: Family inclusion. *Journal of Vocational Rehabilitation, 2*(3), 11–17.

Marshall, L. H., Martin, J. E., Maxson, L., & Jerman, P. (1995). *Choosing employment goals.* Colorado Springs: University of Colorado.

Nisbet, J. (1992). *Natural supports in school, at work, and in the community for people with severe disabilities.* Baltimore: Brookes.

Office for Civil Rights. (1998). *Auxiliary aids and services for postsecondary students with disabilities: Higher education's obligations under Section 504 and Title II of the ADA.* Washington, DC: U.S. Department of Education.

O'Neill, J., Hibbard, M., Brown, M., Jaffe, M., Sliwinski, M., Vandergoot, D., & Weiss, M. (1998). The effect of employment on quality of life and community integration after traumatic brain injury. *Journal of Head Trauma Rehabilitation, 13*(4), 68–79.

Parent, W., Kregel, J., & Wehman, P. (1992). *The Vocational Integration Index: A guide for rehabilitation professionals.* Stoneham, MA: Andover Medical.

Paris, K. A., & Mason, S. A. (1995). *Youth apprenticeship and work-based learning.* Madison: University of Wisconsin, Center on Education and Work.

Prigitano, G. P. (1993). Maintaining work after traumatic brain injury: Experiences from two neuropsychological rehabilitation programs. In D. F. Thomas, F. E. Menz, & D. C. McAlees (Eds.), *Community-based employment following traumatic brain injury* (pp. 179–196). Menomonie: University of Wisconsin–Stout.

Rehabilitation Act of 1973, 29 U.S.C. § 701 *et seq.*

Research and Development Team. (1998). *Keys to unlocking your future.* Kearney, NE: Curtis and Associates.

Sander, A. M., Kreutzer, J. S., Rosenthal, M., Delmonico, R., & Young, E. (1996). A multicenter longitudinal investigation of return to work and community integration following traumatic brain injury. *Journal of Head Trauma Rehabilitation, 11*(5), 70–84.

Senge, P. M., Kleiner, A., Roberts, C., Ross, R. B., & Smith, B. J. (1994). *The fifth discipline fieldbook: Strategies and tools for building a learning organization.* New York: Doubleday.

Swanson, S. (1991). *Is there life after high school? Making decisions about your future.* Minneapolis: Augsburg Fortress.

Wehman, P., & Sherron, P. (1995). *Off to work: A vocational curriculum for individuals with neurological impairment.* Verona, WI: Attainment Company.

Work Incentives Improvement Act of 1999, 42 C.F.R. § 121 *et seq.*

Family Issues

Carolyn Wright and Christine E. Borgelt

Including a family-oriented chapter in a textbook designed to assist speech–language pathologists in their work with survivors of TBI may seem odd; after all, the focus of our training and our energies is on the survivor. However, once professionals take time to ponder the impact of brain injury or observe the rehabilitation process, the importance of families becomes readily apparent. Exemplary professionals not only know content information and have technical skills, but also have exceptional interpersonal skills and an ability to understand and support the feelings of others—including families. Furthermore, appropriate family participation in the survivors' recovery process is of paramount importance, and speech–language pathologists must facilitate that participation. Understanding families' typical reactions to the various stages of recovery can be very helpful toward this goal.

Much of the existing literature about the impact of TBI on families focuses on two issues: (a) how family and support systems cope when a survivor returns home and (b) how rehabilitation teams can educate families about TBI and incorporate them into therapy activities (e.g., Holland & Shigaki, 1998; Kolakowsky-Hayner & Kishore, 1999; McKinlay & Hickox, 1988). Little research has systematically explored families' step-by-step experiences. The goal of this chapter is to address this gap in the literature by presenting information about families' experiences while their loved ones move through various stages of recovery: initial hospitalization, acute rehabilitation, and community reintegration. The information presented comes in a large part from observing and listening as families have shared their experiences rather than from reviewing professional publications. Gaining insight into families' experiences and perceptions by listening to their accounts enhances professional services to the same degree that staying abreast of recent treatment approaches and philosophies refines technical and clinical skills.

Just as every brain injury is unique and results in idiosyncratic patterns of strengths and challenges, every family is unique. Each family reacts in a manner consistent with its coping style and established pattern of functioning. Certainly, not all aspects of the following descriptions will apply to all families, and probably every family will encounter feelings and experiences that extend beyond those presented here. Given this scenario, this chapter focuses on two topics: (a) describing experiences common to many families when brain injury invades their lives and (b) providing information to guide professionals in participating in families' experiences following TBI.

Common Family Experiences

Initial Hospitalization

A severe TBI happens in a fraction of a second, yet its consequences change the future of the injured person and his or her closest relatives more or less permanently (Koskinen, 1998). Initial family experiences following notification that a loved one has sustained a TBI are similar to family experiences associated with other medical or emotional traumas. Pervasive shock and fear are accompanied by impatience with time. Feelings of denial, anger, guilt, anxiety, and depression are frequent (Falvo, 1991). Emergency room and intensive care experiences tend to blur. Time weighs heavily upon the family, yet with each hour, hope becomes a little stronger as the loved one continues to live.

The sparse and sporadic information presented to the family by medical professionals is typically quite technical. Most families process and retain only a small portion of this information (Whelan & Walker, 1989), and this theme continues far into the rehabilitation process. Later, this tendency contributes to friction between formally trained professionals and family members. Especially if an injury is severe, families find themselves feeling isolated as they make immediate decisions (e.g., life supports, emergency surgeries, drug-induced coma) and face the long-term implications and potentially frightening outcomes associated with those decisions.

At this early stage, families fight to save the family member (opting for heroic, life-saving surgeries, for example) without regard for the long-term consequences of what may be a very partial recovery. The prayer is simply, "Please let my daughter live." Bargaining with a higher power is often part of this experience for families: "If only you let her live, I promise I'll. . . ." In the future, these decisions and prayers will be revisited and, depending on the outcome, second-guessed.

An interesting phenomenon begins when the loved one survives. An "against-all-odds" mindset frequently develops; it is not a conscious decision by the family. The experts present information about a survivor's current status and also begin including information about long-term implications. At this time, families are unwilling (or unable) to dwell on possible long-term challenges, instead placing tremendous significance on the immediate status, progress, or short-term accomplishments. The family is thankful for the patient's survival, and professionals perceive them as being relatively happy during these first few days or weeks postinjury (Lezak, 1986). Adding strength to the grateful family mindset is the encouragement received from the experts, friends, extended family, and spiritual supports, all of whom stress the power of positive thinking; the importance of faith and prayer must not be minimized. For the family, this is what they *can* do, *can* contribute, and *can* control. None of us ever knows how influential a positive mindset is in the recovery process.

Acute Rehabilitation

❝ *Surely you aren't really thinking of discharge. He barely recognizes us, let alone anyone else.* ❞
—*Mother of a 22-year-old survivor of TBI*

Trauma and intensive care stays are relatively short; they typically only continue until a patient is medically stable. Families, though, rarely think in terms of length of stay and often have a different definition of medical stability than the medical staff has. Therefore, when discussions regarding discharge occur, families may be taken aback. Shock and surprise at rapid discharge decisions are likely to recur when acute rehabilitation ends.

The manner in which professionals discuss discharge has an enormous influence on families' comfort with impending events. For example, "Your family member is not making progress quickly enough, and your insurance carrier needs to see greater progress for him to stay here," sets off a far different tone than, "Your family member has stabilized nicely, and we should choose the next place for him." Unfortunately, both styles and many variations in between occur regularly.

Families are often asked to select the next stop in the recovery process. They, with the assistance of case managers, may visit rehabilitation facilities or may receive visits from case managers from other facilities. Because of the swirl of this process, families' decisions most often are not based on a good understanding of what to expect during the next phase of rehabilitation. Instead, families make decisions based on factors such as what seems right, what feels best, how wonderful the case manager is, how nice the doctor seems, the reputation of the rehabilitation center, or how close to home the rehabilitation hospital is. Later, family members may second-guess their decision and make comments such as, "If I knew then what I know now, I would have . . . "

Most families are unprepared for the shift from an acute hospital to an acute rehabilitation or subacute setting. Having quickly become accustomed to the close attention, bells and whistles, and high staff-to-patient ratio of

What is a physiatrist?

No, not a psychiatrist, a physiatrist. A physiatrist is a medical doctor who specializes in physical medicine and rehabilitation. Rehabilitation hospitals typically employ physiatrists to work closely with neurologists and neuropsychologists to assist the physical recovery of individuals with neurological injuries such as TBIs, spinal cord injuries, and strokes.

trauma or intensive care settings, many families initially react to an acute rehabilitation setting with thoughts that it is understaffed and may even be "behind the times." At the same time, given the rapid pace of most medical settings, staff frequently forget this may be the first experience a family has had with rehabilitation and may present the routine of the facility but fail to recognize or anticipate family questions and fears. Because family members may feel intimidated about entering yet another unfamiliar, "expert" world, they may not voice their doubts and concerns. This combination of factors sets the stage for poor communication between rehabilitation staff and family members.

Despite their initial concerns, most families eventually gain trust that the doctors, nurses, and therapists know what to do. The confidence that professionals exude is reassuring even though evaluation results may be confusing and technical. At this point, families still process only a portion of what is said to them and, by now, may begin to react strongly to that portion. They also continue to operate consciously or subconsciously under the against-all-odds perspective. Although the rehabilitation doctor or physiatrist may communicate the long-term implications of brain injury and even make statements such as, "Your daughter will likely not walk again," families are still living moment-to-moment and decision-to-decision. Medical and rehabilitation professionals understand that the family has a long road ahead and that the survivor may never return to his or her preinjury status. The family, however, if they understand this at all, certainly has hopes for something greater than the grim scenario presented to them. Families, again drawing hope and optimism from the immediate past (e.g., "She made it through the surgery," "He woke up," "She's nodding at us," "He recognizes us"), muster courage and strength to support therapy efforts—sometimes even more zealously than therapists would wish. Many times the survivor, with the help of therapists and the family, does, indeed, surpass the initial expectations and predictions of professionals. Although both professionals and family members rejoice at such an accomplishment, it has an additional implication for the family's belief system and trust in rehabilitation experts. For the family, the against-all-odds perspective gathers renewed strength and a new twist: Families realize that the experts do not know everything. This can be both disappointing and reassuring. It is disappointing because families so want the experts to know everything; it is reassuring because families realize they are in a world of hopeful possibilities. Once this realization occurs, families may begin contributing frequent ideas and thoughts to the rehabilitation process.

Usually, by this time, the family struggles—covertly or openly—with the unpredictability of rehabilitation and the descriptions or labels that professionals attach to survivors and family members. Differences persist between the perceptions of professionals and those of family members. For example, rehabilitation staff may perceive a survivor as severely impaired, while the family anticipates full recovery within the first year. Then, as physical recovery begins to slow, the family becomes confused and anxious. Further compounding the family's dismay, professionals often attribute this slowdown to the survivor's lack of cooperation and motivation (Lezak, 1986).

Staff perceptions about family members also create opportunities for misinterpretation and conflict. Some family members may be more vocal than others, openly questioning professional opinions and engaging in tearful and angry debates. This openness is frequently misinterpreted as a lack of understanding, a lack of awareness, a lack of acceptance, or even a confrontational attitude toward the rehabilitation staff. In a strange form of irony, rehabilitation staff may view family members who remain silent about their concerns as similarly not understanding or accepting the significance and gravity of the situation. An obvious need exists for family support during rehabilitation, and many researchers stress that families as a whole rather than survivors in isolation should be the focus of education and intervention efforts (Gleckman & Brill, 1995; Junque, Bruna, & Mataro, 1997).

In response to many recent changes in the health care environment and to the trend for hospitals and rehabilitation centers to discharge survivors as soon as possible following injury, Holland and Shigaki (1998) developed a three-phase model to help professionals educate families about TBI and minimize the families' feelings of being overwhelmed with information and responsibility. Holland and Shigaki suggest separating the information provided to families into three phases that coincide with rehabilitation placement. For example, providing a glossary of medical terms and procedures may be appropriate while the survivor is in intensive care; information regarding potential long-term behavioral and emotional changes may be appropriate during the acute rehabilitation phase; and information identifying community support resources may be appropriate at the time the survivor is discharged home. Providing information to families is helpful only when professionals consider current family dynamics and accommodate the family's ability to accept and comprehend the material presented.

Throughout acute rehabilitation, most families only partially understand the impact TBI will have on the rest of their lives. It is at this time, while families are disoriented, that rehabilitation professionals develop interesting—sometimes negative—conceptualizations of the family. The family "bares its soul" to the rehabilitation staff. Family patterns—functional or not—present themselves for the whole rehabilitation world to see; in turn, that world judges those patterns, and rehabilitation decisions are influenced. Families are extremely vulnerable at this time and, except for their against-all-odds mindset, are at the mercy of the staff. Obviously, misperceptions and misinterpretations about how a family functions can have long-lasting impact.

An example of this occurs as families embrace therapy. Often, families are ecstatic about having rehabilitation services twice each day. Yet, at the same time, they may question the content of therapies and wonder whether professionals really know their loved ones or how to work with the effects of brain injury (see the following case example on conflicts between families and professionals). Therapists see this when family members question how particular therapy sessions can possibly be beneficial for their family member. The content may seem such an odd match either for who their family member was prior to injury or for the behavioral mannerisms their family member displays since injury. When families form negative opinions about therapies or question the content, therapists may apply labels to families: *resistant, difficult, demanding*, or *clueless*. Interestingly, families begin to attach the same labels to the therapists. Therapists can go a long way toward alleviating mutual misconceptions and negativity if they keep an open mind and listen to—and truly hear—the family's message (which is not usually meant as an attack on the therapist's competence, but rather an expression of the need for reassurance that the best is being done for their family member).

Community Reintegration

As discharge from the rehabilitation setting nears, another decision looms about where to go next. The same perplexity that arose during the initial hospitalization period may recur at this time. Namely, discharge plans may come as a surprise to the family. One day a family may have thought that rehabilitation

Case Example: Conflicts Between Families and Professionals

Struggles between families and rehabilitation staff often develop over relatively mundane events that can lead to family beliefs that the staff do not sufficiently understand the survivor and his or her therapy needs. The following is an illustration of this phenomenon as related by Bob, the father of a 22-year-old survivor of TBI.

"My son, Jeff, is a complex individual. By all rights and reasons, Jeff should not be alive. A combination of Jeff's strengths and family decisions allowed him to live—and those family decisions are ones I regret much of the time.

"While Jeff was going through the traditional inpatient therapy, he remained volatile and unpredictable. He could not express his thoughts, experiences, or feelings. Confusion with each day seemed to reign. He let us know this frustration through what he could utter: 'Nah nah' (quietly), 'NAH' (a little louder), 'no' (quietly), then 'No NO NO!!!' If we did not pay close attention to his expressions, he had no hesitation about following with a right hook. . . . Look out!

"One day, a well-intentioned, young, traditional speech therapist was proceeding through her speech and cognitive therapy session. She presented Jeff with a tray of objects she wished him to identify as she said each name. I cannot convey to you how quickly my heart fell to my toes or how large the knot in the pit of my stomach grew when I looked at the tray of objects. This bright, attractive therapist working with my son in his area of extreme difficulty—and my bright, attractive but severely impaired son who was now frequently physically aggressive—had among those objects on that tray, a pair of scissors. Oh God, please help us get through this therapy session without injury!"

was progressing nicely; the next day, the case manager or doctor states that discharge will likely occur by the end of the week. The turmoil of impending discharge resurfaces. Home? Whose home? Nursing home? Another specialty program? Rarely do families feel ready to assume this next responsibility. In addition, animosity builds toward *something*—perhaps a doctor and the message that doctor sent, an insurance carrier, a hospital, or a nursing home. Because families have kept faith in immediate outcomes, they inevitably experience distress at the thought of discharge when they still see so much that needs to be accomplished. They are incredulous when the medical world seems ready to give up on their family member.

If the survivor is being discharged to home, structural modifications to the house are likely to be necessary. Families tend to concentrate heavily on these environmental and physical modifications and may not spend as much time reflecting on or preparing for the cognitive, communicative, and behavioral aspects of the transition. This is at least in part because physical disturbances after TBI are usually readily apparent, but changes in personality, emotions, and behavior are less obvious. In the long run, however, these psychosocial changes often prove to be highly disruptive to quality-of-life issues for both the survivor and his or her relatives (Koskinen, 1998). Families are likely to view changes in personality, emotions, and behavior as temporary and tend to minimize the potential effects.

The secret here is not to push families to accept the enormity of an injury's impact. Families are accepting the situation as fast as they can. Hope is carrying them through, and to destroy that is to send the world crashing down around them. Rather, professionals who understand and can anticipate what families may find useful in the future are most helpful. Stebbins and Leung (1998) found that family needs actually "expand" over time rather than "shift."

Learning to negotiate multiple service systems presents one of the greatest challenges to families. To assist with this, professionals must know about and provide easy access to a wide range of supports such as scheduling tips, outpatient services, inpatient specialty programs, phone numbers, and personal resources. They also need information on social and community supports as well as financial resources. At this point, case managers and therapists may provide families with literature about TBI. For some families, the reading material is a wonderful option. For others, the literature is too real, too scary, and too technical—anything but helpful. Quite often, the reading material is best suited for extended family or support system members. The extended support system may find the material helpful in providing them with specific suggestions about ways to be helpful. Without it, many people express a desire to help but are thwarted in their efforts because of not knowing what to say or do. Reading material provides the opportunity to understand and assist the family as they ask questions.

So, what happens following discharge? The array of possibilities includes, but is not limited to (a) doing nothing, (b) looking into day treatment programs, (c) investigating a nursing home placement, (d) pursuing a halfway house placement, and (e) evaluating extended specialty programs. For families who search for more services following acute rehabilitation, the struggles intensify: New placements, new therapists, new doctors, more of the same "Your loved one will probably never . . . " "You must accept . . . "

The challenges a family faces intensify greatly when a survivor is discharged to home—the scenario that occurs for 82% of individuals with acquired brain injury (High, Boake, & Lehmkuhl, 1995). Leaving the hospital or rehabilitation facility means losing ready access to doctors, nurses, therapists, and direct care staff. In addition, families typically find that extended family members and supportive friends resume their normal life patterns when hospitalization ends. Family feelings of loneliness, isolation, and depression are not a surprising consequence. On top of this, the family must adjust to providing care and structure for the injured person. Adjustment of work schedule, developing caregiving skills or hiring caregivers, and reestablishing daily priorities become a work in progress that is subject to change at a moment's notice.

Adjusting the tasks for caregiving and schedule modification becomes the easy part. More difficult is the larger life adjustment of providing care for an individual who was previously independent. This adjustment is a challenge both to noninjured family members and to the injured individual. When the injured family member resists these efforts, an even more challenging situation develops. Researchers have identified behavioral and personality changes as key stressors for family members living with a brain-injured relative (Stebbins & Leung, 1998). However, by surveying families 1 and 5 years following injury, Koskinen (1998) found some relatives reporting that the strain of caring for their family member decreased. Koskinen attributed this finding to individual differences between families, however, and warned against generalization.

As time passes, what initially appeared to be a subtle change in behavior or personality can evolve into a major annoyance to caregivers. The individual discharged from the hospital is quite different from the individual prior to injury, and the persistence of such changes following TBI has been well documented by numerous researchers (e.g., Brooks, Campsie, Symington, Beattie, & McKinlay, 1987; Brooks & McKinlay, 1983; Rosenthal & Young, 1988). The stability and prior functioning of the family system substantially influences its response to the changes (Byng-Hall, 1995). In almost all cases, families begin a grieving process that will continue for years to come—for some, the rest of their lives. Families rejoice that the person lived, but they grieve that this individual is so different from one they knew before. They mourn the loss, and they work at accepting the new person. Often, just as a family begins to reach an acceptance of sorts, a life event occurs that sets them back. For example, a sibling graduates from college and realization hits anew that the survivor will never return to school. Or a family member gleefully announces an engagement, and the family must deal once again with the actuality that the survivor will probably never marry or that the present marriage is unlikely to survive. Living among disability does not always evoke these dour thoughts, however. A family can become more loving, closer, and achieve great feats of empathy and care by living with a person with a disability. Families may come out emotionally strengthened rather than weakened by their experiences with trauma (Byng-Hall, 1995).

Almost constantly, families face the challenge of maintaining balanced lives. Friends who were initially so supportive call and visit less frequently for several reasons: People must resume normal work schedules; friends just do not know what to say or do to be helpful; the injured individual makes others feel uncomfortable; activities that formed the core of a relationship are no longer feasible. The consequent loss of relationships is often so painful to discuss that chasms develop. Social life disappears and is replaced by isolation. Families can no longer attend concerts or sporting events because of the care and supervision they must provide at home. New interests are difficult to develop, and, quite frankly, no time or energy remains.

As reality begins to set in—and for many this is not until 2 or more years following injury—families start realizing that living with TBI is a lifelong challenge. As the 2-year window for recovery elapses, the realization hits that the physical effects of injury—although challenging in their own right—diminish in comparison to the cognitive and behavioral impairments (Brooks et al., 1987; Junque et al., 1997). Families begin second-guessing their previous decisions and recalling some of what the medical professionals were saying during the initial rehabilitation process. Most of the time, this reflection causes more pain and anger than resolution.

> 66 *You know, I should never have said yes to that surgery. But, at the time, that was the only way she could possibly live. How could I live with myself if I had said no? How do I live with myself because I said yes?* 99
> —*Father of a 45-year old survivor who had parts of her frontal and temporal lobes removed following a severe injury sustained in a motor vehicle accident*

When the realities about life after TBI are acknowledged—though not always, as yet, accepted—families turn toward quality-of-life issues. For many, the search begins anew for some sort of solution. Families search for a setting that is neat and clean, that will take care of the loved one, that has terrific direct care staff, and that provides a program to support quality of life. They particularly search for ways to support happiness, social opportunities, and "a life."

This type of search is complicated by three factors: the difficulty of finding such programs, the challenge of securing sufficient funding to purchase them, and the internal family conflicts that inevitably result when making decisions about where loved ones will live and how they will be cared for. By this point, insurance dollars have been exhausted, and families must rely on public money (e.g., Medicaid) for support. Families themselves may be financially strapped, often having taken out huge loans or second mortgages to help provide care. Simultaneously, internal family strife intensifies. Adult siblings or children of the survivor may react adversely to discussions about an alternative placement and, thereby, add to the guilt already experienced by the primary caregiver. Feelings of guilt surface and are expressed in statements such as, "We're giving up," "You're dumping him," and "Why are you getting rid of her?"

Often parents assume long-term caregiving responsibilities for a survivor of TBI but later realize that the individual will outlive them. They must arrange for alternative care provision, guardianship, and placement when they can no longer assume these responsibilities. On the surface, siblings or adult children are the obvious choice. Below the surface, concerns arise about whether those individuals will provide the same care, protection, and support that the parent does. While making plans to have other family members provide for the continued support and care of a survivor, many unresolved issues related to the actions and decisions made by primary caregivers at the time of the injury and in the subsequent years resurface. These unresolved issues are particularly frequent among the siblings of survivors of TBI.

Special Needs of Siblings

Siblings are often the hidden tragedy of TBI. Very little information exists in the professional literature about the impact of having a sibling with TBI (Kneipp, 1996). What is known is that when the survivor is a child the effects on the family system are even more complex than when an adult is injured. The family puts the rest of life on hold while they tend to the injured individual. Initially, siblings go along with the flood of traumatic events fairly well. They listen attentively to their parents and try to understand the enormity of what has happened. They want to be helpful but often do not know what to do. New caregivers enter their lives (e.g., grandparents, other relative, friends), and a regular schedule is attempted. Lots of attention comes their way—at school, at church, at play—but, as time goes on, that attention wanes. The siblings watch their parents spend endless hours at the hospital or make elaborate preparations for bringing the injured sibling home. Practically all discussion centers on the injury and the injured sibling.

Parents place greater expectations and responsibilities on noninjured siblings both while the survivor is in the hospital and upon his or her return home (Kneipp, 1996). This often forces siblings to grow up more quickly than is typical. Parents, certainly without conscious intention, may brush off requests, minimize behaviors, and become impatient with what were once routine interactions; little attention may be paid to homework or extracurricular activities. Some siblings become withdrawn, while others begin to act out. Still others strive to become the "perfect child" and unconsciously try to replace or make up for the parents' lost dreams for the survivor. Over time, spoken and unspoken messages frequently lead siblings to conclude that their behavior does not matter: They will never do anything significant enough to earn more attention than the head injury. Loneliness may set in, but it is a different kind of loneliness than may have been present during the period immediately following the injury. Wherever they turn, nobody understands—not even counselors.

Out of a myriad of reactions siblings have, one of the most frequent is anger. Though this anger may have various targets, siblings are often angry with the survivor. They have thoughts such as, "Look what you've done to our family," or "If you hadn't been drinking . . . " Then, siblings may turn that anger toward their parents with accusations ranging from, "You don't care," to "I have to leave this house; I can't take it anymore."

When parents are remembering their experiences at a much later time, guilt enters the picture. Parents feel guilty for not realizing what was happening to their noninjured children, for not paying more attention, and for angry words spoken in haste. Fortunately, families usually respond well to the reminder that memories do not paint the actual picture of what was happening at the time, and that, given the situation they faced, they made the best possible decisions they could.

Another scenario is common when siblings are teenagers or young adults at the time of an injury. These siblings may be fervent in their belief that their family member will get better. They trust that rehabilitation programs will aid the recovery process, and they have a difficult time accepting that some effects of injury may be permanent. Parents become frustrated at having to discuss repeatedly the long-term implications of TBI. Then, a teenage sibling may accuse the parents of not caring, not thinking positively, or just plain giving up on the injured family member. Relationships between teenagers and parents are usually fragile at best, and a struggle such as this has potential lifelong impact.

> ❝ *Dan's brother doesn't realize Dan is gone, and he's not coming back.* ❞
> —Father of two sons, one injured at 17 and the other 15 at the time of injury

Tips for Working
with Families

The ideas listed in Table 13.1 may be helpful for professionals in their work with the families of survivors. The ideas are not meant to include all possible situations but to serve as general guidelines for establishing positive relationships among professionals and families during a time of tremendous stress. A professional's goal should be to provide terrific services to each family in need.

Summary

In conclusion, no two brain injuries are alike nor do any two families respond to the effects of brain injury in an identical fashion. Patterns of recovery may follow somewhat similar paths, but family responses are likely to vary widely. Rehabilitation professionals deal with the effects of brain injury in a much broader context than each individual family. Professionals typically find it challenging to remain focused on each family as a new system and to recognize what information and services may benefit each unique family system. Often time is an issue—either the rehabilitation stay is short or the number of patients a professional must see precludes individual attention. Nevertheless, each family will proceed through the rehabilitation experience, reacting to trauma, beginning an adjustment process, forming opinions of rehabilitative efforts, and ultimately assuming responsibility for their injured family member. For each family, this becomes a lifelong commitment or adjustment. Professionals, in contrast, have but a few days or weeks to affect this fragile system. With the combination of professional knowledge and skills, an understanding of how families are affected, a willingness to devote time to determining what families are processing, and a touch of creativity, the rehabilitation process can be one of working together to achieve goals. Even though families will continue to be challenging as they attempt to accept how their worlds have changed, rehabilitation professionals must strive to attain "trusted resource" status. As families walk the long walk ahead, they will reflect on the rehabilitation process. Hopefully, they will have positive memories about the helpfulness and guidance they received from rehabilitation professionals during this very difficult time in their lives.

Table 13.1
Tips for Working with Families

- Acknowledge that the family knows their loved one better than anyone else. Listen to their story. You may have heard many stories, but each time you meet a new family, you encounter a new story.

- Listen. This is very important. Most of us think we listen better than we do. We tend to give information, provide explanations, and think we have communicated with the family. Try sometimes to have no answers. Have as a goal, "What can I learn from (not about) this family?"

- Understand how hope helps the family persevere. "Never take away someone's hope; it may be all they have" (Brown, 1991, #139).

- Cry with the family. A particularly touching story or experience is worth a tear or two.

- Talk to the family when times are good, when times are bad, when times are neutral. Have as a goal that the family requests that you call less frequently.

- Invite the family's involvement and know their concerns. If equipment (e.g., wheelchair, walker) is a primary concern, stay on top of the equipment needs. If personal appearance is a primary concern, know about the daily routine.

- Have as a goal that the family sleeps better at night because of the care their loved one receives.

- Laugh with the family. Pick up the phone and call Dad to say, "Guess what Jeff did today?"

- Return phone calls promptly. For the family, you are their lifeline.

- Meet the family at their level. Should we really describe them as "dysfunctional" or "in denial"? Perhaps, but if we went through what they have, most of us would deserve those same descriptions.

- Find out the family's best hope for the future. If the goal appears unrealistic, gently help move them toward reality, but recognize that their hope may be what is holding them together right now. They have a lifetime to deal with the effects of brain injury. They do not have to reach acceptance the first 3 weeks or even the first year following injury. Resolution is a process, not an event.

- Recognize the deep impact TBI has had on the family. How much work have family members missed? Did someone quit his or her job? Is the family capable of experiencing fun and joy?

- Recognize recovery from brain injury is a lifelong process.

- Remember that the family is an important clinical factor in the recovery process for an individual with TBI.

- Develop a list of families who have successfully adjusted to living with brain injury in their family system. Solicit these families to support and share their knowledge with others. Help families get connected with more than just a name. Make connections on the basis of similarities—for example, similar types of injury or similar family structures—whenever possible.

- Remain available during evenings and weekends. This may be the only time the family can get together with you.

Note. Adapted from "A Family Matter," by C. Wright, 2000, *Advance for Providers of Post-Acute Care,* 3(5), p. 42. Copyright 2000 by Merion Publications. Adapted with permission.

References

Brooks, N., Campsie, L., Symington, C., Beattie, A., & McKinlay, W. (1987). The effects of severe head injury on patient and relative within seven years of injury. *Journal of Head Trauma Rehabilitation, 2*, 1–13.

Brooks, N., & McKinlay, W. (1983). Personality and behaviour change after severe blunt head injury: A relative view. *Journal of Neurology, Neurosurgery, and Psychiatry, 46*, 336–344.

Brown, H. J. (1991). *Life's little instruction book.* Nashville: Ruthledge Hill Press.

Byng-Hall, J. (1995). *Rewriting family scripts.* New York: Guilford Press.

Falvo, D. R. (1991). *Medical and psychosocial aspects of chronic illness and disability.* Gaithersburg, MD: Aspen.

Gleckman, A. D., & Brill, S. (1995). The impact of brain injury on family functioning: Implications for subacute rehabilitation programmes. *Brain Injury, 9*, 385–393.

High, W. M., Boake, C., & Lehmkuhl, L. D. (1995). Critical analysis of studies evaluating the effectiveness of rehabilitation after traumatic brain injury. *Journal of Head Trauma Rehabilitation, 10*, 14–26.

Holland, D., & Shigaki, C. L. (1998). Educating families and caretakers of traumatically brain injured patients in the new health care environment: A three phase model and bibliography. *Brain Injury, 12*, 993–1009.

Junque, C., Bruna, O., & Mataro, M. (1997). Information needs of the traumatic brain injury patient's family members regarding the consequences of the injury and associated perception of physical, cognitive, emotional and quality of life changes. *Brain Injury, 11*, 251–258.

Kneipp, S. (1996). Providing support to siblings of children with ABI. In G. H. S. Singer, A. Glang, & J. M. Williams (Eds.), *Children with acquired brain injury: Educating and supporting families* (pp. 137–147). Baltimore: Brookes.

Kolakowsky-Hayner, S. A., & Kishore, R. (1999). Caregiver functioning after traumatic injury. *NeuroRehabilitation, 13*, 27–33.

Koskinen, S. (1998). Quality of life 10 years after a very severe traumatic brain injury (TBI): The perspective of the injured and the closest relative. *Brain Injury, 12*, 631–648.

Lezak, M. D. (1986). Psychological implications of traumatic brain damage for the patient's family. *Rehabilitation Psychology, 31*, 241–250.

McKinlay, W. W., & Hickox, A. (1988). How can families help in the rehabilitation of the head injured? *Journal of Head Trauma Rehabilitation, 3*, 64–72.

Rosenthal, M., & Young, T. (1988). Effective family intervention after traumatic brain injury: Theory and practice. *Journal of Head Trauma Rehabilitation, 3*, 42–50.

Stebbins, P., & Leung, P. (1998). Changing family needs after brain injury. *Journal of Rehabilitation, 64*, 15–22.

Whelan, T. B., & Walker, M. L. (1989). Coping and adjustment of children with neurological disorder. In C. R. Reynolds & E. Fletcher-Janzen (Eds.), *Handbook of clinical child neuropsychology* (pp. 535–555). New York: Plenum Press.

Wright, C. (2000). A family matter. *Advance for Providers of Post-Acute Care, 3*(5), 41–42.

Ethics of Treatment: Do No Harm

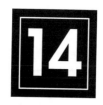

Christine E. Borgelt and Carolyn Wright

Chapter 1 hurled you into the world of a survivor of TBI. You have completed Chapters 2 through 13 to gain information about TBI. You have acquired a fancy new vocabulary, maybe even a fascination with the human brain, and you have examined from a distance what families and survivors of TBI face each and every day. You have, by virtue of completing this textbook, defined yourself as someone with knowledge about TBI. Most likely, you are genuinely interested in helping survivors and their loved ones. Most likely, you are a well-educated, well-intentioned, enthusiastic person with visions of making the world a better place. At a minimum, you may be looking forward to working with challenged individuals who can benefit from your training.

The purpose of this chapter is to make you think beyond your own knowledge and skills—to think beyond your own professional discipline. The purpose is to move you beyond neat and tidy clinical information and to help you understand the lifelong effects that professionals have on survivors of TBI and their families. Our goal now is a simple one: Do no harm.

> *Half of the harm that is done in the world is due to people who want to feel important.*
>
> —Eliot, 1950, p. 111

> *I shall use treatment for the good of the sick to the best of my ability and judgment, and I shall refrain from using it for either harm or wrongdoing.*
>
> —The Oath, from Hippocrates, cited by Levine, 1971, p. 58

Ethics, Experience, and Excellence

Each professional discipline carries its own set of ethical principles. Ethical codes offer a template for interpreting difficult or awkward situations. In a general sense, they protect clients and anticipate professional dilemmas. Professional training programs teach ethical issues in various ways, and a copy of the code of ethics for speech–language pathologists is available from the American Speech-Language-Hearing Association (ASHA, 1994). Familiarity with the ethical standards of your profession is essential for providing excellent service.

Ethical issues come to light through experience. Professional training programs provide the foundation for careers. Knowledge is gained, competencies are passed. All that is left is experience. No degree of clinical knowledge, no training program, no ethical standard, no professional credential, no journal article, no neurological advancement can supplant the value of experience.

Experience teaches that professionals who work with survivors of TBI must embrace the human factor. One brain injury changes the lives of many people forever: individuals, families, friends, and entire communities are affected. TBI challenges the essence of a person by altering characteristics that are uniquely human—memory, understanding of abstract concepts, verbal abilities, focus, and social competence. As a professional, you are challenged to help someone regain or accept himself or herself as a person, including—not in spite of—the effects of a brain injury. Clinical training programs often do not prepare clinicians to consider the essence of someone's person in interventions. (See the following case example on knowing the person.) Brain injury rehabilitation that ignores the uniqueness of a person will be, at best, ineffective and, at worst, harmful.

Rehabilitation: What Is Helping?

Rehabilitation has roots in both the medical and educational worlds. To be effective with survivors of TBI, you need to be aware of your own understanding of "rehabilitation." The language of brain injury rehabilitation is, by definition, quite medical. Families hear many new words—for example, agnosia, dysarthria, aphasia, and ataxia. Medical vocabulary presents the rehabilitation professional as articulate, competent, sophisticated, expert, and even expensive. With enough planning and arrogance, a professional can even intimidate colleagues!

Consider, however, the educational nature of rehabilitation. The goal is to help individuals understand brain injury, recover skills, and regain function. Survivors and families struggle to learn about brain injury and look to professionals to teach them. In that light, a highly medical explanation can sound distant, intimidating, scary, and oddly enough, curable.

A strictly medical approach to brain injury can cause false expectations and prevent survivors and families from asking questions or challenging interventions. Families may become reluctant to contribute knowledge about their loved one. Afraid to speak out, they can become distant from the team. Waiting for an implied cure, they can become disillusioned and angry. At that point,

Case Example: Knowing the Person

Clinically speaking, the issues for Allen's rehabilitation were clear. The professional team had conducted thorough assessments and agreed that a TBI sustained by the young rancher had left him with difficulties in attention, memory, impulse control, gait, and balance. After 3 months of services, family members expressed concern that the therapists had failed to capture their son as a person. Unclear but well intentioned, the therapy staff set about getting to know Allen. They talked with him, talked among themselves, and observed him in numerous settings. They made every effort to get to know this young man better.

After 6 months, Allen's frustrated family said, much less gently, that Allen's lack of progress was because the staff still did not know or care about their son. Upset and defensive, the team regrouped. They compared notes again. They talked among themselves. Finally, they began to get it. They asked questions, and they listened carefully to the responses.

Allen's team asked his wife what he had been like before injury. They wanted to know about Allen when he was a child. Allen's parents told about the activities Allen had enjoyed in childhood and young adulthood. They talked about how much they missed him and how Allen was homesick for his ranching activities and for his teenage niece and nephew.

Therapy changed. The clinical targets—attention, memory, impulse control, gait, and balance—remained the same. But now Allen passed a football around and practiced roping during physical workouts. He taught a supervised class in line dancing. Cognitive staff read Allen's hometown newspaper with him and shopped with him for books on ranching. Allen's niece and nephew attended weekly therapy sessions in the swimming pool, learning about brain injury and how to interact with their uncle. Allen's gait and balance began to improve. He was more willing to participate in therapy, and the team found it easier to redirect Allen.

Allen had survived a horrible injury, and his recovery was slow. But he had begun to recover what he and his family had missed the most: His uniqueness as a person.

Exercise: Take a few minutes in a quiet place. Take a few deep breaths and relax. Think of the person you care about most in the world —a loved one who plays an active role in your everyday life. Think of the things that make that person lovable and loving. Make a mental list of what it is that makes your relationship special.

Imagine that the person you love most in the world has just sustained a severe TBI. You can neither control nor predict the outcomes. You will be living with this for the next 42 years. It is a horrible, unpleasant image, but the families of your clients live this reality. For you, the feelings and image will go away.

When you are past the flood of emotions that accompany the image, consider what you would want from professionals working with your loved one. How would you like them to describe your loved one's deficits? Which of your loved one's special traits are you willing to live without? What traits would be most important for your loved one to recover? At what point in your loved one's recovery would you be willing to give up on progress?

Even if you bring to your professional work a personal understanding of head injury, your experience will not have been the same as the family's sitting in your office. You have not been in their shoes, have not heard their whole story, and may not understand where they are in the recovery process.

Even though families look to you for expertise, listen for opportunities to learn about the person who has survived TBI and to offer gentle teaching. Most important, look for opportunities to ask questions, and value opportunities to simply be silent and listen. (Adapted from staff development materials, Quality Living, Inc., Omaha, NE.)

someone on the team usually decides that the family has one of several "D-seases": They are "dysfunctional," in "denial," or "difficult"—all because the professionals were focused on their roles as experts instead of their potential as teachers.

The medical and educational roots of rehabilitation can be effectively blended. TBI rehabilitation demands a delicate balance of competent professional and gentle teacher in the context of knowing a survivor as a person. Dunst and Trivette (1988) observed,

> The extent to which help-seeking and help-giving have either positive or negative consequences depends on the intertwining of a host of intrapersonal and interpersonal factors. These include one's perception of the need for help, the manner in which help is offered, the source of help, the response costs involved in accepting help, and the sense of indebtedness the recipient feels toward the help provider. (p. 343)

Traumatic Brain Injury: A Unique Vulnerability

Individuals with TBI are uniquely vulnerable. In subtle or startling ways, they are constantly reminded of their deficits. The condition is chronic but never static. Awareness and adjustment issues come with the territory. Life becomes very unpredictable. Guilt and relief confound the grief process. Often, medical decisions become a way of life. Resources are constantly challenged. Social connections diminish. Declines or improvements in one area can alter functioning in another area.

With every family milestone—a wedding, graduation, or birth—comes the reminder of what one may never attain. Family members adjust in their own way, at their own pace. They may have painful memories of early recovery that are completely forgotten by their injured loved one. The world following TBI can be lonely, confusing, and uncertain.

Working with survivors of TBI and their caregivers can be immensely gratifying, humbling, and heartwarming. Every day offers rich opportunities to experience the depth of the human spirit. An appreciation of the unique vulnerability, along with competence and creativity, can produce very real differences in the quality of life for the people you serve.

If you are considering a career in brain injury, ask yourself these questions: Do you enjoy unpredictability? Are you flexible? Can you take solid clinical knowledge and adapt that to a person who may be very different from yourself? Are you a team player? Do you enjoy staying abreast of rapidly changing research? Do you know how to say, "I don't know"? Do you like people? Are you a natural teacher? Can you laugh easily?

The complexities of brain injury require a comprehensive approach to intervention. Coordinated efforts involving the injured person, caregivers, relevant professionals, and social supports establish an environment in which real-life interventions

Reflections of a Rehabilitation Novice

I was only a few weeks into my new career in brain injury rehabilitation. I went, somewhat overwhelmed, to the director of clinical services. I reflected on my brief orientation to residential rehabilitation.

I wanted to understand how a person with a very intact sense of humor could have such severe cognitive deficits;

I struggled with my own emotions after seeing a beautiful, feisty young mother who had been anoxic following cardiac arrest;

I was embarrassed when I could not understand someone who was trying so hard to be understood;

I was humbled when that person smiled and gave me another chance;

I had met families desperate to care for their loved ones at home, knowing that they did not have the physical or emotional resources to do so;

I had seen families exhausted from years of hope;

I wondered when to stay silent, as family members angrily told of other settings where they had been under-promised, over-promised, but mainly unheard.

The director of clinical services gave me a puzzled look until I blurted out, "How do you do rehabilitation when the potential to do harm is so great?" Little did I know, I had taken the first step toward understanding TBI.

can lead to long-term gains. Professionals pulling together can create a balanced environment that supports the unique vulnerability associated with brain injury.

Opportunities To Do Harm

Professionals who dedicate years to training rarely enter a work situation with the expectation of doing harm. Many might find the idea that competent professionals can do harm to be offensive. The distinction between the task and the process of interventions may be helpful here. As professionals coordinate their efforts, the task at hand may be their entire focus. For example, the task may be to help a person correctly identify coworkers' names; or the task may be to remember when and how to feed the family dog; or the task may be taking notes during a college lecture. Whatever the task, interactions among team members, the survivor, and the family constitute the process. The task is *what* you are attempting to achieve with your client. The process is *how* you and your team work to achieve that goal.

Chapters 2 through 13 have supplied a basis for *what* you do when working with people with TBI. Staying current on research, having data to support your interventions, and accepting feedback from other team members on the accuracy of your observations can go a long way to prevent unintentional harm based on what you are doing. The final section of this chapter is provocative, personal, and practical. The goal is to make you consider the how of your interventions. Please take time to contemplate a few of the major pitfalls through which professionals may inadvertently do harm.

Overpromising

The same traits—caring, compassion, and a desire to help—that bring talented people to brain injury work can be traits that create false hope, anger, and disappointment. Consider that you are working with a family member whose youngest son, at age 30, sustained a severe injury in a motor vehicle accident. The mother has seen fluctuating progress over the 6 months since the accident. A medical setback has the entire team discouraged and the family questioning the skill of the professionals. During a weekly staffing, the exhausted mother states, "I just want him to get better. I don't know how much longer I can take this." Without hesitating, the member of the team sitting closest to the mother reaches out to touch her forearm and says gently, "Don't worry. Your son will get better. We'll see to it." Three months later, the family is more angry and confused. Medical setbacks have continued, and the early gains their son achieved have been lost. The family had held on to the well-intentioned 10-second gesture of a warm and caring professional who overpromised that the team would make their son better. Other messages of support may have been more appropriate. Developing such scripts ahead of time can prepare you to maintain your caring without delivering false expectations. What the professional did in the above scenario was well timed and touching, but how the caring was conveyed left room for improvement.

Underpromising

In an era of litigation, some professionals worry excessively about liability. A fear of overpromising and being hauled into court can restrain us from offering hope, even when best professional judgment indicates that improved outcomes are expected for a survivor. Rick was 14 years old when he was injured in a car accident. His father, Jack, conveyed the following frustration with professionals providing information about Rick's recovery:

> I think professionals tend to—because of liability or whatever the reason may be—tend to be overly pessimistic, and I think that they need to be a little bit encouraging, too. Say it can be one way or the other, but don't make any promises. But give them [the family] the positive side as well as the negative side to some extent. (Borgelt, Carrington Rotto, & Hux, 1998)

The nature of brain injury challenges professionals to be accurate while helping people to maintain a sense of hope and future.

Political Correctness

Brain injury frequently leads to an inability to monitor what one says. Survivors who have lost the ability to screen their thoughts become socially isolated. The novice professional may have difficulty distancing personal values of politically correct social behavior from the content of a conversation with a survivor. If you work with survivors of TBI, it is very, very likely that you will encounter comments that you find personally offensive. Describing that behavior as malicious or unacceptable does little to teach your client how to regain social skills. Be careful not to create a punitive atmosphere while describing behavioral changes associated with TBI. Family members, and perhaps the survivor, may be aware of the offensive nature of these unfiltered comments. They may already be embarrassed and afraid of how people will judge the family. Reinforcing that embarrassment will only further distance the family from the team. To avoid doing harm, look for ways to educate, followed by strategies for coping with communication challenges.

Behavior as Communication

Humans are by nature psychologists. We read a newspaper story of a mother who drowned her children, and we apply motive to her behavior. Children tantrum at the grocery checkout stand, and we silently question the parenting skills of the customer in front of us. We hear that a professional athlete was arrested, and we discuss at the coffee machine why so many athletes engage in violent acts. Magazines and newspapers are filled with examples of human behavior that we interpret based on personal biases. In short, most of us have opinions about why a person in a certain situation behaved in a certain way.

Consider the example of a man in his mid-20s who sustained considerable injury while riding his motorcycle. Several years postinjury, he had a vocabulary of only four nonsense words. He looked healthy but had very limited memory and practically no way to communicate his needs. He required residential services for structure and because of his unpredictable behavior. Many evenings, during his shower, he would throw unexplained "tantrums." For no apparent reason, after the water began running, he would yell and bang on the shower walls. His behavior was "out of control." He was "agitated," "acting out," and "unmanageable." Maybe some even thought he was "psychotic." An astute caregiver noticed that each time this man became upset in the shower, someone in the bathroom next door had just flushed the toilet. Yelling and banging were attempts to communicate that the shower water was too hot. A simple intervention to lock the staff bathroom during shower time eliminated the yelling.

Working with survivors of TBI requires an understanding of your own biases about human behavior. Beware of interpreting behavior without data. Opinions without data can do harm.

Missing the Context

Chapters 10 through 12 presented various contexts—social, educational, and vocational—in which communication difficulties can affect functioning. Cultural contexts are also important in developing effective interventions.

A husband worked with a team to establish discharge goals for his young wife. The rehabilitation team was comprised of talented, assertive, competent professionals. The family and survivor set goals that included returning home—a realistic goal given certain accommodations. Several team members became fond of the young woman who was struggling to resume her roles of homemaker and mother. In this family's culture, the husband was the unquestioned head of the household. Team members who cared for the young woman struggled with their own opinions that the husband should be more supportive of his wife and more willing to care for the children. The husband had difficulty accepting expert advice from the women on the team, having lived all his life in a patriarchal social structure. The question for the rehabilitation team became whether they were trying to rehabilitate the young woman into someone she had not been before injury. The challenge for the team was to put aside personal biases. They observed the family setting and developed an appreciation for the social context into which this young woman eventually returned.

School and work reentry involve this same analysis. What are the resources of the school team? Where can classroom modifications be made most easily? What are the barriers to reentering the educational system? In vocational settings, what can we learn from employers as we develop treatment plans? Who will the key support people be at work? What education do they need about TBI?

Not Listening

We invest a lot of energy into our professional training programs. We are enthusiastic and passionate about helping people. So, when teammates or families want our input, we are ready to share. We impress ourselves with what we have to say.

Survivors of TBI and their families will be only negatively impressed if we are so busy talking that we forget to listen. If you find yourself in a meeting about brain injury where you are dominating the conversation and have asked no questions, mentally step back and analyze your interactions. This will help you know what a family hears. As one family member put it, "The best professionals are the ones who listen" (Borgelt et al., 1998).

Summary

Communication difficulties present tremendous challenges following brain injury. Survivors and their families look to professional teams for answers, strategies, hope, and support. Rehabilitation is a process that begins with establishing relationships with both survivors and fellow team members. Often a professional's contact with a client is a small window in time compared to the lifelong challenges the survivor faces. As we develop a healthy awareness of our own biases, we avoid doing harm along the way. If we maintain our ability to see the person instead of the injury, we can even help to restore a sense of hope and future. Please, do no harm.

References

American Speech-Language-Hearing Association. (1994). Code of ethics. *Asha, 36,* 1–2.

Borgelt, C. E., Carrington Rotto, P., & Hux, K. (1998). *TBI: A case study* [Videotape]. Available from American Psychological Association Division 16, Washington, DC.

Dunst, C. J., & Trivette, C. M. (1988). Helping, helplessness, and harm. In J. C. Witt, S. N. Elliott, & F. M. Gresham (Eds.), *Handbook of behavior therapy in education* (pp. 343–376). New York: Plenum Press.

Eliot, T. S. (1950). *The cocktail party.* New York: Harcourt, Brace, & Co.

Levine, E. B. (1971). *Hippocrates.* New York: Twayne.

Index

About the Editor

Karen Hux, PhD, is an associate professor of communication disorders at the University of Nebraska–Lincoln. Her work has focused on helping survivors of traumatic brain injury and their families deal with the multiple cognitive, communicative, social, and emotional consequences of injury. She lives in Lincoln, Nebraska, with her daughter.